ANNALS *of* THE NEW YORK ACADEMY OF SCIENCES

DIRECTOR AND EXECUTIVE EDITOR
Douglas Braaten

ASSISTANT EDITOR
Joseph Abrajano

PROJECT MANAGER
Steven E. Bohall

PROJECT COORDINATOR
Ralph W. Brown

CREATIVE DIRECTOR
Ash Ayman Shairzay

The New York Academy of Sciences
7 World Trade Center
250 Greenwich Street, 40th Floor
New York, NY 10007-2157

annals@nyas.org
www.nyas.org/annals

The New York Academy of Sciences

Published by Blackwell Publishing
On behalf of the New York Academy of Sciences

Boston, Massachusetts
2010

ANNALS *of* THE NEW YORK ACADEMY OF SCIENCES

VOLUME 1199

ISSUE

Neuroprotective Agents

Ninth International Conference

ISSUE EDITORS

Russell J. Andrews, William Slikker, Jr., Bruce Trembly, and Tucker A. Patterson

This volume presents papers stemming from the "Ninth International Conference on Neuroprotective Agents," held on September 7–11, 2008 at the Marine Biological Laboratory, Woods Hole, Massachusetts.

TABLE OF CONTENTS

Ann. N.Y. Acad. Sci. ISSN 0077-8923

ANNALS OF THE NEW YORK ACADEMY OF SCIENCES
Issue: *Neuroprotective Agents*

Metabolic syndrome, age-associated neuroendocrine disorders, and dysregulation of tryptophan—kynurenine metabolism

Gregory F. Oxenkrug
Tufts University/Tufts Medical Center, Boston, Massachusetts
Address for correspondence: Gregory F. Oxenkrug, Director, Psychiatry and Inflammation Program, Department of Psychiatry, Tufts University School of Medicine and Tufts Medical Center, Boston, MA 02111. goxenkrug@tuftsmedicalcenter.org

The neuroendocrine theory of aging identified a cluster of conditions (hypertension, obesity, dyslipidemia, diabetes type 2, menopause, late onset depression, vascular cognitive impairment, impairment of immune defense, and some forms of cancer, e.g., breast and prostate) as age-associated neuroendocrine disorders (AAND). Obesity, dyslipidemia, hypertension, and type 2 diabetes were later described as metabolic syndromes (MetS). Chronic inflammation is currently considered as a common feature of MetS/AAND. One of the mechanisms by which chronic inflammation might trigger and/or maintain the development of MetS/AAND is transcriptional induction of indoleamine 2,3-dioxygenase (IDO), rate-limiting enzyme of tryptophan (TRY)–kynurenine (KYN) pathway, by pro-inflammatory cytokines (PIC). Activation of IDO shifts TRY metabolism from serotonin synthesis to formation of "kynurenines." Diminished serotonin production is associated with mental depression while increased formation of kynurenines might contribute to development of MetS/AAND via their apoptotic, neurotoxic, and pro-oxidative effects, and upregulation of inducible nitric oxide synthase, phospholipase A2, arachidonic acid, prostaglandin, 5-lipoxygenase, and leukotriene cascade. The combined presence of high producers of alleles of polymorphic PIC genes (e.g., interferon-gamma and tumor necrosis factor alpha) might account for the genetic predisposition to high levels of PIC production, leading to "superinduction" of IDO. The other rate-limiting enzyme of the TRY–KYN pathway, TRY 2,3-dioxygenase, is activated by substrate (TRY) and cortisol. Therefore, KYN–TRY metabolism might be the meeting point for gene-environment interaction and a new target for prevention and treatment of MetS/AAND.

Keywords: metabolic syndrome; age-associated neuroendocrine disorders; tryptophan; kynurenine; cytokines; inflammation

Metabolic syndrome and age-associated neuroendocrine disorders

The neuroendocrine theory of aging suggests the common mechanisms of developmental (prereproductive) and aging (postreproductive) processes and identified a cluster of conditions (hypertension, obesity, dyslipidemia, diabetes type 2, menopause, late onset depression, vascular cognitive impairment, impairment of immune defense, and some forms of cancer), as age-associated neuroendocrine disorders (AAND).[1–4] Obesity, dyslipidemia, hypertension, and type 2 diabetes were later described as metabolic syndrome (MetS). MetS affects approximately 20–30% of the middle-aged population, and represents an increased risk to cardiovascular disorders, the leading cause of death in the United States.[5]

As shown in Table 1, several other conditions, such as immunosuppression, climacteric (menopause), hypercorticolism (increased secretion of cortisol), cancrophilia (increased prevalence of some types of cancers), and late onset depression are components of AAND and MetS. Vascular cognitive impairment might be included in the clusters of MetS and AAND as well.[6] It is noteworthy

doi: 10.1111/j.1749-6632.2009.05356.x

Table 1. MetS/AAND and kynurenine metabolism: references to the published reports

Metabolic syndrome	Age-associated neuroendocrine disorders	TRY–KYN metabolism	Cytokine levels	Gene polymorphisms
Dyslipidemia	Atherosclerosis	55–57	62–64	
Obesity	Obesity	58–60	67–72	79–81
Hypertension	Hypertension		66	88–91
Insulin resistance	Pre-diabetes (type 2 diabetes)			85
	Climacteric (menopause)		73–76	
	Hypercorticolism (in increased cortisol)	93,94	95	88
	Late-onset depression	6,13,95	78,95,101	82–84
	Cancrophilia			87
	Vascular cognitive impairment	6	6	6
	Aging	22,61,77		92

that the prevalence of MetS increases with age.[7,8] VM Dilman suggested that there should be a common causative mechanism for the development of AAND.[1–3] Similarly, there was a gradual realization that MetS is a syndrome with a central unifying etiological factor expressed as its various components.[5] Although inflammatory processes are not included in the current definition of MetS, low grade inflammation was suggested as a causative and contributing factor for MetS.[5,8] C-reactive protein, free fatty acids (FFA), and pro-inflammatory type Th-1 cytokines (PIC), for example, TNF-alpha, interleukins (IL) -1 and -6, were considered as inflammatory mediators of MetS.[5,7–9]

This paper reviews the data suggesting that one of the mechanisms by which chronic inflammation might contribute to the development of MetS/AAND is upregulation of kynurenine (KYN) pathway of tryptophan (TRY) metabolism.

Metabolism of tryptophan

TRY is an essential (for humans) amino acid with two non-protein metabolic pathways: methoxyindole and KYN (Fig. 1). One of the factors influencing availability of TRY as a substrate of both pathways is plasma free tryptophan.[10] FFAs release plasma TRY from their bond with albumin.[11]

Methoxyindole pathway

The methoxyindole pathway leads to formation of serotonin (5-HT) and melatonin (Fig. 1).

The rate-limiting step of the 5-HT biosynthesis is hydroxylation of TRY catalyzed by TRY-hydroxylase with the formation of 5-hydroxytryptophan. The subsequent decarboxylation results in the formation of 5-HT. Availability of TRY as a substrate is one of the rate-limiting factors of 5-HT biosynthesis because less than 5% of TRY is metabolized along this pathway.[10]

5-HT is a substrate for melatonin biosynthesis. The rate-limiting step of melatonin biosynthesis is 5-HT-*N*-acetylation resulting in the formation of *N*-acetyl-serotonin (NAS) with subsequent O-methylation into 5-methoxy-*N*-acetyltryptamine (melatonin).[6]

The deficient production of 5-HT, NAS, and melatonin contribute to depressed mood,[12,13] disturbances of sleep[14] and circadian rhythms.[15]

Tryptophan–kynurenine pathway

About 95% of TRY is metabolized by the TRY–KYN pathway. It involves the cleavage of the indole ring of TRY resulting in the formation of *N*-formylkynurenine followed by kynurenine in an ensuing step (Fig. 1).[10,16]

The rate-limiting enzyme of KYN formation from TRY is indoleamine 2,3-dioxygenase (IDO) that is ubiquitously distributed in mammals, except the liver, in astrocytes, microglia, microvascular endothelial cells, and macrophages.[17] The other enzyme able to break TRY's indole ring is TRY 2,3-dioxygenase (TDO). TDO is found in bacteria and the liver, kidney, and brain of mammals.[16,18]

IDO is a monomeric enzyme and has broader substrate specificity than TDO. IDO reacts with either oxygen or superoxide and other indoleamines, including D-tryptophan, D- and

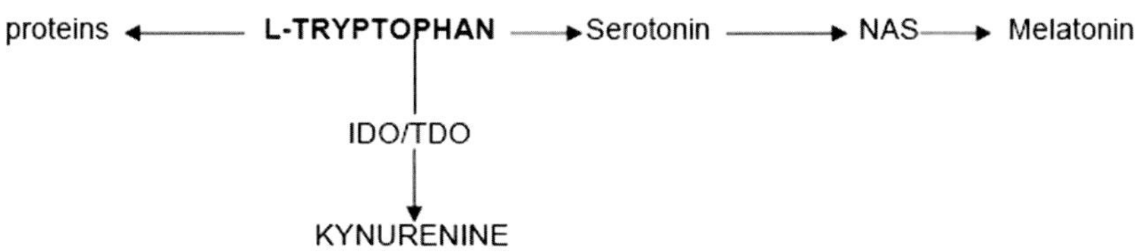

Figure 1. Major pathways of tryptophan metabolism. IDO: indoleamine 2,3-dioxygenase; TDO: tryptophan 2,3-dioxygenase; NAS: *N*-acetylserotonin.

L-5-hydroxytryptophan, 5-HT, and tryptamine. TDO is a homotetrameric enzyme and displays high substrate specificity.[18]

IDO is induced by PIC while TDO is activated by TRY and stress hormones (see below). A decrease of TDO activity occurs concomitantly with IDO induction, suggesting a coordinate shift in TRY metabolism from the liver to extrahepatic tissues during an immune response.[19]

KYN inhibits TRY transport via the blood-brain barrier, stimulates IDO activity and exerts anxiogenic activity in animal models of anxiety.[20]

Post-kynurenine metabolism

Kynurenine is further metabolized along the two distinct routes competing for KYN as a substrate:

(a) KYN, kynurenic acid (KYNA) pathway; and
(b) KYN, nicotinamide adenine dinucleotide (NAD) pathway (Fig. 2).

KYN–KYN acid pathway

The KYN–KYNA pathway is regulated by kynurenine aminotransferases (KAT I, II, III). KAT I and II are the major biosynthetic enzymes of KYNA in the brain with KAT II being the most abundant in rat and human brain and KAT III most abundant in mouse brain.[16]

The end product of this pathway is KYNA, the only known endogenous *N*-methyl-D-aspartate (NMDA) receptor antagonist.[16] KYNA, similarly to the exogenous NMDA antagonists, ketamine and MK-801, may have psychotomimetic effects.[25,26] The function of KYNA, however, is not limited to NMDA receptors. KYNA is an antagonist to alpha 7 nicotinic acetylcholine receptors (alpha7nAChRs), and has higher affinity for alpha7nAChRs than to NMDA receptors. KYNA-induced inhibition of alpha7nAChRs on glutamatergic afferents reduces basal extracellular dopamine levels in the rat striatum.[21] KYNA, as an alpha7nAChR antagonist, might contribute to cognitive impairment

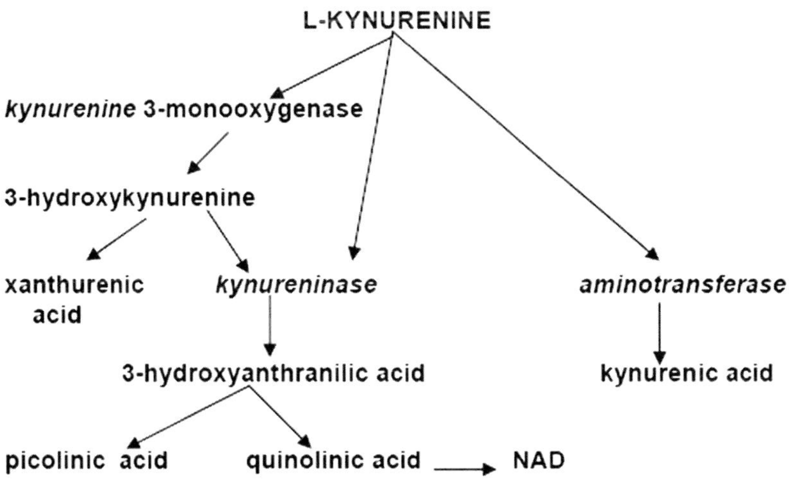

Figure 2. Competitive pathways of kynurenine metabolism. TRY: tryptophan; 5-HT: serotonin; NAT: *N*-acetyltransferase; NAS: *N*-acetylserotonin; NAD: nicotinamide adenine dinucleotide.

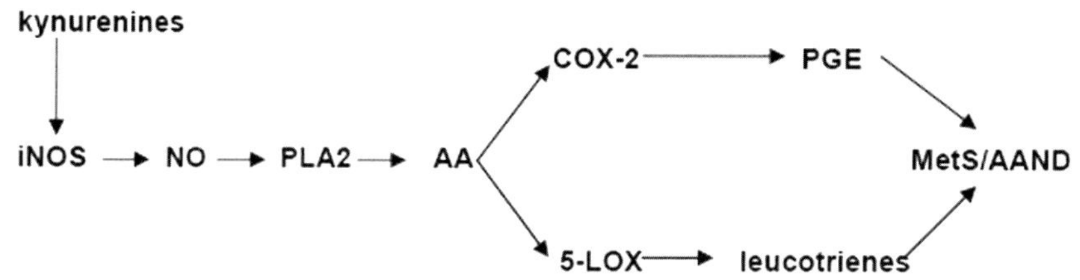

Figure 3. IDO and metabolic syndrome/age-associated neuroendocrine disorders. iNOS: inducible nitric oxide synthase; NO: nitric oxide; PLA: phospholipase A2; AA: arachidonic acid; COX: cyclooxygenase; 5-LOX: arachidonate 5-lipoxygenase; PGE: prostaglandines; MetS: metabolic syndrome; AAND: age-associated neuroendocrine disorders.

observed in depression, schizophrenia, dementia, obesity, hypertension, Down's syndrome, and Crohn's, Huntington's, Parkinson' syndrome, and diseases.[21–24]

In addition, KYNA has signaling functions through activation of its recently identified receptor, GPR35. GPR35 is predominantly detected in immune cells and the gastrointestinal tract, and might be involved in nociceptive perception.[27] KYNA might have an anti-inflammatory effect by inhibition of lipopolysaccharide-induced tumor necrosis factor (TNF)-alpha secretion in peripheral blood mononuclear cells.[28]

The KYN–nicotinamide adenine dinucleotide pathway

The major enzymes of the KYN–NAD pathway are KYN-3-monooxygenase and kynureninase.[16] The end product of this pathway is NAD. Among more than 30 intermediate metabolites (collectively named "kynurenines") are NMDA agonists (quinolinic and picolinic acids) and free radical generators (3-hydroxykynurenine and 3-hydroxyanthranilic acids).[6,10,29] KYN and 3-hydroxykynurenine and 3-hydroxyanthranilic acids induce apoptosis.[17] One of the major metabolites of this pathway, 3-hydroxykynurenine, is a potential neurotoxin involved in several neurodegenerative disorders.[16] The other metabolite, xanthurenic acid, reacts with insulin with formation of a complex antigenetically indistinguishable from insulin.[30] Formation of insulin/xanthurenic acid complex might result in decreased sensitivity to insulin, that is, with insulin resistance typical for MetS/AAND.[30] Quinolinic and picolinic acids exert anxiogenic effects in animal models.[31–33] Quinolinic and picolinic acids stimulate inducible nitric oxide synthase (iNOS) and together with 3-hydroxykynurenine and 3-hydroxyanthranilic acids might increase lipid peroxidation, and trigger an arachidonic acid cascade resulting in the increased production of inflammatory factors: prostaglandins, via activation of cycloxygenase (COX) and leucotrienes, via activation of arachidonate 5-lipoxygenase (5-LOX)[6,34] (Fig. 3).

The pathway of the inflammatory enzyme 5-LOX was suggested as a putative common mechanism that is affected by aging and may link depression and atherosclerosis.[35] Association between depressive symptoms and the progression of subclinical atherosclerosis was shown in a progressive 3-year study of healthy, older individuals. Higher levels of depressive symptoms (e.g., ahedonia, fatigue, and sleep/appetite disturbance) at baseline were associated with a greater 3-year change in carotid intima-media thickness. The authors suggested that a likely explanation for the observed association between depressive symptoms and atherosclerosis is that both are triggered and/or maintained by a common biological mechanism.[35,36]

Regulation of KYN–NAD pathway

Hormonal regulation of KYN–NAD pathway. Considering the possibility of kynurenines impact on aging and menopause, it is noteworthy to mention the data on the effects of hormones on post-KYN pathways of TRY metabolism. Affymetrix array analysis shows that estradiol and progesterone caused a significant sixfold decrease in the key enzyme of KYN–NAD pathway, kynurenine 3-mono-oxygenase, in macaque dorsal raphe region.[37] Decreased excretion of 3-hydroxykynurenine, xanthurenic, 3-hydroxyanthranilic, and quinolinic acids was reported in women on oral contraceptive.[38] Estrogens inhibit the other key enzyme of KYN–NAD pathway, kynureninase, in postmenopausal women. This effect might be mediated through decreased availability of vitamin B6, the coenzyme of kynureninase,[39] and quinolinic acid decarboxylase.[40] It is noteworthy that estrogens but not testosterone inhibit lipid peroxidation[41] that might be the result of kynurenines-induced activation of iNOS[34] (Fig. 3).

Cytokines regulation of KYN–NAD pathway. Interferon-gamma (IFNG) stimulates both key enzymes of the KYN–NAD pathway, kynurenine mono-oxygenase and kynureninase, in immortalized murine macrophages.[42]

Cross-talk between the methoxyindole and kynurenine pathways of tryptophan metabolism. 5-HT (not competitively) and NAS and melatonin (competitively) inhibit TDO[43] while KYNA, similarly to the exogenous NMDA antagonist, ketamine, may inhibit 5-HT-*N*-acetylation, the rate-limiting step of melatonin biosynthesis.[44]

Regulation of rate-limiting enzymes of TRY–KYN pathway

Regulation of tryptophan 2,3-dioxygenase

Substrate activation. TDO is activated by its substrate, TRY.[10] Although administration of low to moderate doses of TRY stimulates 5-HT synthesis, administration of excessive doses of TRY results in decreased 5-HT synthesis due to TRY-induced TDO activation and KYN competition for TRY transport via the blood-brain-barrier.[6,45,46]

Hormonal activation. Cortisol activates TDO and increases KYN production.[47] Literature data regarding the effect of estrogens and testosterone on TDO is controversial: both adrenalectomy and ovariectomy reduced TDO activity in homogenates of liver from mature rats. However, administration of estrogens and testosterone had no effect on TDO[6] although they inhibited activity of the key enzymes of the KYN–NAD pathway.[37–40]

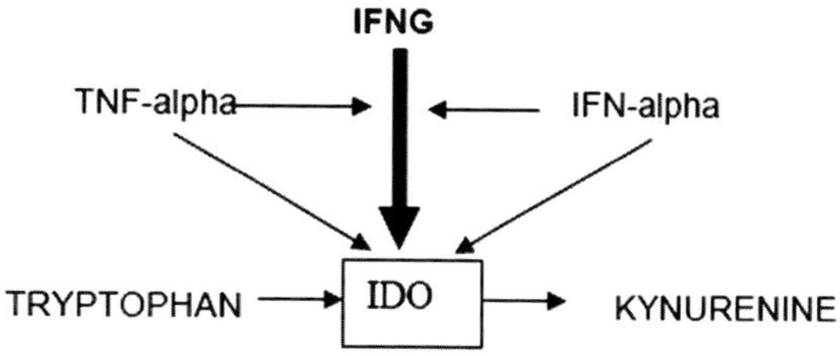

Figure 4. Cytokines and regulation of IDO. IFNG: interferone-gamma; IFN-alpha: interferone-alpha; TNF-alpha: tumor necrosis factor-alpha; IDO: indoleamine 2,3-dioxygenase.

Regulation of indoleamine 2,3-dioxygenase

Cytokines and IDO. IDO is a cytokine-inducible enzyme (Fig. 4).

IFN-gamma. Pro-inflammatory cytokines (including, most notably, interferons) transcriptionally induce IDO in a variety of immune cells (e.g., monocyte-derived macrophages and microglia). IFNG is the strongest known inducer of IDO.[46] Besides IDO, IFNG stimulates activity of 3-hydroxylase and kynureninase in immortalized murine macrophages.[42]

IFN-alpha. Systemically administrated IFN-alpha passes the blood-brain barrier and reaches effective concentrations acting on microglial cells as well as macrophage receptors. IFN-alpha has much weaker direct IDO stimulating effect than IFNG but might increase IDO activity by stimulating the production of IFNG and TNF-alpha[46] (Fig. 4).

It is noteworthy that IFN-alpha treatment resulted in psychiatric side effects in 30% of involved patients because of upregulation of TRY–KYN metabolism.[46]

TNF-alpha. TNF-alpha stimulates IDO activity and enhances (up to 300%) IFNG-induced IDO expression.[48] The induction of IDO by the bacterial endotoxin lipopolysaccharide was IFNG-independent and might be mediated by Toll-like receptors.[49]

Other proinflammatory molecules, such as IL-1, IL-12, Il-18, PGE_2 synergistically with IFNG induce IDO activity.[50]

Hormones and cytokines-induced activation of IDO. Although IDO is mainly induced by cytokines, experimental data pointed to possible hormonal influences on IDO activity. The expression

Table 2. High and low producer genotype groups

Cytokine gene	IFNG	TNF-alpha
Promoter site position	+874	−308
Single-base substitution	T → A	G → A
High producer allele	T	A
Low producer allele	A	G

of the IFNG gene may be subject to direct hormonal control: receptors of prolactin and IFNG share their structure and signal transduction pathway. Prolactin by itself has little or no effect on IDO but potentiates INFG-induced IDO activation in CD14-positive cells.[51] Estrogen increased the activity of the IFNG promoter in lymphoid cells.[52]

Application of hydrocortisone and dexamethasone in human astrocytoma cells and in native human astrocytes resulted in "super-induction" of IDO (by 300%).[6]

Cytokine gene polymorphism and IDO

IFNG production is influenced by polymorphic IFNG (+874) gene with high (T) and low (A) producer alleles (Table 2). Mean concentration of IFNG cytokine released by stimulated peripheral blood mononuclear cells is higher in healthy carriers of T than in carriers of A allele.[53] Because IFNG induces IDO activity one might suggest that high producer alleles would be associated with higher IDO activity than low producer alleles. Indeed, in healthy women in Finland, high producer T allele of IFNG (+874) gene was associated with increased IDO activity (i.e., elevated plasma KYN/TRY ratios) in comparison with the presence of low producer A allele.[54] Therefore, TRY–KYN metabolism might be genetically controlled by IFNG gene via regulation of IDO activity.

TNF-alpha production is influenced by the TNF-alpha (-308 A/G) polymorphic gene. In healthy individuals high producer A allele of TNF-alpha (−308) gene was associated with high production of TNF.[49] Because TNF-alpha stimulates IDO and potentiates IFNG-induced stimulation of IDO.[48] TNF-alpha (−308) high producer (A) allele might strengthen the association between IFNG (+874) high producer (T) and IDO upregulation.[6]

Kynurenines, pro-inflammatory cytokines, and gene polymorphism in metabolic syndrome/age-associated neuroendocrine disorders

The data on the activity of IDO, production of PIC, and polymorphisms of PIC genes is available for most (but not all) components of MetS/AAND (Table 1).

Production of kynurenines and MetS/AAND

The ratio of KYN to TRY, KYN/TRY, is widely used in clinical studies as an index of IDO activity. In 986 young adults and in 921 older (46–76 years) subjects IDO activity correlated significantly with several risk factors for atherosclerosis, that is, with age, carotid artery intima/media thickness, low density lipoprotein, body mass index, weakly with C-reactive protein and inversely with high density lipoprotein and triglycerides in females, whereas in males, IDO activity correlated significantly with C-reactive protein and inversely with high density lipoprotein.[55,56] Increased KYN/TRY ratio was found in a significant proportion of coronary heart disease patients.[57]

Free TRY was decreased in the plasma of obese rats.[58] Plasma TRY concentrations were decreased in obese subjects independently of weight reduction or dietary intake.[59] Preoperative KYN/TRY ratio in morbidly obese patients was significantly increased compared to the control group (41.6 ± 20.1 versus 26.5 ± 5.1 mmol/mol), and postoperative weight reduction did not normalize KYN/TRY ratio (37.9 ± 14.0 mmol/mol). In addition, these TRY metabolic changes may subsequently reduce 5-HT production and cause mood disturbances, depression, and impaired satiety ultimately leading to increased caloric uptake and obesity.[60]

IDO activity increases with aging.[54] High baseline IDO activity predicted lethality in a prospective study of elderly subjects.[61]

KYNA production was found to increase with aging in human subjects, and in Down's syndrome (accelerated aging) patients.[22]

Production of pro-inflammatory cytokines

Th1 response and its mediators: IFNG, TNF-alpha, IL-1, -12 and -18 have a proatherogenic effect[62] that can be prevented in mice by administration of IFNG inhibitory protein, sIFNGR.[63]

Elevated myocardial TNF-alpha was associated with hypertension and/or cardiac remodeling in rats.[64]

High levels of TNF-alpha were associated with the presence of MetS and the number of metabolic syndrome components in 1,914 individuals aged 70–79 years without cardiovascular disease or type 2 diabetes.[65] The lipopolysaccharide-stimulated secretion of TNF-alpha and IL-1beta was significantly increased in peripheral blood monocytes from hypertensive patients in comparison with healthy individuals.[66]

Recent studies suggest a role for IFNG in regulation of the inflammatory response that accompanies obesity. White adipose tissue secretes IFNG, inducible protein 10, and PIC, such as TNF-alpha, IL-1 and IL-6.[67] Obese mice produced more IFNG than controls and had deficient IFNG receptors.[68] Injection of TNF-alpha or IL-6 to pregnant rats resulted in 30–40% increase in adipose tissue weight in their offspring.[69]

Secretion of IFNG was significantly higher in the obese than in the control subjects that might be partly dependent on the action of leptin, an adipocyte-secreted hormone, that shifts T-helper (Th) cells toward a Th1 phenotype. In obese children, a shift to Th1-cytokine profile is dominated by the production of IFNG and is related to insulin resistance.[70] Pro-inflammatory cytokines exacerbate insulin resistance and augment MetS.[71]

TNF-alpha seems to impair insulin action, and thus, contributes to the development of type 2 diabetes.[72]

Menopause is a core component of AAND[1–3] but its association with MetS has been recognized only recently. Cross-sectional[73] and prospective[74] studies suggest the prevalence of MetS increases from pre- to postmenopause, independent of age and known cardiovascular diseases risk factors. Production of IFNG in women in their 40s and in postmenopausal women was significantly higher compared with that of younger women.[75]

Aging is characterized by increased IFNG and TNF-alpha production. Age-dependent increase in IFNG and TNF-alpha and a reduction in IL-2 levels, with minor changes in the remaining studied cytokines was found in senescence-accelerated mice.[76] Age-associated increases in nitric oxide levels of senescence-accelerated mice[76] might depend on IFNG-induced activation of iNOS mediated by kynurenines.[6,34]

Down's syndrome, a condition with accelerated aging, was associated with higher percentages of IFNG-producing cells in comparison with mentally retarded (15.9 ± 1.3, 7.9 ± 0.6, 4.8 ± 0.3) and healthy controls (15.6 ± 1.9, 7.2 ± 1.1, 4.6 ± 0.6)[77] consistent with increased KYNA levels in Down's syndrome patients.[22]

Late onset depression is considered as a component of AAND[4] and is associated with the increased production of IFNG, IL-6, and other PIC.[78]

Genetic studies and Mets/AAND

TNF-alpha (−308) (A/G). Linkage and association studies have suggested that a region of human chromosome 6 containing TNF-alpha gene is involved in the pathogenesis of obesity and obesity-associated hypertension.[79] High producer (A) allele of TNF-alpha (−308) gene was positively associated with obesity (total of 3,562 individuals), systolic arterial blood pressure (a total of 1,624 individuals), and plasma insulin levels (total of 3,720 subjects), and increased the risk of developing these conditions by 23%.[80]

Obese patients with high producer allele (A) of TNF-alpha (−308) gene had higher baseline and after treatment weight than carriers of low producer (G) alleles. The authors concluded that weight loss is associated with different changes depending on TNF-alpha genotype—carriers of low producer alleles have a better metabolic response than carriers with high producer alleles.[81]

Increased frequency of TNF-alpha -308A allele (high producer) was reported in Korean subjects with major depression,[82] in Korean bipolar I depressed patients,[83] and in Polish subjects with personal and family history of bipolar affective disorder.[84]

IFNG (+874) (T/A). Contrary to our hypothesis the frequency of the low IFNG (+874) production allele (A) was significantly higher in type 2 diabetics compared to controls.[85] It is noteworthy, that in contrast with healthy controls[54] there was no association between high producer alleles and high production of IFNG among type 2 diabetes patients probably due to the activity of molecules directly or indirectly inhibiting IFNG production.[85]

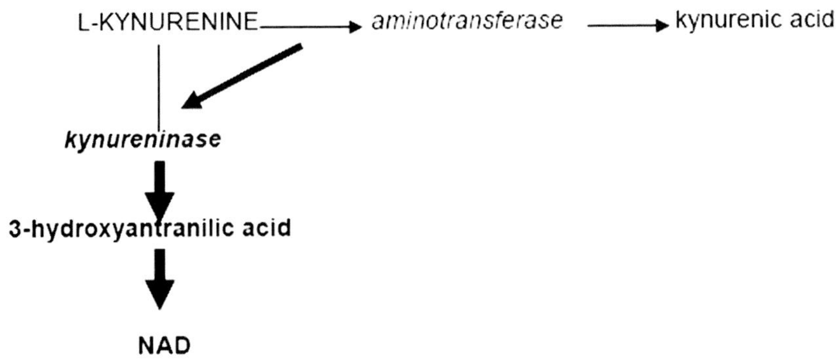

Figure 5. Hypothetical shift of post-kynurenine metabolism from KYN–KYNA to KYN–NAD pathways in hypertension. NAD: nicotinamide adenine dinucleotide.

Increased incidence of breast cancer is a part of AAND.[3,86] Frequency of IFNG (+874) T/T (high producer allele) genotype was significantly higher in breast cancer patients (n = 223) compared to those of controls (n = 267) suggesting that carriers of IFNG (+874) T/T genotype may be at increased risk of breast cancer development. There were no differences in the TNF-alpha and TNF-beta alleles and genotypes frequencies between breast cancer patients and control subjects.[87]

Human hypertension was found to be associated with -930(A/G) polymorphism in the p22 (phox) promoter that contains IFNG site.[88]

Post-KYN metabolism was found to be disturbed in SHR rats. The missense mutation of KAT, the key enzyme of the KYN–KYNA pathway,[89] and increased mRNA expression of kynureninase,[90] the key enzyme of the KYN–NAD pathway, were discovered in SHR. This might shift KYN metabolism from the KYN–KYNA toward the KYN–NAD pathway (Fig. 5).[90] It is noteworthy that spontaneously hypertensive rats are characterized, not only by high blood pressure, but by other components of the MetS/AAND cluster: diabetes, atherosclerosis, obesity, and immunodeficiency.[90]

Association between polymorphism of the human kynureninase gene and essential hypertension was confirmed in Han Chinese population.[91]

The high producer allele (+874T) of the IFNG gene was associated with high lethality in elderly subjects.[92]

Gene–environmental interaction and TRY–KYN metabolism

The increased formation of kynurenines that triggers the chain of biochemical events contributing to the development of Mets/AAND (Fig. 4) might be the result of gene-environmental interaction.

Genetic predetermination of the development of MetS/AAND

The review of available data (see above) suggests that most of the components of MetS/AAND are associated with increased IDO activity, increased production of PIC (in particular, IFNG and TNF-alpha) and high frequency of high producer alleles of genes impacting PIC production. This paper proposes that the risk of MetS/AAND development might be genetically predetermined by the combined presence of high producer alleles of PIC (at least, IFNG and TNF-alpha) resulting in high levels of PIC, and, consequently, in "superinduction" of IDO and shifting of TRY metabolism from methoxyindoles to the KYN pathway.

Environmental impact on TRY–KYN metabolism

Stress and TRY–KYN metabolism. As mentioned above, the other enzyme of the TRY–KYN pathway, TDO, is regulated by substrate and stress hormones but not by PIC. Increased cortisol production (e.g., as in aging and stress)[4,93,94] might, therefore, stimulate TDO and upregulate the KYN pathway of TRY metabolism.[6,47] In addition, cortisol might augment IFNG-induced activation of IDO[6] while PIC may cause hypothalamic-pituitary-axis (HPA) hyperactivity by disturbing the negative feedback inhibition of circulating corticosteroids on the HPA axis[95] (Fig. 6).

Therefore, genetic (mediated via IDO) and environmental (mediated via TDO) factors might

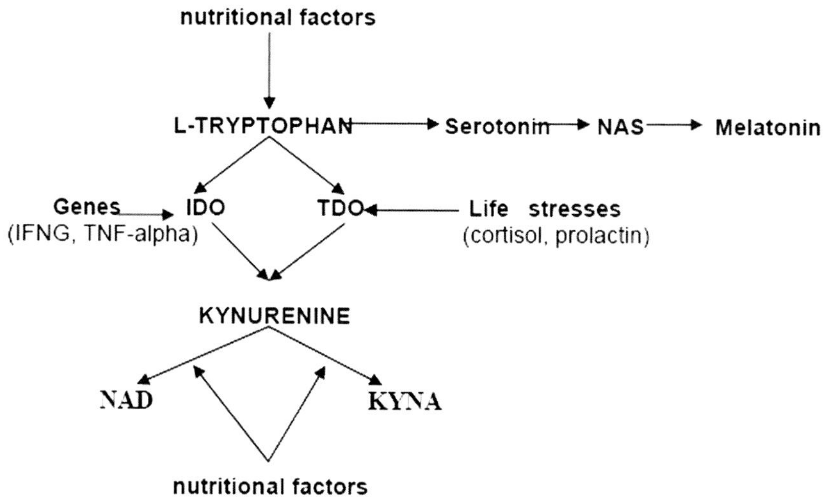

Figure 6. Genetic and environmental impacts on tryptophan metabolism. NAS: *N*-acetylserotonin; IFNG: interferon-gamma; TNF: tumor necrosis factor; IDO: indoleamine 2,3-dioxygenase; TDO: tryptophan 2,3-dioxygenase; NAD: nicotinamide adenine dinucleotide; KYNA: kynurenic acid.

augment each other in activation of the KYN pathway of TRY metabolism: stress superimposed on inflammation, or inflammation superimposed on hyperactivated HPA might trigger increased production of kynurenines (Fig. 6).

Nutritional factors and TRY–KYN metabolism. The concept of gene-environment interaction[96] might be applied to TRY–KYN metabolism as well. Firstly, availability of TRY is influenced by diet because TRY is an essential amino acid for humans. Secondly, TRY release from bond with protein depends on FFA level.[11] TRY deficiency results in pellagra (and pellagric dementia), and might affect IDO-regulated immune status.[97] IFNG production might be affected by micronutrients, for example, zinc.[98]

Both branches of post-KYN metabolism are affected by vitamin B6, the coenzyme of kynureninase[39] and quinolinic acid decarboxylase.[40] It is noteworthy that plasma pyridoxyl-5′-phosphate concentrations were significantly associated with depressive feelings in the elderly population.[99]

Limitations

One of the assumptions of the present hypothesis is that carriers of high producer alleles of cytokine genes have higher production of cytokines than carriers of low promoter alleles. These relationships were reported for healthy volunteers but might be complicated in MetS/AAND, for example, type 2 diabetes.[85] Similarly, association of high producer alleles for the IFNG (+874) gene and high IDO activity was observed in healthy volunteers[54] but no studies done in MetS/AAND.

TRY–KYN metabolism as a new target for prevention and treatment of MetS/AAND

Genotype assessment might help identify subjects-at-risk for the development of MetS/AAND.

Potential pharmacological interventions in identified subjects may include:

(a) inhibition of cytokine production by antibodies to TNF-alpha (e.g., etanercept, infiximab) and IFNG,[100] and by antidepressants, e.g., selective 5-HT inhibitor, fluoxetine,[101] and dopamine enhancer, wellbutrin;[102]
(b) inhibition of IDO activity by MAO inhibitors,[45] minocycline[103] and 1-methyl-L-TRY;[104]
(c) inhibition of TDO by NAS and melatonin;[43]
(d) administration of antibodies to KYN, KYNA, and 3-hydroxyanthranilic acid ;
(e) administration of methoxyindoles (melatonin and NAS) that modulate the

TRY–KYN pathway due to their inhibitory effect on production of cortisol[105] and pro-inflammatory cytokines.[106–108] Methoxyindoles (melatonin, in particular) might attenuate excitatory, glutamate-mediated responses triggered by KYN pathway metabolites;[109,110]

(f) administration of melatonin agonists, e.g., Ramelteon that attenuates age-associated hypertension and body weight gain.[111]

Acknowledgment

The ideas expressed in this review were inspired by my mentors, Professor Vladimir Dilman (1925–1994), who authored the hypothesis of age-associated neuroendocrine disorders, and Professor Slava Lapin, who initiated the studies of neurotropic activities of kynurenines.

Conflicts of interest

The author declares no conflicts of interest.

References

1. Dilman, V.M. 1954. The origin of climacteric and age-associated elevation of blood pressure, cholesterol level and body weight. PhD Thesis, Leinigrad, Russia.
2. Dilman, V.M. 1971. Age-associated elevation of hypothalamic threshold to feedback control, and its role in development, ageing, and disease. *Lancet* **1:** 1211–1219.
3. Dilman, V.M. 1994. *Development, Aging and Disease: A New Rationale for an Intervention Strategy*. Harvard Acad. Publ. Chur, Switzerland.
4. Dilman, V.M., I.P. Lapin & G.F. Oxenkrug. 1979. Serotonin and aging. In *Serotonin in Health and Disease*, Vol. 5. Essman, W., Ed.: 111–123. Spectrum Press, NY-London.
5. Fulop, T. *et al.* 2006. The metabolic syndrome. *Pathologie Biologie* **54:** 375–386.
6. Oxenkrug, G.F. 2007. Genetic and hormonal regulation of the kynurenine pathway of tryptophan metabolism: new target for clinical intervention in vascular dementia, depression and aging. *Ann. N.Y. Acad. Sci.* **1122:** 35–49.
7. Holvoet, P. 2008. Relations between metabolic syndrome, oxidative stress and inflammation and cardiovascular disease. *Verh. K. Acad. Geneeskd. Belg.* **70:** 193–219.
8. Sutherland, J.P. *et al.* 2004. The metabolic syndrome and inflammation. *Metab. Syndr. Relat. Disord.* **2:** 82–104.
9. Ridker, P.M. 2007. Inflammatory biomarkers and risks of myocardial infarction, stroke, diabetes, and total mortality: implications for longevity. *Nutr. Rev.* **65**(12 Pt 2): S253–S259.
10. Gál, E.M. & A.D. Sherman. 1980. L-kynurenine: its synthesis and possible regulatory function in brain. *Neurochem. Res.* **5:** 223–239.
11. Curzon, G. 1996. Brain tryptophan. Normal and disturbed control. *Adv. Exp. Med. Biol.* **398:** 27–34.
12. Lapin, I. P. & G.F. Oxenkrug. 1969. Intensification of the central serotoninergic processes as a possible determinant of the thymoleptic effect. *Lancet* **1:** 32–39.
13. Oxenkrug, G.F. 2010. Tryptophan–kynurenine metabolism as a common mediator of genetic and environmental impacts in major depressive disorder: "the serotonin hypothesis" revisited 40 years later. *Israel J. Psychiatry* (in press).
14. Brzezinski, A. *et al.* 2005. Effects of exogenous melatonin on sleep: a meta-analysis. *Sleep Med. Rev.* **9:** 41–50.
15. Oxenkrug, G.F. & P.J. Requintina. 2003. Melatonin and jet lag syndrome: experimental model and clinical implications. *CNS Spectrums.* **8:** 139–148.
16. Schwarcz, R. & R. Pellicciari. Manipulation of brain kynurenines: glial targets, neuronal effects, and clinical opportunities. *J. Pharmacol. Exp. Ther.* **303:** 1–10.
17. Rongvaux, A. *et al.* 2003. Reconstructing eukaryotic NAD metabolism. *Bioessays* **25:** 683–690.
18. Dang, Y. *et al.* 2000. Comparative effects of oxygen on indoleamine 2,3-dioxygenase and tryptophan 2,3-dioxygenase of the kynurenine pathway. *Free Radic. Biol. Med.* **28:** 615–624.
19. Takikawa, O. *et al.* 1986. Tryptophan degradation in mice initiated by indoleamine 2,3-dioxygenase. *J. Biol. Chem.* **261:** 3648–3653.
20. Lapin, I.P. 1996. Kynurenines and anxiety. *Adv. Exp. Med. Biol.* **398:** 191–194.
21. Wu, H.Q. *et al.* 2007. Kynurenic acid leads, dopamine follows: a new case of volume transmission in the brain? *J. Neural Transm.* **114:** 33–41.
22. Baran, H. *et al.* 1996. Increased kynurenic acid levels and decreased brain kynurenine aminotransferase I in patients with Down syndrome. *Life Sci.* **58:** 1891–1899.
23. Connick, J.H. *et al.* 1989. Increase in kynurenic acid in Huntington's disease motor cortex. *J. Neurochem.* **52:** 985–987.

24. Elias, M.F. *et al.* 2003. Lower cognitive function in the presence of obesity and hypertension: the Framingham. *Int. J. Obes. Relat. Metab. Disord.* **27:** 260–268.
25. Krystal, J.H. *et al.* 1994. Subanesthetic effects of the noncompetitive NMDA antagonist, ketamine, in humans. Psychotomimetic, perceptual, cognitive, and neuroendocrine responses. *Arch. Gen. Psychiatry* **51:** 199–214.
26. Zarate, C.A. *et al.* 2005. An open-label trial of the glutamate-modulating agent riluzole in combination with lithium for the treatment of bipolar depression. *Biol. Psychiatry* **57:** 430–432.
27. Kuc, D. *et al.* 2008. Micromolar concentration of kynurenic acid in rat small intestine. *Amino Acids* **35:** 503–505.
28. Wang, J. *et al.* 2006. Kynurenic acid as a ligand for orphan G protein-coupled receptor GPR35. *J. Biol. Chem.* **281:** 22021–22028.
29. Oxenkrug, G.F. & I.P. Lapin. 1975. Kynurenine pathway of the metabolism of tryptophan and its possible neuropharmacologic role. In *Chemistry and Pharmacology of Indole Compounds.* V. Yakovelev, Ed.: 5–18. Stinza. Kishinev.
30. Kotake, Y. *et al.* 1975. Abnormal tryptophan metabolism and experimental diabetes by xanthurenic acid. *Acta Vitamin Enzymol. (Milano)* **29:** 236–240.
31. Lapin, I.P. 1978. Convulsions and tremor in immature rats after intraperitoneal injection of kynurenine and its metabolites. *Pharmacol. Res. Comm.* **10:** 81–84.
32. Lapin, I.P. 2005. Neurokynurenines (NEKY) as common neurochemical links of stress and anxiety. *Adv. Exp. Med. Biol.* **527:** 121–125.
33. Lapin, I.P. 1998. Antagonism of kynurenic acid to anxiogens in mice. *Life Sci.* **63:** PL231–PL236.
34. Melillo, G. *et al.* 1994. Regulation of nitric-oxide synthase mRNA expression by interferon-gamma and picolinic acid. *J. Biol. Chem.* **269:** 8128–8133.
35. Stewart, J.C. *et al.* 2007. Negative emotions and 3-year progression of subclinical atherosclerosis. *Arch. Gen. Psychiatry* **64:** 225–233.
36. Manev, G. & R. Manev. 2007. 5-lipoxygenase as a possible biological link between depressive symptoms and atherosclerosis. *Arch. Gen. Psychiatry* **64:** 1333.
37. Reddy, A.P. & C.L. Bethea. 2005. Preliminary array analysis reveals novel genes regulated by ovarian steroids in the monkey raphe region. *Psychopharmacology (Berl)* **180:** 125–140.
38. Green, A.R. *et al.* 1978. Metabolism of an oral tryptophan load by women and evidence against the induction of tryptophan pyrrolase by oral contraceptives. *Br. J. Clin. Pharmacol.* **5:** 233–241.
39. Wolf, H. *et al.* 1980. Effect of natural oestrogens on tryptophan metabolism: evidence for interference of oestrogens with kynureninase. *Scand. J. Clin. Lab. Invest.* **40:** 15–22.
40. Moursi, G.E. *et al.* 1970. The influence of sex, age, synthetic oestrogens, progestogens and oral contraceptives on the excretion of urinary tryptophan metabolites. *Bull. World Health Organ.* **43:** 651–661.
41. Requintina, P.J. & G.F. Oxenkrug. 2005. The *in vitro* effect of testosterone and estradiol on the iron-induced lipid peroxidation in rat brain and kidney tissues. *Ann. N. Y. Acad. Sci.* **1053:** 400–404.
42. Alberati-Giani, D. *et al.* 1997. Differential regulation of indoleamine 2,3-dioxygenase expression by nitric oxide and inflammatory mediators in IFN-gamma-activated murine macrophages and microglial cells. *J. Immunol.* **159:** 419–426.
43. Walsh, H.A. & S. Daya. 1997. Inhibition of hepatic tryptophan-2,3-dioxygenase: superior potency of melatonin over serotonin. *J. Pineal Res.* **23:** 20–23.
44. Zawilska, J.B. *et al.* 1997. Suppressive effect of NMDA receptor antagonist MK-801 on nocturnal serotonin N-acetyltransferase activity in the rat pineal gland. *Pol. J. Pharmacol.* **49:** 479–483.
45. Samsonova, M.L. & G.F. Oxenkrug. 1972. Inhibition of substrate induction of TRY-pyrrolase in liver and increase in the content in 5-HT in brain under action of inhibitors of MAO. *Vopr. Med. Khim.* **17:** 198–201.
46. Taylor, M.W. & G.S. Feng. Relationship between interferon-gamma, indoleamine 2,3-dioxygenase, and tryptophan catabolism. *FASEB J.* **5:** 2516–2522.
47. Rubin, R.T. *et al.* 1966. Corticosteroid responses to limbic stimulation in man: localization of stimulus sites. *Science* **153:** 767–768.
48. Robinson, C. *et al.* 2005. The role of IFN-gamma and TNF-alpha-responsive regulatory elements in the synergistic induction of indoleamine dioxygenase. *J. Interferon Cytokine Res.* **25:** 20–30.
49. Wilson, A.G. *et al.* 1993. An allelic polymorphism within the human tumor necrosis factor-alpha promoter region is strongly associated with HLA A1, B8, and DR3 alleles. *J. Exp. Med.* **177:** 557–560.
50. Liebau, C. *et al.* 2002. Interleukin-12 and interleukin-18 induce indoleamine 2,3-dioxygenase (IDO) activity in human osteosarcoma cell lines independently from interferon-gamma. *Anticancer Res.* **22:** 931–936.
51. Kawaguchi, R. *et al.* 2005. Prolactin (PRL) upregulates indoleamine 2,3-dioxygenase (IDO) expression in

CD14+ cells. *Nihon. Rinsho. Meneki. Gakkai. Kaishi.* **228:** 407–412.
52. Gonsky, R. 2006. An IFNG SNP with an estrogen-like response element selectively enhances promoter expression in peripheral but not lamina propria T cells. *Genes Immun.* **7:** 342–351.
53. Pravica, V. *et al.* 2000. A single nucleotide polymorphism in the first intron of the human INFG gene: absolute correlation with a polymorphic CA micro marker of high INFG gene. *Hum. Immunol.* **61:** 8333–8366.
54. Raitala, A. *et al.* 2005. Association of interferon-gamma +874(T/A) single nucleotide polymorphism with the rate of tryptophan catabolism in healthy individuals. *Scand. J. Immunol.* **61:** 387–390.
55. Pertovaara, M. *et al.* 2007. Indoleamine 2,3-dioxygenase enzyme activity correlates with risk factors for atherosclerosis: the Cardiovascular Risk in Young Finns Study. *Clin. Exp. Immunol.* **148:** 106–111.
56. Niinisalo, P. *et al.* 2008. Indoleamine 2,3-dioxygenase activity associates with cardiovascular risk factors: the Health 2000 study. *Scand. J. Clin. Lab. Invest.* **68:** 767–70.
57. Wirleitner, B. *et al.* 2003. Immune activation and degradation of tryptophan in coronary heart disease. *Eur. J. Clin. Invest.* **33:** 550–554.
58. Finkelstein, J.A. 1982. Brain serotonergic activity and plasma amino acid levels in genetically obese Zucker rats. *Pharmacol. Biochem. Behav.* **17:** 939–944.
59. Brandacher, G. *et al.* 2007. Chronic immune activation underlies morbid obesity: is IDO a key player? *Curr. Drug Metab.* **8:** 289–295.
60. Brandacher, G. *et al.* 2006. Bariatric surgery cannot prevent tryptophan depletion due to chronic immune activation in morbidly obese patients. *Obes. Surg.* **16:** 541–548.
61. Pertovaara, M. *et al.* 2006. Indoleamine 2,3-dioxygenase activity in nonagenarians is markedly increased and predicts mortality. *Mech. Ageing Dev.* **127:** 497–499.
62. Jawień, J. 2008. New insights into immunological aspects of atherosclerosis. *Pol. Arch. Med. Wewn.* **118:** 127–131.
63. Koga, M. *et al.* 2007. Postnatal blocking of interferon-gamma function prevented atherosclerotic plaque formation in apolipoprotein E-knockout mice. *Hypertens Res.* **30:** 259–267.
64. Bergman, M.R. *et al.* 1999. Myocardial tumor necrosis factor-alpha secretion in hypertensive and heart failure-prone rats. *Am. J. Physiol.* **277**(2 Pt 2): H543–H550.
65. You, T. *et al.* 2008. The metabolic syndrome is associated with circulating adipokines in older adults across a wide range of adiposity. *J. Gerontol. A Biol. Sci. Med Sci.* **63:** 414–419.
66. Dorffel, Y. *et al.* 1999. Preactivated peripheral blood monocytes in patients with essential hypertension. *Hypertension* **34:** 113–117.
67. Meier, C.A. & S. Thalman. 2007. White adipose tissue, inflammation and atherosclerosis. *Bull. Acad. Natl. Med.* **191:** 897–908.
68. Rocha, V.Z. *et al.* 2008. Interferon-gamma, a Th1 cytokine, regulates fat inflammation: a role for adaptive immunity in obesity. *Circ. Res.* **103:** 467–476.
69. Dahlgren, J. *et al.* 2001. Prenatal cytokine exposure results in obesity and gender-specific programming. *Am. J. Physiol. Endocrinol. Metab.* **281:** E326–E334.
70. Pacifico, L. *et al.* 2006. Increased T-helper interferon-gamma-secreting cells in obese children. *Eur. J. Endocrinol.* **154:** 691–697.
71. Lann, D. & D. LeRoith. 2007. Insulin resistance as the underlying cause for the metabolic syndrome. *Med. Clin. North Am.* **91:** 1063–1077.
72. Susa, S. *et al.* 2008. A functional polymorphism of the TNF-alpha gene that is associated with type 2 DM. *Biochem. Biophys. Res. Commun.* **369:** 943–947.
73. Janssen, I. *et al.* 2008. Menopause and the metabolic syndrome: The Study of Women's Health Across the Nation. *Arch. Intern. Med.* **168:** 1568–1575.
74. Carr, M.C. 2003. The emergence of the metabolic syndrome with menopause. *J. Clin. Endocrinol. Metab.* **88:** 2404–2411.
75. Deguchi, K. *et al.* 2001. Postmenopausal changes in production of type 1 and type 2 cytokines and the effects of hormone replacement therapy. *Menopause* **8:** 266–273.
76. Rodríguez, M.I. *et al.* 2007. Chronic melatonin treatment reduces the age-dependent inflammatory process in senescence-accelerated mice. *J. Pineal Res.* **42:** 272–279.
77. Franciotta, D. *et al.* 2006. Interferon-gamma- and interleukin-4-producing T cells in Down's syndrome. *Neurosci. Lett.* **395:** 67–70.
78. Schiepers, O.J. *et al.* 2005. Cytokines and major depression. *Prog. Neuropsychopharmacol. Biol. Psychiatry* **29:** 201–217.
79. Pausova, Z. *et al.* 2003. Segment of rat chromosome 20 regulates diet-induced augmentations in adiposity, glucose intolerance, and blood pressure. *Hypertension* **41:** 1047–1055.
80. Sookoian, S.C. *et al.* 2005. Meta-analysis on the G-308A tumor necrosis factor alpha gene variant and

phenotypes associated with the metabolic syndrome. *Obes. Res.* **13:** 2122–2131.

81. de Luis, D.A. *et al.* 2007. Influence of G308A polymorphism of tumor necrosis factor alpha gene on insulin resistance in obese patients after weight loss. *Med. Clin. (Barc).* **129:** 401–404.
82. Jun, T.Y. *et al.* 2003. Possible association between -G308A tumour necrosis factor-alpha gene polymorphism and major depressive disorder in the Korean population. *Psychiatr. Genet.* **13:** 179–181.
83. Pae, C.U. *et al.* 2004. Tumor necrosis factor alpha gene-G308A polymorphism associated with bipolar I disorder in the Korean population. *Psychiatry Res.* **125:** 65–68.
84. Czerski, P.M. *et al.* 2008. Association of tumor necrosis factor -308G/A promoter polymorphism with schizophrenia and bipolar affective disorder in a Polish population. *Neuropsychobiology* **57:** 88–94.
85. Tsiavou, A. *et al.* 2005. Correlation between intracellular interferon-gamma production by CD4+ and CD8 +lymphocytes and IFN-gamma gene polymorphism in patients with type 2 diabetes mellitus and latent autoimmune diabetes of adults (LADA). *Cytokine* **31:** 135–141.
86. Oxenkrug, G.F. 2005. Antidepressant effect of N-acetylserotonin in relation to aging, hypertension and cancer. In *Hormones, Age and Cancer*. L. Berstein, Ed.: 140–158. Nauka. St. Petersburg.
87. Kamali-Sarvestani, E. *et al.* 2005. Polymorphism in the genes of alpha and beta tumor necrosis factors (TNF-alpha and TNF-beta) and gamma interferon (IFN-gamma) among Iranian women with breast cancer. *Cancer Lett.* **223:** 113–119.
88. Moreno, M.U. *et al.* 2003. Preliminary characterization of the promoter of the human p22(phox) gene: identification of a new polymorphism associated with hypertension. *FEBS Lett.* **542:** 27–31.
89. Kwok, J.B. *et al.* 2002. A missense mutation in kynurenine aminotransferase-1 in spontaneously hypertensive rats. *J. Biol. Chem.* **277:** 35779–35782.
90. Mizutani, K. *et al.* 2002. Kynureninase is a novel candidate gene for hypertension in spontaneously hypertensive rats. *Hypertens Res.* **25:** 135–140.
91. Zhang, Y. *et al.* 2005. [A polymorphism of kynureninase gene in a hypertensive candidate chromosomal region is associated with essential hypertension]. *Zhonghua Xin Xue Guan Bing Za Zhi* **33:** 588–691.
92. Lio, D. *et al.* 2002. Allele frequencies of +874T-A single nucleotide polymorphism at the first intron of interferon-gamma gene in a group Italian centernarians. *Exp. Gerontol.* **37:** 315–319.
93. Oxenkrug, G.F. *et al.* 1983. Aging and cortisol resistance to supression by dexamethasone: a positive correlation. *Psychiatry Res.* **10:** 125–130.
94. Oxenkrug, G.F. *et al.* 1984. Dexamethasone suppression test: experimental model in rats and effect of age. *Biol. Psychiat.* **19:** 413–416.
95. Leonard, B. 2006. The HPA and immune axes in stress: the involvement of the serotonergic system. *Neuroimmunomodulation* **13:** 268–276.
96. Ordovas, J. 2007. Diet/genetic interactions and their effects on inflammatory markers. *Nutr. Rev.* **65:** S203–207.
97. Penberthy, W.T. 2007. Pharmacological targeting of IDO-mediated tolerance for treating autoimmune disease. *Curr. Drug Metab.* **8:** 245–266.
98. Hamer, D.H. *et al.* 2009. Micronutrient deficiencies are associated with impaired immune response and higher burden of respiratory infections in elderly ecuadorians. *J. Nutr.* **139:** 113–119.
99. Merete, C. *et al.* 2008. Vitamin B6 is associated with depressive symptomatology in Massachusetts elders. *J. Am. Coll. Nutr.* **27:** 421–427.
100. Skurkovich, B. & S. Skurkovich. 2006. Inhibition of IFN-gamma as a method of treatment of various autoimmune diseases, including skin diseases. *Ernst Schering Res. Found. Workshop.* **56:** 1–27.
101. Kenis, G. & M. Maes. Effects of antidepressants on the production of cytokines. *Int. J. Neuropsychopharmacol.* **5:** 401–412.
102. Brustolim, D. *et al.* 2006. A new chapter opens in anti-inflammatory treatments: the antidepressant bupropion lowers production of tumor necrosis factor-alpha and interferon-gamma in mice. *Int. Immunopharmacol.* **6:** 903–909.
103. Ryu, J. K. *et al.* 2006. Combined minocycline plus pyruvate treatment enhances effects of each agent to inhibit inflammation, oxidative damage, and neuronal loss in an excitotoxic animal model of Huntington's disease. *Neuroscience* **141:** 1835–1848.
104. Cady, S.G. & Sono M. 1991. 1-Methyl-DL-tryptophan, beta-(3-benzofuranyl)-DL-alanine (the oxygen analog of tryptophan), and beta-[3-benzo(b)thienyl]-DL-alanine (the sulfur analog of tryptophan) are competitive inhibitors for indoleamine 2,3-dioxygenase. *Arch. Biochem. Biophys.* **291:** 326–333.
105. Oxenkrug, G.F. *et al.* 1984. Effects of pinealectomy and aging on the serum corticosterone circadian rhythm in rats. *J. Pineal Res.* **1:** 181–185.
106. Perianayagam, M.C. *et al.* 2005. Immune modulating effects of melatonin, N- acetyl serotonin and

N-acetyl dopamine. *Ann. N.Y. Acad. Sci.* **1053:** 386–393.

107. Requintina, P.J. & G.F. Oxenkrug. 2003. Differential effects of lipopolysaccharide on lipid peroxidation in F344N, SHR rats and BALB/C mice and protection of melatonin and NAS against its toxicity. *Ann. N.Y. Acad. Sci.* **993:** 325–333.
108. Bachurin, S. *et al.* 1999. N-acetylserotonin, melatonin and their derivatives improve cognition and protect against beta-amyloid-induced neurotoxicity. *Ann. N.Y. Acad. Sci.* **890:** 155–166.
109. Lapin, I.P. *et al.* 1998. Anticonvulsant activity of melatonin against seizures induced by quinolinate, kainate, glutamate, NMDA and pentylenetetrazole in mice. *J. Pineal Res.* **24:** 215–218.
110. Prakhie, I.V. & G.F. Oxenkrug. 1998. The effect of nifedipine, Ca ++antagonist, on activity of MAO inhibitors, N-acetylserotonin and melatonin in the mouse tail suspension test. *Intern. J. Neuropsychopharmac.* **1:** 35–40.
111. Oxenkrug, G.F. & P. Summergrad. 2010. Ramelteon attenuates age-associated hypertension and weight gain in spontaneously hypertensive rats. *Ann. N.Y. Acad. Sci.* **1191:** 114–120.

Ann. N.Y. Acad. Sci. ISSN 0077-8923

ANNALS OF THE NEW YORK ACADEMY OF SCIENCES
Issue: *Neuroprotective Agents*

Diabetes aggravates heat stress-induced blood-brain barrier breakdown, reduction in cerebral blood flow, edema formation, and brain pathology

Possible neuroprotection with growth hormone

Dafin F. Muresanu,[1] Aruna Sharma,[2] and Hari Shanker Sharma[2]

[1]Department of Neurology, University of Medicine and Pharmacy "Iuliu Hatieganu", Cluj-Napoca, Romania. [2]Department of Surgical Sciences, Anesthesiology & Intensive Care Medicine, University Hospital, Uppsala University, Sweden

Address for correspondence: Hari Shanker Sharma, PhD (BHU), Dr. Med Sci (UU), Professor of Neurobiology (MRC), Docent in Neuroanatomy (UU); Frödingsgatan 12:28, SE-75421 Uppsala, Sweden. Sharma@surgsci.uu.se

The possibility that diabetes influences the outcome of heat stress-induced brain pathology was examined in our experimental rat model. Because growth hormone (GH) deficiency is an important factor in diabetes, the possible neuroprotective role of GH supplements was also examined in diabetic rats following heat stress. Rats receiving streptozotocine once daily for three days (50 mg/kg, i.p.) and allowed to survive four weeks resulted in diabetes (blood glucose level 18 and 20 mMol/L) compared to controls (blood glucose 4–6 mMol/L). Control or diabetic rats when subjected to four hours' heat stress at 38° C in a biological oxygen demand incubator (BOD) showed profound disruption of the blood-brain barrier (BBB), reduction in cerebral blood flow (CBF), brain edema formation, and cell injury. These effects were most pronounced in diabetic rats. Pretreatment with GH (50 μg/kg/min for 10 min before heat stress) significantly attenuated brain pathology in normal animals subjected to hyperthermia. On the other hand, almost a double dose of the growth hormone (80 to 120 μg/g/min for 10 min) is needed in diabetic rats to induce considerable neuroprotection following heat stress. These observations are the first to suggest that diabetic rats are more vulnerable to heat stress-induced brain pathology and further show that the efficacy of neuroprotective drugs is also severely reduced in diabetic rats. Taken together, our results demonstrate that the dosage of neuroprotective drugs requires adjustment to enhance neuroprotection depending on the patient's endocrine or metabolic status, for example, diabetes mellitus, a finding not reported earlier.

Keywords: heat stress; diabetes mellitus; neuropathology; hyperthermia; blood-brain barrier; cerebral blood flow; brain edema; hippocampus; growth hormone; neuroprotection

Introduction

The incidence of heat stroke associated with heat stress has increased remarkably during summer months recently among European populations, probably due to global warming.[1–3] However, it is still unclear whether populations suffering from various disorders of endocrine metabolism, for example, diabetes mellitus, are equally or more sensitive to heat stroke-induced pathophysiology. There are reasons to believe that diabetes mellitus itself could influence the blood-brain barrier (BBB) permeability.[4–8] However, this issue is still controversial (see Ref. 7). An increase in the BBB function will allow leakage of serum proteins that could result in brain edema formation.[9] Thus, it is quite likely that hyperglycemia associated with diabetes mellitus may alter the brain microvasculature leading to brain edema formation through modification of the BBB function.

Few studies indicate that patients with diabetes are more sensitive to changes in environmental temperatures.[10–12] Thus, it is possible that diabetic animals could be more sensitive to heat-induced hyperthermia and brain dysfunctions. Because chronic renal hypertension exacerbates the BBB disruption,

doi: 10.1111/j.1749-6632.2009.05328.x

brain edema formation and cell injury in a rat model of heat stroke,[13] a possibility exists that diabetic rats may also show altered responsiveness of BBB function following heat stress.

Several clinical and experimental studies show that diabetes is able to attenuate the release and sensitivity of growth hormone.[14–16] A reduction in growth hormone or its effect on the biological system in diabetes mellitus could be instrumental in influencing brain dysfunction and related disorders. Thus, a possibility exists that exogenous supplement of growth hormone may improve brain functions in diabetic animals.

The present investigation was undertaken to understand the brain pathophysiology of hyperthermia in an experimental diabetic rat model. Furthermore, the role of growth hormone deficiency in diabetes-induced brain function was also examined following exogenous supplement of growth hormone in our rat model.[14] In view of the fact that the microvascular responsiveness is known to be altered in chronic hyperglycemic episodes in several diabetic models,[15–18] we wanted to see whether the diabetic rats require any adjustment of the growth hormone dosage to induce neuroprotection as compared to normal animals following heat stress.

Materials and methods

Animals

Experiments were carried out on inbred Charles Foster male rats (200–300 g) housed at a controlled ambient temperature (21 ± 1° C) with 12-h light and 12-h dark schedule. The tap water and food were supplied *ad libitum* before the experiments. All experimental procedures and handling of animals were carried out according to National Institute of Health (NIH) guidelines for Handling and Care of Experimental animals to minimize their sufferings. These experimental conditions were approved by Local Institutional Ethics Committee.

Treatment with streptozotocine

Rats were treated with Streptozotocine (Sigma Chemical Co., St. Louis, MO) in a dose of 25 to 75 mg/kg, i.p. per day for 3 days and animals were allowed to survive 4 weeks for the development of chronic diabetes-like conditions (see Table 1). Streptozotocine was prepared freshly each time and dissolved in 0.9% saline with a slightly acidic pH (5.6) immediately before injection in order to avoid denaturation of the compound that could occur within 10 to 15 min in solution.[19–21] The blood glucose from tail vein was measured every day using an automatic blood glucose analyzer (Abbott, London, United Kingdom).

Only those animals were used in the experiments that did not develop BBB leakage due to diabetic complications and were not entered into a moribund state due to excessive hyperglycemia. We found that 50 mg/kg, i.p. of streptozotocine for 3 consecutive days is sufficient enough to develop a mild hyperglycemia and did not induce other

Table 1. Effect of streptozotocine on blood glucose level, blood-brain barrier permeability, and brain edema formation in rats after four weeks of survival

Experiment type	n	Blood glucose mMol/L	BBB permeability Evans blue leakage	Brain edema visual swelling
Streptozotocine (i.p.) per day for 3 days				
25 mg/kg	8	$12 \pm 4^{**}$	nil	nil
50 mg/kg	12	$18 \pm 4^{**}$	nil	nil
75 mg/kg	12	$32 \pm 5^{**}$	++	+++
0.9% saline (i.p.) per day for 3 days	10	5 ± 2	nil	nil
0.9% saline (pH 5.6, i.p.) per day for 3 days	12	6 ± 2	nil	nil

Values are mean ± SD. $^{**} = P < 0.01$, Student's unpaired t-test.

complications of the diabetes, for example, brain swelling or BBB dysfunction. Those animals that showed a blood glucose level > 20 mMol/L were not used for further experiments (see Table 1). These diabetic animals were maintained properly in their cages (placed individually) and care was taken to check each animal for any complications every 6 h during 8:00 AM until 10:00 PM as standard procedure.

Exposure to heat stress

Diabetic or normal rats (saline treated) were exposed to 4 h heat stress at 38° C in a biological oxygen demand (BOD) incubator (relative humidity 45–47%; and wind velocity 20–25 cm/s) as described earlier.[22,23]

Treatment with growth hormone

Rats made diabetic or normal animals were treated with rat growth hormone (Gift from Prof. Fred Nyberg, Uppsala University) in a dose of 50 μg/kg to 120 μg/kg/min for 10 min intravenously (30 min before heat stress) through a polyethylene cannula (PE 10) implanted aseptically into their right jugular vein 1 week before the experiments.[22–25]

Parameters measured

The following parameters were measured in normal, heat-stressed, and diabetic rats exposed to hyperthermia using standard procedures.

Thermal stress symptoms

Changes in rectal temperature, behavioral salivation and prostration were examined in rats as thermal stress symptoms. The rectal temperature was measured using thermistor probes (Yellow Springs, OH) connected to telethermometer (Aplab Electronics, London, United Kingdom). The magnitude and severity of heat stress was assessed using the intensity of salivation occurring around snouts of rats during heat exposure.[23] Also heat-induced prostration was used to indicate heat exhaustion symptoms.[22,23]

Blood-brain barrier permeability

The BBB was measured using two protein tracers, that is, Evans blue albumin (2% of a 0.3 mL/100 g sterile solution) and radioiodine (^{131}Iodine 10 μCi/100 g rat) administered together in the right jugular vein immediately after termination of heat stress. These tracers when administered into the circulation will bind serum proteins (largely albumin, EBA about 68% and ^{131}Iodine about 56%) and thus, their leakage in brain represents extravasation of serum protein complex (see Refs. 22, 26, 27). The tracers were allowed to circulate 10 min after administration and then the animals were anesthetized with equithesin (1 to 2 mL/kg, i.p.).[22]

Brain edema formation

Brain edema formation was measured using brain water content determinations.[22,23,28] For this purpose, under equithesin anesthesia, small tissue pieces from brain were taken out immediately after heat stress, and large superficial blood vessels or blood clots, if any, were removed. The brain samples were weighed and placed in an oven at 90° C to obtain the dry weight of these samples. Water content was calculated from the differences between wet and dry weight of samples.[23]

Cerebral blood flow

In a separate group of animals, local cerebral blood flow (CBF) was examined using ^{125}I radiolabelled (^{125}Iodine) carbonized microspheres (o.d. 15 ± 0.6 μm) as described earlier.[29] About 1 million microspheres were administered retrogradely toward the heart through the left common carotid artery, and the peripheral arterial blood samples were collected from the right femoral artery at the regular intervals of 30 s starting from 30 s before microsphere administration until 90 s after completion of the injection.[22,23,28,29] The reference arterial blood was withdrawn from femoral artery at the rate of 0.8 mL/min.[29] At the end of 90 s after microsphere administration, the brains were removed and tissue samples were dissected out (sample size about 135 to 250 mg) and the radioactivity was counted in a Gamma counter (Packard Instruments, Meriden, CT). The whole blood radioactivity from the samples withdrawn was also determined. The CBF was calculated from the radioactivity seen in the brain in relation to radioactivity present in reference blood samples at the time of decapitation using standard formula (see Ref. 29).

Histopathology

In separate groups of rats brain pathology was determined using standard procedures. After heat stress, these animals were perfused with 0.9% saline through cardiac puncture followed by 4% buffered paraformaldehyde at 100 torr perfusion pressure (see Refs. 22, 23). After perfusion, the brains were dissected out and kept in the same fixative at 4° C in a refrigerator for 1 week. After that, small tissue pieces from various brain regions were cut and embedded in paraffin. About 3 μm thick paraffin sections were obtained and processed for Nissl and Haematoxylin and Eosin staining using standard protocol (see Ref. 30).

Statistical analyses

ANOVA followed by Dunnet's test for multiple group comparison with one control and unpaired Student's *t*-tests were used to evaluate statistical significance of the data obtained. A *P*-value < 0.05 was considered significant.

Results

Streptozotocine-induced diabetes

Streptozotocine in a dose range of 25 mg to 75 mg/kg intraperitoneally administered once daily for 3 days induced diabetes (blood glucose level 18 to 20 mMol/L) in rats after 4 weeks that was quite comparable to those seen in clinical situations (see Table 1). In our experiments, 50 mg/kg i.p. dose of streptozotocine was found optimal to produce considerable hyperglycemia in rats without opening of the BBB permeability to Evans blue or inducing any brain swelling at 4 weeks after its administration (Table 1). In these animals development of diabetes was gradual and blood glucose levels did not reach beyond 30 mMol/L during 4 weeks of survival (Table 1). On the other hand, a lower dose of streptozotocine (25 mg) was not sufficient enough to induce profound hyperglycemia over 4 weeks (Table 1). However, a 75 mg dose of streptozotocine resulted in the death of several rats due to severe hyperglycemia during the 4 weeks of survival period (Table 1). Thus, we used the 50 mg/kg dose of streptozotocine to induce diabetes in rats, quite comparable to that seen in the clinical situation for our investigation in heat stress.

Administration of normal saline or saline with a slightly acidic pH (5.6) that is used to dissolve streptozotocine did not alter either the blood glucose levels in rats or induce any changes in the BBB permeability to Evans blue dye or brain edema formation (Table 1).

Thermal stress symptoms

Normal animals when subjected to 4 h heat stress showed profound hyperthermia, salivation, and signs of behavioral prostration (Table 2). Diabetic animals when subjected to identical heat stress exhibited much higher thermal stress symptoms than the normal animals (Table 2). In diabetic animals the body temperature showed a significantly higher increase (mean 41.86°) than normal animals (mean 41.06° C) after 4 h heat stress (Table 2). The magnitude and intensity of salivation and behavioral prostration were also greater in diabetic rats

Table 2. Effect of growth hormone on gross brain pathology in normal and diabetic rats

		BBB permeability (Evans blue leakage)		Brain edema (visual swelling)	
Type of experiment	*n*	Normal	Diabetic	Normal	Diabetic
Control		nil	nil	nil	nil
4 h heat stress (HS)		++++	++++++	++++	++++++
Growth hormone 10 min					
10 μg/min		++++	+++++++	++++	++++++
20 μg/min		++++	++++++	++++	++++++
50 μg/min		+	+++++	+	+++++
80 μg/min		+/−	++++	+/−	++++
120 μg/min		nil	++	nil	++

Growth hormone was infused intravenously 30 min before heat stress. Animals were subjected to four h heat stress at 38° C in a BOD incubator. For details, see text.
Nil = absent; + = present; +/− = faint; ++ = mild; ++++ = moderate; +++++ = high; ++++++ = very high.

Table 3. Effect of heat stress on thermal stress symptoms and cortical blood-brain barrier permeability, cerebral blood flow, brain edema, and brain pathology following heat stress in normal and in diabetic rats

		Heat stress 4 h 38° C			
		Untreated		Growth hormone treatment 10 min	
Type of experiment	Control	Normal	Diabetic	Normal 50 μg/min	Diabetic 80 μg/min
A. Thermal stress symptoms $n = 6$		**whole body symptoms**			
Rectal T° C	37.04 ± 0.023	41.06 ± 0.12**	41.86 ± 0.23**a	40.34 ± 0.19*a	40.67 ± 0.21*b
Salivation	nil	++++	++++++	+++	+++
Prostration	nil	+++	+++++	++	++
B. Blood-brain barrier permeability $n = 8$		**cerebral cortex**			
Evans blue albumin mg %	0.26 ± 0.07	1.89 ± 0.12**	2.34 ± 0.23**a	0.67 ± 0.21**a	0.84 ± 0.32**b
[131]Iodine %	0.30 ± 0.08	2.34 ± 0.19**	3.12 ± 0.31**a	0.87 ± 0.17**a	0.98 ± 0.32**b
C. Cerebral blood flow $n = 6$					
ml/g/min	1.15 ± 0.07	0.82 ± 0.07**	0.74 ± 0.04**a	0.89 ± 0.03**a	0.88 ± 0.06**b
D. Brain edema $n = 8$					
Water content %	74.56 ± 0.34	78.46 ± 0.54**	80.34 ± 0.21**a	76.04 ± 0.22**a	77.09 ± 0.10**b
E. Brain pathology $n = 6$					
Distorted neurons nr	3 ± 4	112 ± 23**	189 ± 28**a	56 ± 19**a	78 ± 24**b

Values are mean ± SD. * = $P < 0.05$; ** = $P < 0.01$ compared with control group; a = $P < 0.05$ compared with untreated heat-stressed rats; b = $P < 0.05$, compared with diabetic heat-stressed rats. ANOVA followed by Dunnet's test for multiple group comparison.

compared to normal animals following heat stress (Table 2).

BBB permeability

Normal animals at 4 h heat stress showed a marked increase in the BBB permeability to protein tracers, that is, Evans blue and radioiodine (Table 2). This increase in the BBB permeability to Evans blue and radioiodine was further aggravated in diabetic rats after identical heat exposure (Table 2). Analysis of regional changes in the BBB showed extravasation of radioiodine in all the 10 brain regions examined in normal animals after heat stress. The most marked increase in radioiodine extravasation from the control rats (not exposed to heat stress) was seen in cortical and subcortical regions. Brain stem showed only a mild but significant increase in the BBB breakdown to radioiodine (Table 3). In diabetic rats, extravasation of radioiodine in these brain regions was significantly higher compared to normal animals after heat stress, except in hypothalamus and in brain stem (Table 3). The most marked increase in BBB permeability to iodine in diabetic rats was seen largely in the cortical brain areas and in the cerebellum (Table 3).

Cerebral blood flow

Normal animals after 4 h heat stress exhibited a significant reduction in the CBF compared to rats kept at room temperature (Table 2). This decrease in CBF was most pronounced when diabetic rats were exposed to identical periods of heat stress (Table 2). Regional analysis of CBF showed a mild to moderate decrease by heat stress in all the 10 brain regions examined in normal animals (Table 3). The most marked decrease in the CBF (20 to 40%) was seen in cortical areas of the brain followed by hippocampus. Thalamus, hypothalamus, and brain stem showed much less decrease in the CBF after heat stress. Diabetic rats showed an even greater decrease in the CBF compared with normal rats after heat stress (Table 2). This decrease in regional CBF was greater in almost all brain areas in diabetic animals compared to normal rats under identical heat exposure

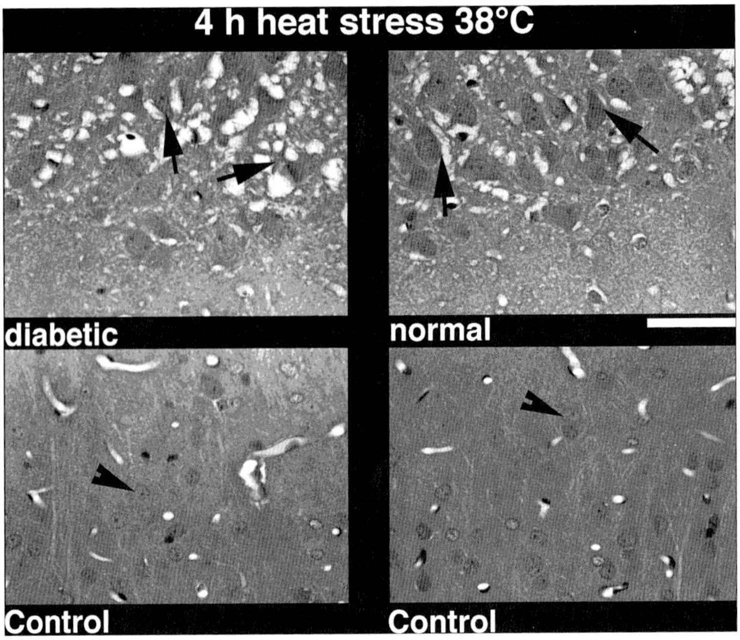

Figure 1. Excessive neuronal damage (*arrows, left upper panel*) in diabetic rats after 4 h heat stress as compared to normal animals (*right upper panel*). Diabetic rats before heat stress show only mild changes in the neuronal density (*left lower panel*) compared to normal rats kept at room temperature (*right lower panel*). Bar: 35 μm.

(Table 3). In general, the reduction in CBF was most prominent in cortical areas followed by hippocampus and thalamus. Hypothalamus and brain stem did not show much reduction in CBF after heat exposure (Table 3). However, the magnitude of this CBF decrease was not correlated with the intensity of BBB breakdown in these brain regions either in normal rats or in diabetic animals after heat exposure.

Brain edema

Heat stress induced profound development of brain edema at 4 h in normal animals as compared to the control group kept at room temperature (Table 2). The magnitude of edema formation examined using changes in brain water content was much greater in diabetic rats after heat exposure as compared to normal animals following identical heat exposure (Table 2).

Brain pathology

Four h heat stress resulted in marked neuronal damage in normal animals (Table 2). The magnitude and intensity of these neuronal damages were most pronounced in diabetic rats after heat stress (Table 2). Regional analysis of neuronal damage showed profound neuronal distortion and cell death in almost all brain regions showing breakdown of the BBB permeability. A representative example of neuronal damage in heat stress in the cerebral cortex of normal animals showed profound neuronal distortion, neurodegeneration, sponginess, and edema. Many neuronal nuclei are dark stained and seen with eccentric nucleoli in heat-stressed rats (Fig. 1). Diabetic rats show widespread areas of neuronal damage in which several dark and distorted neurons are seen in the neuropil. The magnitude of sponginess, edema, and neuronal damage was greater in diabetic rats following heat stress as compared to normal animals after identical heat exposure (Fig. 1).

Treatment with growth hormone

Growth hormone when administered into normal rats intravenously in the range of 10 to 120 μg/kg/min for 10 min showed pronounced neuroprotective effects in heat-stressed animals (see Table 4). In normal animals subjected to heat stress, 50 μg/kg/min for 10 min infusion of growth hormone was found very effective in inducing neuroprotection (Table 4). However, diabetic rats required

Ann. N.Y. Acad. Sci. 1199 (2010) 15–26 © 2010 New York Academy of Sciences.

Table 4. Regional blood-brain barrier (BBB) and cerebral blood flow (CBF) following heat stress in normal and diabetic rats

	Control		4 h heat stress			
			Normal		Diabetic	
Brain regions	BBB [131] iodine % $n = 6$	CBF ml/g/min $n = 6$	BBB [131] iodine % $n = 8$	CBF ml/g/min $n = 8$	BBB [131] iodine % $n = 12$	CBF ml/g/min $n = 12$
1. Frontal cortex	0.23 ± 0.04	1.12 ± 0.05	0.78 ± 0.10**	0.89 ± 0.02*	0.98 ± 0.08**b	0.78 ± 0.08**b
2. Parietal cortex	0.28 ± 0.06	1.08 ± 0.06	1.10 ± 0.08**	0.80 ± 0.03**	1.18 ± 0.04**	0.76 ± 0.08**b
3. Occipital cortex	0.26 ± 0.05	1.14 ± 0.04	1.34 ± 0.10**	0.78 ± 0.04**	1.56 ± 0.12*b	0.70 ± 0.06**
4. Temporal cortex	0.24 ± 0.08	1.06 ± 0.04	0.98 ± 0.06**	0.82 ± 0.06**	1.21 ± 0.08**b	0.73 ± 0.05**b
5. Cingulate cortex	0.18 ± 0.09	1.04 ± 0.06	1.03 ± 0.04**	0.80 ± 0.09*	1.23 ± 0.04**b	0.74 ± 0.03**b
6. Hippocampus	0.30 ± 0.08	0.91 ± 0.02	0.98 ± 0.03**	0.78 ± 0.02*	1.14 ± 0.03*b	0.70 ± 0.04**b
7. Cerebellum	0.11 ± 0.04	0.98 ± 0.03	1.01 ± 0.04**	0.74 ± 0.02*	1.34 ± 0.10**b	0.70 ± 0.02**
8. Thalamus	0.34 ± 0.09	0.89 ± 0.08	0.97 ± 0.08**	0.88 ± 0.10	0.89 ± 0.10*b	0.78 ± 0.08**b
9. Hypothalamus	0.36 ± 0.11	0.87 ± 0.04	0.89 ± 0.10**	0.80 ± 0.13	0.88 ± 0.12**	0.75 ± 0.03**
10. Brain stem	0.18 ± 0.08	0.78 ± 0.04	0.67 ± 0.07**	0.70 ± 0.10	0.64 ± 0.14**	0.73 ± 0.04**

Values are mean ± SD. * = $P < 0.05$, ** = $P < 0.01$ compared with control group; b = $P < 0.05$, compared with diabetic heat-stressed rats. ANOVA followed by Dunnet's test for multiple group comparison.

almost a double dose of the growth hormone (80 to 120 μg/kg/min for 10 min) to induce considerable neuroprotection in heat stress (Tables 2 and 4). Thus, most investigations on brain pathology were made with 50 μg/kg growth hormone in normal rats and 80 μg/kg growth hormone in diabetic rats in heat stress (See Tables 2, 4, and 5).

Thermal stress symptoms. Growth hormone in a dose of 50 μg/kg/min for 10 min significantly attenuated thermal stress symptoms following 4 h heat exposure in normal rats (Table 2). However, 80 μg/kg dose of growth hormone is needed in diabetic rats to reduce thermal stress symptoms after heat exposure (Table 2).

BBB permeability. The BBB permeability to Evans blue albumin and radioiodine was significantly reduced in normal animals after heat exposure when growth hormone was administered in a dose of 50 μg/kg/min for 10 min, 30 min before heat stress. However, this dose of growth hormone was ineffective in influencing BBB dysfunction in diabetic rats following heat stress. In diabetic animals an 80 μg/kg/min dose of growth hormone was needed to reduce BBB dysfunction to protein tracers effectively after heat stress (Table 2). In these doses, growth hormone was also seen to effectively reduce the regional BBB permeability in diabetic rats (Table 5). Thus, 50 μg/kg/min growth hormone effectively attenuated BBB permeability to radioiodine in several brain regions after 4 h heat stress in normal animals, whereas 80 μg/kg/min growth hormone was able to effectively reduce the regional BBB changes to radioiodine in diabetic rats after heat stress (Table 5).

Cerebral blood flow. In normal animals growth hormone in a dose of 50 μg/kg/min for 10 min if given 30 min before heat stress remarkably improved the CBF at 4 h heat exposure (Table 2). However, to achieve similar effects on CBF in diabetic rats in heat stress 80 μg/kg growth hormone infusion is needed for 10 min before heat stress (Table 2). Regional blood flow changes also show that growth hormone (50 μg/kg/min) is able to markedly improve CBF in normal animals after 4 h heat stress, a feature that is seen in diabetic animals only after administration of 80 μg/kg/min for 10 min in heat stress (Table 5).

Brain edema formation. In normal animals, 50 μg/kg/min growth hormone was able to significantly reduce the brain edema formation at 4 h

Table 5. Effects of growth hormone treatment on regional blood-brain barrier (BBB), cerebral blood flow (CBF), and brain pathology following heat stress in normal and diabetic rats

		4 h heat stress at 38° C growth hormone treated					
		Normal rats 50 μg/min		Diabetic rats 80 μg/min		Normal rats 50 μg/min	Diabetic rats 80 μg/min
Brain regions	n	BBB [131] iodine %	CBF ml/g/min	BBB [131] iodine %	CBF ml/g/min	neuronal injury	neuronal injury
1. Frontal cortex		0.56 ± 0.10**a	0.95 ± 0.06*a	0.87 ± 0.08*b	0.86 ± 0.06*b	56 ± 12*	87 ± 23*b
2. Parietal cortex		0.69 ± 0.10**a	0.88 ± 0.04*a	0.88 ± 0.10**b	0.84 ± 0.05*b	64 ± 18*	95 ± 10*b
3. Occipital cortex		0.62 ± 0.08**a	86 ± 0.04*a	0.90 ± 0.10*b	0.76 ± 0.05*b	68 ± 23*	89 ± 10*b
4. Temporal cortex		0.60 ± 0.08*a	0.89 ± 0.08*a	0.76 ± 0.10*b	0.80 ± 0.08*b	38 ± 8*	49 ± 9*b
5. Cingulate cortex		0.56 ± 0.08**a	0.90 ± 0.05*a	0.78 ± 0.04**b	0.80 ± 0.03*b	49 ± 14*	64 ± 21*b
6. Hippocampus		0.56 ± 0.08**a	0.82 ± 0.04*a	0.70 ± 0.07**b	0.75 ± 0.03*b	69 ± 14*	89 ± 22*
7. Cerebellum		0.48 ± 0.10**a	0.85 ± 0.08**a	0.65 ± 0.13**b	0.83 ± 0.04*b	86 ± 34*	97 ± 23*
8. Thalamus		0.54 ± 0.08**a	0.87 ± 0.03	0.67 ± 0.10*a	0.74 ± 0.09*	56 ± 12*	67 ± 23*b
9. Hypothalamus		0.65 ± 0.12**a	0.85 ± 0.08	0.74 ± 0.07*a	0.80 ± 0.03	46 ± 13*	62 ± 18*b
10. Brain stem		0.38 ± 0.03**a	0.76 ± 0.07	0.48 ± 010*	0.70 ± 0.06	24 ± 10*	36 ± 18*b

Values are mean ± SD. * = $P < 0.05$, ** = $P < 0.01$ compared with control group; a = $P < 0.05$ compared from untreated heat-stressed rats; b = $P < 0.05$, compared from diabetic heat-stressed rats. ANOVA followed by Dunnet's test for multiple group comparison. For details, see text.

after heat stress (Table 2). However, in diabetic rats 80 μg/kg/min growth hormone is needed to induce similar reduction in brain edema formation at 4 h heat stress (Table 2).

Brain pathology. Fifty μg/kg/min growth hormone administered 30 min before heat stress induces significant neuroprotection in different regions of the brain at 4 h (Tables 2 and 5). However, to achieve similar neuroprotection in diabetic rats, 80 μg/kg/min for 10 min growth hormone is needed (Table 2). Regional changes in neuronal damage show that heat stress in normal animals results in average 150 to 280 distorted or damaged neurons in the cortex followed by 120 to 150 neurons in hippocampus and about 180 to 260 neurons in cerebellum, thalamus, and hypothalamus (results not shown). Diabetic animals resulted in higher number of neuronal damage following 4 h heat stress. As a result, diabetic rats show about 240 to 390 neuronal damage in cortex, about 180 to 260 in hippocampus, and 310 to 450 neurons in thalamus, hypothalamus, and brain stem (results not shown). Pretreatment with growth hormone (50 μg/kg/min) markedly reduced the number of damaged neurons in normal animals after 4 h heat stress (Table 5), whereas 80 μg/kg/min growth hormone was required to induce similar neuroprotection in heat stress in diabetic rats (Table 5).

Discussion

The salient new finding of this investigation is that diabetic rats when subjected to heat stress show exacerbation of thermal stress symptoms, BBB breakdown, brain edema, and brain pathology compared to normal animals exposed to identical heat stress. These observations are the first to show that diabetic animals are more susceptible to heat stress-induced brain damage. It appears that diabetic patients are likely at greater risk for thermal stress-induced brain pathology especially during hot summer seasons. This indicates that to provide better patient care in diabetic subjects their exposure to hot environments should be restricted to avoid unnecessary heat-related brain dysfunction.

The other novel finding in this investigation is less responsiveness of growth hormone treatment to achieving neuroprotection in heat stress-induced brain pathology in diabetic rats compared to normal animals. This suggests that diabetic animals are less responsive to neurotherapeutic agents, a feature not reported earlier. In our investigations, diabetic rats require almost double the dose of growth hormone to alleviate heat-induced symptoms and brain pathology. This suggests that the dose of drug treatments for treating different brain diseases may vary in normal subjects and in diabetic patients. Accordingly, to minimize heat-induced brain pathology in diabetic subjects, higher drug doses are needed as compared to normal subjects. This observation is in line with our previous report in which growth hormone treatment failed to induce neuroprotection in hypertensive rats but normal animals showed good neuroprotection with the same amount of the growth hormone.[22]

The significance of these findings is that during clinical trials, the drug dose may be adjusted in subjects depending on their co-morbidities, for example, alterations in their endocrine or cardiovascular status. Our observations could thus explain why some of the neuroprotective agents failed to show good results in clinical cases of stroke or CNS trauma. It appears the patients with comorbidities, such as diabetes or chronic hypertension, may also have been given the same amount of drug doses as compared to normal patients suffering from stroke or trauma. In future clinical trials, the endocrine and cardiovascular status of patients with brain disorders should be taken into account for the adjustment of drug doses to achieve neuroprotection.

It is interesting to note that on the one hand diabetic rats are more sensitive to heat-induced BBB permeability disturbances, brain edema, and cell injuries, while on the other hand, these diabetic animals are less responsive to growth hormone-induced neuroprotection. The basic mechanisms of these two aspects of diabetic animals in heat stress are unclear from this investigation.

We used streptozotocine 50 mg/kg i.p. for 3 consecutive days to induce diabetes in rats at 4 weeks (see Refs. 18–21). Our dose and treatment schedule of streptozotocine to induce diabetes is a mild one compared to other studies in which a single dose of high amount of streptozotocine was given intravenously (60 to 75 mg/kg).[20,21] This high dose of streptozotocine may induce diabetes within 3 to 14 days. Also, in these animals, blood glucose could reach beyond 20 mMol/L in many animals. However, we wanted to induce a mild and gradual increase in blood glucose that could be comparable to clinical situations. The gradual increase in blood glucose to a level of 18 to 20 mMol/L in 4 weeks in the present investigation is very close to that seen in chronic diabetic patients.[20,21] We feel that our diabetic model is comparable to other animal models of diabetes and represents a clear picture of the diabetic patient in relation to hyperglycemia.

Because diabetic rats showed exacerbation of hyperthermia after heat exposure compared to normal animals, it appears that increased blood and brain temperature may also influence greater BBB dysfunction in these rats. Hyperthermia is known to induce release of various neurochemical mediators of BBB dysfunction, for example, serotonin, prostaglandins, histamine, opioid peptides, catecholamines, cytokines, and many other vasoactive factors (see Refs. 1–3, 22, 23, 26, 30). It is likely that more severe hyperthermia could induce greater release of these neurochemicals or vasoactive substances in the circulation and in the brain.[2,3] High concentrations of these neurochemicals may act on the cerebral microvessels on the luminal and/or on the abluminal side of the endothelial cells to increase greater BBB permeability.[2–4,22–26,28–30]

Cerebral microvessels contain various neurochemical transmitter receptors and/or transporters on both the luminal and abluminal sides of the endothelial cells.[2,3,31,32] High concentrations of these neurochemicals will activate these receptors and/or transporters on the cerebral microvessels (see Refs. 28–30). As a result, increased synthesis and release of cAMP and cGMP could occur within the brain microvessels (see Refs. 29, 33, 34). An increased production of cAMP and cGMP is likely to induce breakdown of the BBB either directly or through production of nitric oxide (see Refs. 35–38). Increased production of nitric oxide, the free radical per se will damage the endothelial cells causing breakdown of the BBB function.[37,38]

Alternatively, in diabetic rats hyperglycemia and its influence on cerebral microvessels may also enhance oxidative stress including nitric oxide production to induce BBB dysfunction following heat stress. That hyperglycemia in itself in normal animals did not induce BBB breakdown suggests that additional heat stress is needed to amplify the hyperglycemic and/or oxidative stress to enhance BBB disruption.[4–8] In addition, high blood and brain temperatures may directly affect the cerebral microcirculation, leading to heat-induced degeneration of microvessels causing a greater degree of the vascular permeability to protein tracers.

There are reasons to believe that diabetes itself reduces the release and activity of growth hormone in human cases.[14–16] Additional supplement of growth hormone could help in reducing hyperglycemia-induced cell damage or oxidative stress.[22,24,25] For this reason, we supplemented growth hormone in diabetic rats to see if the hormone is able to attenuate brain pathology in heat stress. Our results show that almost double the dose of growth hormone is needed to achieve neuroprotection in diabetic animals following heat exposure (see Refs. 22, 24). The inability of growth hormone to induce neuroprotection in diabetic rats may be due to altered sensitivity of growth hormone to microvessels in these animals.[14,15] Alternatively, hyperglycemia-induced functional changes in the microvessels, for example, oxidative stress, generation of free radicals or nitric oxide production, and related alterations in membrane transporter or receptor function might have altered the therapeutic actions of growth hormone on the cerebral microvessels.[17–21] Massive reduction in CBF in diabetic rats following hyperthermia in comparison to normal animals is in line with this idea (see Ref. 20).

Growth hormone is a well known neuroprotective agent in trauma and in hyperthermia.[22–24] Thus, repeated topical application of growth hormone following spinal cord injury markedly attenuates breakdown of the BBB permeability, spinal cord edema, and cell injury.[24] Furthermore, growth hormone was also able to reduce heat stress-induced BBB disruption and brain pathology in normal rats.[22] These observations suggest that growth hormone could improve cellular membrane function and reduce cellular and/or molecular stress when administered in excess quantity in pathological situations.[22–24] It appears that growth hormone may work as a neurotrophic factor in the microvessels strengthening the cell membrane structure and function in hyperthermia or trauma.[39,40] Exogenous supplement of growth hormone results in less BBB disruption in trauma and hyperthermia (see Refs. 22–24, 39, 40). Obviously, a reduction in BBB permeability to proteins is likely to reduce edema formation and cell injury (see Refs. 36–38).

We observed a greater permeation of radioiodine in several brain regions following heat stress in diabetic or normal rats compared to Evans blue. This difference in Evans blue and radioiodine extravasation could be due to differences in the type or sizes of the proteins to which they bind in circulation (see Ref. 23). Obviously, a greater binding of Evans blue to albumin (68%) compared to radioiodine (56%) will result in a smaller iodine–protein complex, resulting in widespread extravasation of the radiotracer as compared to the Evans blue–albumin complex (see Refs. 26–29). However, profound reduction in the BBB to both tracers by growth hormone in normal and diabetic rats suggest that membrane stabilization effects of growth hormone could definitely reduce the permeation of large and small sized tracers in the brains of heat-stressed animals.

Conclusion

In conclusion, our observations clearly show that diabetic animals are more sensitive to heat stress-induced brain damage. Furthermore, growth hormone could induce profound neuroprotection in animals, if administered in high doses as compared to normal animals. These observations suggest that diabetes dramatically alters the cerebral microvascular function in heat stress. Thus, in clinical situations the dosage of neuroprotective drugs may need to be adjusted to enhance neuroprotection depending on the patient's endocrine or metabolic status, such as diabetes mellitus, a feature not described earlier.

Acknowledgments

This investigation is supported by Grants from Swedish Medical Research Council (nr. 2710, HSS); Göran Gustafsson Foundation, Stockholm, Sweden (HSS); Alexander von Humboldt Foundation, Bonn, Germany (HSS); Society for Study on Neuroplasticity and Neuroregeneration (SSNN), Romania (HSS); Global College of Neuroprotection and Neuroregeneration (GCNN, UK); Ebewe Neuro Pharma, Austria (HSS); Astra-Zeneca, Mölndal, Sweden (HSS); StressGen Research Foundation, Canada (HSS); Ministry of Science & Technology, Govt. of India, New Delhi (HSS); Indian Council of Medical Research (ICMR), New Delhi (HSS). The skillful technical assistance of Kärstin Flink, Kerstin Rystedt (Uppsala); Franziska Drum, Angela Ludwig

(Berlin), and secretarial assistance of Ulla Lindholm is highly appreciated.

Conflicts of interest

The authors have no conflict of interest with any of the organizations listed above.

References

1. Sharma, H.S. Neurobiology of hyperthermia. In *Prog. Brain Res.*, Vol. 162. H.S. Sharma, Ed.: 1–616. Elsevier. North Holland, Amsterdam.
2. Sharma, H.S. 2007. Methods to produce hyperthermia-induced brain dysfunction. *Prog. Brain Res.* **162:** 173–199. Review.
3. Sharma, H.S. 2006. Hyperthermia influences excitatory and inhibitory amino acid neurotransmitters in the central nervous system. An experimental study in the rat using behavioural, biochemical, pharmacological, and morphological approaches. *J. Neural. Transm.* **113:** 497–519.
4. Huber, J.D. 2008. Diabetes, cognitive function, and the blood-brain barrier. *Curr. Pharm. Des.* **14:** 1594–600. Review.
5. Liu, H., X. Liu, L. Jia, *et al.* 2008. Insulin therapy restores impaired function and expression of P-glycoprotein in blood-brain barrier of experimental diabetes. *Biochem. Pharmacol.* **75:** 1649–1658.
6. Hawkins, B.T., T.F. Lundeen, K.M. Norwood, *et al.* 2007. Increased blood-brain barrier permeability and altered tight junctions in experimental diabetes in the rat: contribution of hyperglycaemia and matrix metalloproteinases. *Diabetologia* **50:** 202–211. Epub 2006 Dec 2.
7. Hawkins, B.T., S.M. Ocheltree, K.M. Norwood, *et al.* 2007. Decreased blood-brain barrier permeability to fluorescein in streptozotocin-treated rats. *Neurosci Lett.* **411:** 1–5. Epub 2006 Nov 15.
8. Huber, J.D., R.L. VanGilder & K.A. Houser. 2006. Streptozotocin-induced diabetes progressively increases blood-brain barrier permeability in specific brain regions in rats. *Am. J. Physiol. Heart Circ. Physiol.* **291:** H2660–H2668. Epub 2006 Sep 1.
9. Sharma, H.S., J. Westman & F. Nyberg. 1998. Pathophysiology of brain edema and cell changes following hyperthermic brain injury. *Prog. Brain Res.* **115:** 351–412. Review.
10. Jamal, Z. & E.D. Saggerson. 1988. Factors influencing the altered thermogenic response of rat brown adipose tissue in streptozotocin-diabetes. *Biochem. J.* **249:** 415–421.
11. Pabbidi, R.M., S.Q. Yu, S. Peng, *et al.* 2008. Influence of TRPV1 on diabetes-induced alterations in thermal pain sensitivity. *Mol. Pain* **4:** 9.
12. Batista, F., M.S. Pinzur & C.A. Nery. 2005. Cutaneous thermal sensitivity in diabetic neuropathy. *Foot Ankle Int.* **26:** 927–931.
13. Muresanu, D.F. & H.S. Sharma. 2007. Chronic hypertension aggravates heat stress induced cognitive dysfunction and brain pathology: an experimental study in the rat, using growth hormone therapy for possible neuroprotection. *Ann. N.Y. Acad. Sci.* **1122:** 1–22.
14. Irie, M., Y. Itoh, Y. Miyashita, *et al.* 2004. Complications in adults with growth hormone deficiency—a survey study in Japan. *Endocr. J.* **51:** 479–485.
15. Møller, N. & J.O. Jørgensen. 2009. Effects of growth hormone on glucose, lipid and protein metabolism in human subjects. *Endocr. Rev.* [Epub ahead of print]
16. Cenci, M.C., F.L. Conceição, D.V. Soares, *et al.* 2008. Impact of 5 years of growth hormone replacement therapy on cardiovascular risk factors in growth hormone-deficient adults. *Metabolism* **57:** 121–129.
17. Melamed, E. 1976. Reactive hyperglycaemia in patients with acute stroke. *J. Neurol. Sci.* **29:** 267–275.
18. Mooradian, A.D. 1997. Pathophysiology of central nervous system complications in diabetes mellitus. *Clin. Neurosci.* **4:** 322–326.
19. Ding, C., Q. He & P.A. Li. 2004. Activation of cell death pathway after a brief period of global ischemia in diabetic and non-diabetic animals. *Exp. Neurol.* **188:** 421–429.
20. Duckrow, R.B., D.C. Beard & R.W. Brennan. 1987. Regional cerebral blood flow decreases during chronic and acute hyperglycemia. *Stroke* **18:** 52–58.
21. Mayer, G., R. Nitsch & S. Hoyer. 1990. Effects of changes in peripheral and cerebral glucose metabolism on locomotor activity, learning and memory in adult male rats. *Brain Res.* **532:** 95–100.
22. Muresanu, D.F. & H.S. Sharma. 2007. Chronic hypertension aggravates heat stress induced cognitive dysfunction and brain pathology: an experimental study in the rat, using growth hormone therapy for possible neuroprotection. *Ann. N.Y. Acad. Sci.* **1122:** 1–22.
23. Sharma, H.S. 2007. Methods to produce hyperthermia-induced brain dysfunction. *Prog. Brain Res.* **162:** 173–99. Review.
24. Mustafa, A., H.S. Sharma, Y. Olsson, *et al.* 1995. Vascular permeability to growth hormone in the rat central nervous system after focal spinal cord injury. Influence of a new anti-oxidant H 290/51 and 15. *Neurosci. Res.* **23:** 185–194.

25. Nyberg, F. & H.S. Sharma. 2002. Repeated topical application of growth hormone attenuates blood-spinal cord barrier permeability and edema formation following spinal cord injury: an experimental study in the rat using Evans blue, ([125])I-sodium and lanthanum tracers. *Amino Acids* **23:** 231–239.
26. Sharma, H.S., J. Westman, J. Cervós-Navarro, *et al.* 1997. Opioid receptor antagonists attenuate heat stress-induced reduction in cerebral blood flow, increased blood-brain barrier permeability, vasogenic edema and cell changes in the rat. *Ann. N.Y. Acad. Sci.* **813:** 559–571.
27. Sharma, H.S., J. Westman, J.C. Navarro, *et al.* 1995. Probable involvement of serotonin in the increased permeability of the blood-brain barrier by forced swimming. An experimental study using Evans blue and 131I-sodium tracers in the rat. *Behav. Brain Res.* **72:** 189–196.
28. Sharma, H.S., Y. Olsson, F. Nyberg, *et al.* 1993. Prostaglandins modulate alterations of microvascular permeability, blood flow, edema and serotonin levels following spinal cord injury: an experimental study in the rat. *Neuroscience* **57:** 443–449.
29. Sharma, H.S., Y. Olsson & P.K. Dey. 1990. Changes in blood-brain barrier and cerebral blood flow following elevation of circulating serotonin level in anesthetized rats. *Brain Res.* **517:** 215–223.
30. Sharma, H.S. & J. Cervós-Navarro. 1990. Brain oedema and cellular changes induced by acute heat stress in young rats. *Acta. Neurochir. Suppl. (Wien).* **51:** 383–386.
31. Poller, B., H. Gutmann, S. Krähenbühl, *et al.* 2008. The human brain endothelial cell line hCMEC/D3 as a human blood-brain barrier model for drug transport studies. *J. Neurochem.* **107:** 1358–1368.
32. Gosselet, F., P. Candela, E. Sevin, *et al.* 2009. Transcriptional profiles of receptors and transporters involved in brain cholesterol homeostasis at the blood-brain barrier: use of an *in vitro* model. *Brain Res.* **1249:** 34–42. Epub 2008 Oct.
33. Soma, T., H. Chiba, Y. Kato-Mori, *et al.* 2004. Thr(207) of claudin-5 is involved in size-selective loosening of the endothelial barrier by cyclic AMP. *Exp. Cell Res.* **300:** 202–212.
34. Esposito, P., S. Basu, R. Letourneau, *et al.* 2003. Corticotropin-releasing factor (CRF) can directly affect brain microvessel endothelial cells. *Brain Res.* **968:** 192–198.
35. Sharma, H.S. & P. Alm. 2002. Nitric oxide synthase inhibitors influence dynorphin A (1–17) immunoreactivity in the rat brain following hyperthermia. *Amino Acids* **23:** 247–259.
36. Sharma, H.S., P. Alm & J. Westman. 1998. Nitric oxide and carbon monoxide in the brain pathology of heat stress. *Prog. Brain Res.* **115:** 297–333. Review.
37. Sharma, H.S. & P. Alm. 2004. Role of nitric oxide on the blood-brain and spinal cord barriers. In *Blood-Spinal Cord and Brain Barriers in Health and Disease.* H.S. Sharma & J. Westman, Eds.: 191–229. Elsevier, Oxford, San Diego, Boston.
38. Sharma, H.S. 2004. Blood-brain and spinal cord barriers in stress. In *Blood-Spinal Cord and Brain Barriers in Health and Disease.* H.S. Sharma & J. Westman, Eds.: 231–298. Elsevier Inc. USA.
39. Sharma, H.S. 2007. A select combination of neurotrophins enhances neuroprotection and functional recovery following spinal cord injury. *Ann. N.Y. Acad. Sci.* **1122:** 95–111.
40. Sharma, H.S. 2007. Neurotrophic factors in combination: a possible new therapeutic strategy to influence pathophysiology of spinal cord injury and repair mechanisms. *Curr. Pharm. Des.* **13:** 1841–1874. Review.

Ann. N.Y. Acad. Sci. ISSN 0077-8923

ANNALS OF THE NEW YORK ACADEMY OF SCIENCES
Issue: *Neuroprotective Agents*

Arsenite induces oxidative injury in rat brain

Synergistic effect of iron

Su-Feng Fan,*[1] Pei-Ling Chao,*[1] and Anya Maan-Yuh Lin[1,2]

[1]Department of Medical Research and Education, Taipei Veterans General Hospital, Taipei, Taiwan. [2]Department of Pharmacology, National Yang-Ming University, Taipei, Taiwan

Address for correspondence: Anya Maan-Yuh Lin, Department of Pharmacology, National Yang-Ming University, Taipei, Taiwan. myalin@vghtpe.gov.tw

*These authors contributed equally to this work.

Sodium arsenite (arsenite)-induced neurotoxicity and its interaction with ferrous citrate (iron) was investigated in rat brain. *In vitro* data showed that arsenite (1–10 μmol/L) concentration dependently increased lipid peroxidation and the potency of arsenite was less than that of iron. The oxidative activity of arsenite, sodium arsenate (arsenate), monomethylarsonic acid (MMA), and dimethylarsinic acid (DMA) were evaluated by inducing lipid peroxidation in cortical homogenates, and the potency for this effect was as follows: arsenite > arsenate > MMA and DMA. Several well-known antioxidants, including glutathione, melatonin, and β-estradiol inhibited arsenite-induced lipid peroxidation in a concentration-dependent manner. Our *in vivo* study employed intranigral infusion of arsenite (5 nmol) in the substantia nigra (SN) of anesthetized rats. Four hours to 7 days after infusion, lipid peroxidation was elevated while glutathione was depleted in the infused SN. The dopamine content in the striatum ipsilateral to arsenite-infused SN was first elevated 24 h and then decreased 7 days after intranigral infusion of arsenite. Using pretreatment of L-buthionine-[S,R]-sulfoximine (L-BSO, i.c.v.) to reduce glutathione content in rat brain, arsenite-induced oxidative injury was augmented. Low doses of arsenite (1.5 nmol) and iron (3 nmol) alone induced minimal oxidative injury; however, co-infusion of arsenite and iron augmented neurotoxicity, including elevated lipid peroxidation and reduced striatal dopamine content. Moreover, expression of heme oxygenase-1, α-synuclein aggregation, and DNA fragmentation were significantly enhanced in SN co-infused with low doses of arsenite and iron. Taken together, our study demonstrates that arsenite was less potent than iron in inducing oxidative stress. Furthermore, concomitant arsenite and iron potentiated oxidative injury in the nigrostriatal dopaminergic system, indicating that interaction of metals plays a more clinically-relevant role in pathophysiology of central nervous system neurodegeneration.

Keywords: arsenite; iron; neurotoxicity

Introduction

Due to the environmental pollution from contaminated ground water, contaminated food, and industrial wastes, the central nervous system (CNS) is one of the organs accumulating a significant amount of heavy metals and metalloid, including arsenic.[1–5] In addition, arsenic trioxide is currently used in the clinic for the treatment of acute promyelocytic leukemia[6,7] and more and more human clinical trials try to search for therapeutic use of arsenic trioxide for the treatment of cancers.[8,9] Neurotoxicity, including numbness, paresthesia of the distal extremities, insomnia, and convulsion are frequent complaints in patients treated with arsenic trioxide[8,9]; therefore, it is very important to delineate the neurotoxic effect due to arsenic in the peripheral nervous system (PNS) and CNS. In the PNS, sodium arsenite (arsenite) has been shown to inhibit axonal growth in the dorsal root ganglion (DRG) explants.[10] Furthermore, apoptosis is reportedly involved in the arsenite-treated DRG explants[11,12] or DRG of rats receiving oral arsenite (unpublished data). In the CNS, arsenic-induced deficits include a reduction in locomotor activity, sleep disturbances, auditory–evoked potential, and learning and

doi: 10.1111/j.1749-6632.2009.05170.x

memory deficits.[1,3] Moreover, systemic administration of arsenic decreased levels of dopamine and norepinephrine in several brain regions, including basal ganglia.[4] Our previous studies have demonstrated that intranigral infusion of arsenite induced apoptosis and necrosis[13,14] and systemic melatonin was found to attenuate arsenite-induced neurotoxicity in the nigrostriatal dopaminergic system.[14]

Apart from arsenic, iron, an essential cofactor for many proteins involved in physiological functions, reportedly accumulates with age in CNS, including substantia nigra (SN) and locus coeruleus.[15] Furthermore, clinical studies have revealed an overload of iron in the CNS of patients with Parkinson's disease.[16] Iron, known as a Fenton reagent, has been shown to induce oxidative stress by forming free radicals which attack macromolecules including lipids and proteins and thus result in cell death.[16–19] The interaction of iron and dopamine, the primary neurotransmitter of the nigrostriatal system, has been proposed to induce abnormal protein aggregation as one possible mechanism of Parkinsonism.[16–21] In support to this notion, *in vivo* studies using intranigral infusion of iron demonstrated oxidative injury, including elevation in lipid peroxidation and depletion in striatal dopamine content.[22–24]

More than one transition metal has been reported to be overloaded in the same brain regions,[1,16] therefore, the interaction of these potentially detrimental metals has been proposed for the pathophysiology of CNS neurodegenerative diseases.[1,25–30] For example, co-exposure of arsenic and manganese or arsenic and lead is found to augment neurotoxicity in the CNS.[25–27] Furthermore, concomitant treatment of manganese and lead or manganese and iron actually aggravated the behavioral deficits of treated rats.[28–30] In the present study, several questions were addressed: (1) Compared with iron and other arsenics, is iron or arsenite the most potent in inducing oxidative stress? (2) Does arsenite-induced neurotoxicity change if antioxidative defensive systems are deteriorated in the brain? and (3) Does arsenite enhance the neurotoxicity of iron in the nigrostriatal dopaminergic system? The potentiation by arsenite and iron may be more clinically relevant in the pathophysiology of CNS neurodegenerative diseases.

Materials and methods

Animals

Adult, male Sprague–Dawley rats, weighing 250–350 g, were used. These animals were maintained according to the guidelines established in the *Guide for the Care and Use of Laboratory Animals* prepared by the Committee on Care and Use of Laboratory Animals of the Institute of Laboratory Animal Resources Commission on Life Sciences, National Research Council, U.S.A. (1985). The use of animals has been approved by the Institutional Animal Care and Use Committee of Taipei Veterans General Hospital, Taipei, Taiwan, R.O.C.

In vitro studies using cortical homogenates

Cortical samples were homogenized in chilled Ringer's solution (50 mg/mL) and incubated at 37° C for 15 h with saline, arsenite, sodium arsenate (arsenate) or monomethyl arsenate (MMA), dimethyl arsenate (DMA) and ferrous citrate (iron) which were purchased from Sigma (St. Louis, MO). A 400 μL sample was transferred to an eppendorf tube containing 300 μL chloroform and 100 μL methanol. The slurry was mixed and kept on ice for 15 min. After centrifugation (8000 *g* for 5 min), an aliquot of chloroform extract was transferred to another tube containing 100 μL methanol. Lipid peroxidation expressed as relative fluorescence unit (RFU) was determined by measuring the levels of malondialdehyde and its dihydropyridine polymers, which emit fluorescence at 426 nm when activated by UV at 356 nm.[31]

Chronic surgery and drug infusion

Rats were anesthetized with chloral hydrate (450 mg/kg, i.p., Sigma) and placed in a stereotaxic instrument (David Kopf Instruments, Palo Alto, CA). After skin incision and exposure of the parietal bone, holes were drilled above the cortical surface for intranigral infusion of drugs. One μL filtered Kreb's Ringer solution of arsenite (1.5–5 nmol), iron (3 nmol) or a mixture of arsenite (1.5 nmol) and iron (3 nmol) was infused stereotaxically into SN[32] (coordinates: 3.2 mm anterior and 2 mm above the interaural zero; 2.1 mm lateral to the midline; 3.5 mm below the incisor bar). Drug solutions were infused at a rate of 0.2 μL/min through a 30 gauge stainless steel needle. The

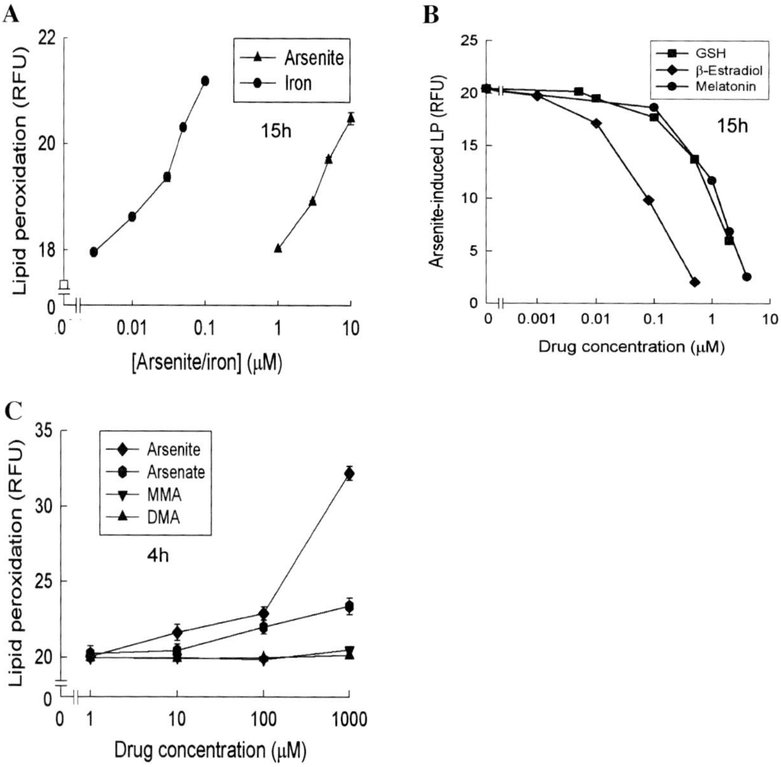

Figure 1. Arsenics induced oxidative stress *in vitro.* (A) Incubation of arsenite or iron increased lipid peroxidation in cortical homogenates. After 15 h incubation at 37° C, the lipid peroxidation of cortical homogenates was measured and reported as relative fluorescence unit (RFU). (B) Melatonin, β-estradiol, and GSH concentration dependently attenuated arsenite-induced lipid peroxidation. After 15 h incubation at 37° C, the lipid peroxidation of cortical homogenates was measured and reported as RFU. (C) The oxidative capacity of arsenite, arsenate, monomethyl arsenate (MMA), and dimethyl arsenate (DMA) was compared by measuring lipid peroxidation in cortical homogenates. After 4 h incubation at 37° C, the cortical lipid peroxidation was measured and reported as RFU. Values are the mean ± S.E.M. ($n = 3$) from a representative experiment that was replicated with similar results.

injection needle was held in place for an additional 3 min following drug infusion. After surgery, rats were allowed to recover from anesthesia and were placed in their home cages (for 4 h to 7 days) until sacrificed.

Fluorescence assay of lipid peroxidation in substantia nigra

At the end of each *in vivo* experiment, rats were sacrificed by decapitation. Dissected SNs were homogenized in chilled 400 μL chloroform and 200 μL methanol. After centrifugation, an aliquot of the chloroform and methanol layer was scanned using a spectrofluorometer (Aminco Bowman-2, Thermo Fisher Scientific Inc., Waltham, MA). The relative fluorescent intensities of samples in a cuvette were measured as mentioned above.

High pressure liquid chromatography electrochemical analysis of striatal dopamine content

Rats were decapitated and striata were dissected and immediately frozen in liquid nitrogen and stored at −70° C until analysis. An HPLC (CC5/PM80, Bioanalytical Systems Inc., West Lafayette, IN) with electrochemical detection (LC-4C, Bioanalytical Systems Inc., West Lafayette, IN) procedure was used to quantify dopamine content in rat striatum. Applied potential was 0.75 volt versus Ag/AgCl. Mobile phase (liter) contained 2.1 g heptanesulfonic

Table 1. A time-dependent effect of arsenite-induced oxidative injury in the nigrostriatal dopaminergic system of rat brain

Drugs infused (time after infusion)	LP in SN (RFU)	Striatal DA level (pmole/mg tissue)	GSH in SN (μg/mg tissue)
Intact control	3.10 ± 0.10	79.0 ± 2.9	29.7 ± 0.3
As (4 h)	5.49 ± 048*	88.6 ± 6.9	23.4 ± 1.2*
As (24 h)	9.80 ± 1.23*	92.9 ± 4.0*	13.6 ± 1.1*
As (48 h)	9.32 ± 2.22*	54.8 ± 15.0	16.5 ± 2.5*
As (7 d)	6.47 ± 0.47*	31.2 ± 5.8*	20.7 ± 1.7*

Arsenite (5 nmol) was locally infused in substantia nigra (SN) of anesthetized rats. Lipid peroxidation (LP) in SN was reported as relative fluorescence unit (RFU) and striatal dopamine (DA) content was detected by HPLC-ECD. GSH = glutathione. Numbers in parentheses indicate the number of SN from anesthetized rats. Values are the mean ± S.E.M. (n = 5–6). *, $P < 0.05$ in the arsenite group compared with the intact control by one way ANOVA followed by a Bonferroni multiple-comparisons procedure as a post hoc analysis.

acid, 3.5 mL triethylamine, 3 mL phosphoric acid, 0.1 g NaEDTA and 170 mL acetonitrile. The retention time for dopamine was about 7.5 min.[33]

Measurement of glutathione content in SN

Glutathione (GSH) levels were determined according to the method of Griffith.[34] Frozen SN tissue was thawed in 5 volumes of ice-cold 0.2 N perchloric acid and homogenized by sonication. Tissue homogenates were centrifuged at 12,000 g for 15 min. Aliquots of the supernatants were added to 0.1 mol/L phosphate buffer saline (PBS, pH 7.5) containing 0.6 mmol/L 5,5′-dithiobis(2-nitrobenzoic acid) and 0.2 mg/mL nicotinamide adenine dinucleotide phosphate to make a total volume of 980 μL. After mixing, GSH reductase (20 U/mL, 20 μL) was added to initiate the assay. The formation of 5-thio-2-nitrobenzoic acid was measured spectrophotometrically at 412 nm for 2 min. The amount of total GSH was determined from a standard curve with known amounts of GSH standard.

Western blot analysis of heme oxygenase-1 and α-synuclein

At the end of experiment, rats were decapitated 48 h after arsenite infusion. Dissected SNs were homogenized with a sonicator in 40 μL ice-cold protease inhibitor cocktail (Calbiochem., San Diego, CA). After homogenization, the lysates were centrifuged at 12,000 g for 30 min at 4° C. The supernatant was frozen in liquid nitrogen and stored at −80° C. The protein samples were run on 7–15% sodium dodecyl sulfate-polyacrylamide gel electrophoresis and then transferred onto a nitrocellulose membrane (Biorad, Hercules, CA) at 80 V for 75 min. Blots were probed with primary antibodies against HO-1 and α-synuclein at 4° C for 45 min. After primary antibody incubation, the membrane was washed and incubated with horseradish peroxidase-conjugated goat antimouse IgG (Chemicon, Temecula, CA) for 40 min at room temperature. The immunoreaction was visualized using Amersham enhanced chemiluminescence (Amersham Pharmacia Biotech, Piscataway, NJ). After this detection, the bound primary and secondary antibodies were stripped by incubating the membrane in stripping buffer (Tris-base 63 mM, 0.7% 2-mercaptoethanol, 2% sodium dodecyl sulfate) at 50° C for 30 min. The membrane was re-probed with b-actin antibody (as loading controls). The densities of blots were analyzed using a scanning densitometer which was operated by Scanner Control software (Molecular Dynamics, Sunnyvale, CA). Results were obtained by calculating the density using Imagequant software (Amersham Biosciences, Pittsburg, PA) and reported as relative optical density of the specific proteins.

Detection of DNA fragmentation

Seventy-two h after arsenite infusion, rats were decapitated. The total DNA of frozen SN was extracted according to the procedures reported previously.[35] Nucleosomal DNA ladders were detected by the DNA ladder assay kit (Maxim Biotech., San Francisco, CA) and separated by electrophoresis.

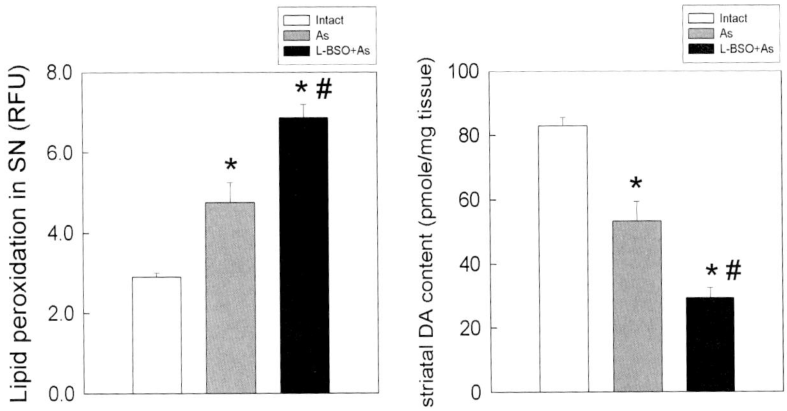

Figure 2. Effect of L-buthionine-[S,R]-sulfoximine (L-BSO) on arsenite-induced oxidative injury *in vivo*. Twenty-four h after intracerebroventricular infusion of L-BSO, arsenite was locally infused in substantia nigra (SN) of chloral hydrate anesthetized rats. Seven days after intranigral infusion of arsenite (3 nmol), lipid peroxidation in SN was reported as relative fluorescence unit (RFU) and the striatal dopamine content was detected by HPLC-ECD. *, $P < 0.05$ in the arsenite-infused SN compared with that in the intact SN. #, $P < 0.05$ in the arsenite-infused SN of L-BSO-pretreated group compared with that in the vehicle-treated group. Values are the mean ± S.E.M. ($n = 4$–5) from a representative experiment that was replicated with similar results.

Intracerebroventricular infusion of L-buthionine-[S,R]-sulfoximine

Rats were divided into two groups. One received an intracerebroventricular infusion (coordinates: 0.8 mm posterior to bregma; 1.5 mm lateral to the midline; 3.6 mm below the cortical surface; 3.5 mm below the incisor bar) of L-BSO (15 μL, 120 mg/mL; Sigma, Sigma) and the other group received an equal amount of Ringer's solution. Twenty-four h after L-BSO, rats were re-anesthetized and arsenite (3 nmol) was infused in SN. Seven days after arsenite infusion, rats were sacrificed and biochemical assays were performed.

Statistics

Statistical comparisons were made as indicated either using unpaired t-test or one way ANOVA followed by a Bonferroni multiple-comparisons procedure as a post hoc analysis.

Results and discussion

Arsenite increased lipid peroxidation in cortical homogenates: *in vitro* study

Several lines of evidence have supported the finding that oxidative stress is involved in arsenic-induced cytotoxicity.[36–40] First, arsenic-induced overproduction of free radicals include nitric oxide,[36] peroxynitrite,[38] hydrogen peroxide,[39] and hydroxyl radicals[40] that result in oxidative-related products, including lipid peroxidation, DNA damage, and protein nitrosylation in the arsenic-induced cytotoxicity.[11–14,36–42] In the present *in vitro* study, arsenite-induced oxidative stress was investigated using cortical homogenates. After a 15 h incubation, lipid peroxidation of cortical homogenates was elevated from 0.76 ± 0.02 RFU at 0° C to 17.3 ± 0.5 RFU at 37° C ($n = 6$, $P < 0.01$). Incubation with arsenite (1–10 μmol/L) further increased the formation of peroxidized lipids of cortical homogenates in a concentration-dependent manner (Fig. 1A). Compared with iron, the oxidative potency of arsenite was approximately 200-fold less potent than iron in inducing lipid peroxidation (Fig. 1A). In addition to vitamin C and E[43], GSH, β-estradiol, and melatonin inhibited arsenite-induced lipid peroxidation in a concentration-dependent manner (Fig. 1B). These data consistently indicate that arsenite can induce oxidative stress and antioxidative treatments may be therapeutically useful.[12,14,37,43]

Trivalent arsenic compounds are reportedly more potent in inducing cytotoxicity, including free radical generation and inhibition of enzyme activity.[39,44] In the present study, the oxidative capacity of arsenite, arsenate, MMA, and DMA was compared.

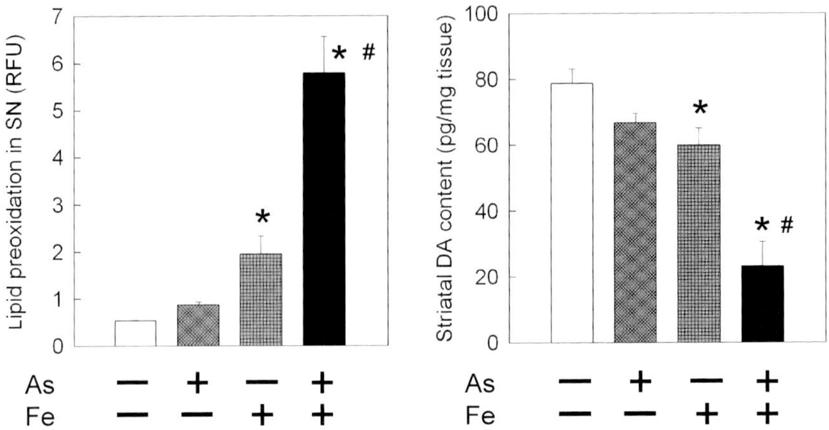

Figure 3. Synergistic effect by co-infusion of arsenite and iron on oxidative injury in rat brain. Seven days after intranigral infusion of arsenite (As, 1.5 nmol) or ferrous citrate (iron, 3 nmol) or a mixture of arsenite and iron, striatal dopamine content was detected by HPLC-ECD and lipid peroxidation in substantia nigra (SN) was reported as relative fluorescence unit (RFU). *, $P < 0.05$ in the iron group compared with that of the intact control. #, $P < 0.05$ in the As+iron group compared with that of the iron group. Values are the mean ± S.E.M. ($n = 4$–5) from a representative experiment that was replicated with similar results.

After incubation at 37° C for 4 h, arsenite was most potent in inducing oxidative stress followed by arsenate, while neither MMA nor DMA induced significant lipid peroxidation of cortical homogenates (Fig. 1C). Consistent with our previous study, when using equal amount of arsenic compounds, arsenite was found to be better than arsenate, MMA, and DMA at inducing HO-1 and heat shock protein-70 expression in DRG explants.[11] Furthermore, only arsenite is reportedly capable of activating procaspase 3 and 12 in the treated DRG explants.[11] Both the previous and present studies demonstrate that arsenite is the most potent arsenic compound in inducing oxidative stress.

Arsenite-induced oxidative injury *in vivo*

In the Parkinsonian studies, local infusion of iron or zinc in SN[22–24] has been employed to mimic the neurodegeneration found in patients overloaded with transition metals.[16] In the present study, arsenite was locally infused in SN and arsenite-induced oxidative injury was observed in a time-dependent manner (Table 1). Four hours after arsenite infusion (5 nmol), lipid peroxidation was abruptly elevated and GSH content was slightly depleted in the infused SN; no significant change in dopamine levels in the striatum ipsilateral to arsenite-infused SN was observed (Table 1). Twenty-four h after arsenite infusion, a maximal elevation in lipid peroxidation and reduction in GSH was demonstrated in the infused SN. At the same time, the striatal dopamine content was significantly increased (Table 1). Seven days after arsenite infusion, arsenite-elevated lipid peroxidation was reduced but was still significantly higher. Furthermore, GSH in the infused SN was still lower than the control whereas striatal dopamine levels ipsilateral to the infused SN were only 40% of the control (Table 1). Consistent with our previous study, which showed the involvement of apoptosis and necrosis in the arsenite-induced neurotoxicity,[13,14] the present study demonstrated that intranigral infusion of arsenite first induced lipid peroxidation followed by GSH depletion in SN; anterograde neurodegeneration of the dopaminergic axons in the ipsilateral striatum required at least 2 days.

Augmentation by L-buthionine-[S,R]-sulfoximine of arsenite-induced oxidative injury

In Parkinsonism and during the aging process there is a reduction in antioxidative defensive systems.[45–47] To experimentally mimic this effect, intracerebroventricular infusion of L-BSO which inhibits γ-glutamylcysteine synthetase, was employed to reduce GSH in CNS. Twenty-four h after L-BSO infusion, GSH content in rat brain was depleted (data not shown); arsenite (3 nmol) was then locally infused in SN. Seven days after arsenite infusion, arsenite-induced oxidative injury was enhanced in the L-BSO-pretreated rats, including arsenite-elevated lipid peroxidation in the infused SN and arsenite-depleted striatal dopamine content (Fig. 2). This is consistent with the previous investigations in which L-BSO potentiated arsenite-induced toxicity in liver[48] and in lung epithelial cells.[49] From our previous and present studies, the potentiation by L-BSO of arsenite, zinc,[23] and iron[50]-induced neurotoxicity strongly suggests that a compromised antioxidative defense system may aggravate neurotoxicity induced by metals in patients with neurodegenerative diseases or during the aging process.

Potentiation of oxidative injury by co-infusion of arsenite and iron

We also examined the effects of low doses of arsenite (1.5 nmol) and iron (3 nmol), which are likely to be more pathologically relevant. Compared with the minimal oxidative injury by arsenite or iron alone, co-infusion of arsenite and iron significantly augmented the lipid peroxidation in the infused SN and depleted the striatal dopamine content (Fig. 3). Furthermore, HO-1 expression, a chaperone protein, and α-synuclein aggregation, a pathological marker commonly found in the CNS neurodegenerative diseases,[51–53] were enhanced in SN co-infused with arsenite and iron (Fig. 4A). The DNA laddering assay demonstrated significant DNA fragmentation when arsenite and iron were simultaneously infused in SN (Fig. 4B). One explanation is that low doses of arsenite, instead of directly inducing weak oxidative stress, may indirectly interact with iron. In support to this notion, arsenic species have been reported to release iron from its binding proteins[54]; in this case, it is possible that released iron, which was found to be more potent than arsenite in inducing oxidative stress, would augment oxidative injury when coexisting in CNS.

In conclusion, among the arsenic compounds, our study showed that arsenite possesses the most potent oxidative activity; however, the oxidative capacity of arsenite was less than that of iron. Furthermore, a reduced antioxidative defense system may aggravate the arsenite-induced neurotoxicity in the nigrostriatal dopaminergic system. Along with iron, zinc, and manganese, the oxidative injury induced by arsenite and iron further suggests a pathophysiological role of the interaction of metals in CNS neurodegeneration.

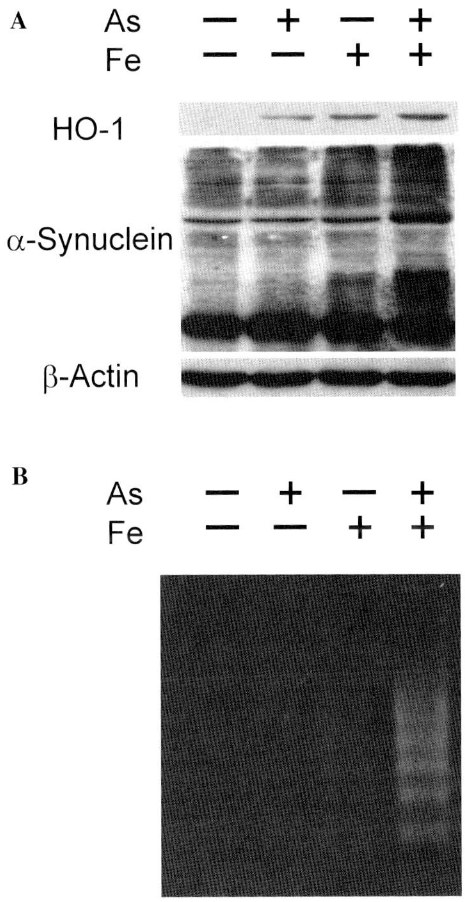

Figure 4. Synergistic effect by co-infusion of arsenite and iron on neurotoxicity in rat brain. (A) Forty-eight hours after intranigral infusion of arsenite (As, 1.5 nmol) or iron (3 nmol) or a mixture of arsenite and iron, the expression of HO-1 and α-synuclein aggregation was detected in the infused substantia nigra (SN) using Western blot assay. (B) Seventy-two h after intranigral infusion, DNA fragmentation was measured in the infused SN using DNA laddering assay. Lane 1: intact SN; Lane 2, arsenite-infused SN; Lane 3, iron-infused SN; Lane 4, SN co-infused with arsenite and iron. Results were repeated with three independent experiments.

Acknowledgments

The authors expresses their gratitude to Dr. L.T. Ho, the director of the Department of Medical Research and Education, Veterans General Hospital–Taipei and Drs. C.Y. Chai and T.C. Lee at the Institute of Biomedical Sciences, Academia Sinica, for their encouragement and generous gifts of arsenic compounds. Special thanks are due to Dr. R.K. Freund at the University of Colorado–Denver, Aurora, CO for editing this paper. This study was supported by NSC97-2420-B-075-017 and VGH97-373, Taipei, Taiwan, R.O.C.

Conflicts of interest

The authors declare no conflicts of interest.

References

1. Wright, R.O. & A. Baccarelli. 2007. Metals and neurotoxicology. *J. Nutr.* **137:** 2809–2813.
2. Hall, A.H. 2002. Chronic arsenic poisoning. *Toxicol. Lett.* **128:** 69–72.
3. Bolla-Wilson, K. & M.L. Bleecker. 1987. Neuropsychological impairment following inorganic arsenic exposure. *J. Occup. Med.* **29:** 500–503.
4. Itoh, T. *et al.* 1990. The effect of arsenic trioxide on brain monoamine metabolism and locomotor activity of mice. *Toxicol. Lett.* **54:** 345–353.
5. Rodriguez, V.M., M.E. Jimenez-Capdeville & M. Giordano. 2003. The effects of arsenic exposure on the nervous system. *Toxicol. Lett.* **145:** 1–18.
6. Soignet, S.L., P. Maslak & Z.G. Wang. 1998. Complete remission after treatment of acute promyelocytic leukemia with arsenic trioxide. *N. Eng. J Med.* **339:** 1341–1348.
7. Shen, Z.X. *et al.* 1997. Use of arsenic trioxide (As2O3) in the treatment of acute promyelocytic leukemia (APL): II. Clinical efficacy and pharmacokinetics in relapsed patients. *Blood* **89:** 3354–3360.
8. Lin, C.C. *et al.* 2007. Arsenic trioxide in patients with hepatocellular carcinoma: a phase II trial. *Invest. New Drug* **25:** 77–84.
9. Kim, K.B. *et al.* 2005. A phase II trial of arsenic trioxide in patients with metastatic melanoma. *Cancer* **104:** 1687–1692.
10. Windebank, A.J. 1986. Specific inhibition of myelination by lead *in vitro*; Comparison with arsenic, thallium, and mercury. *Exp Neurol.* **94:** 203–212.
11. Chao, Y.H. *et al.* 2008. Arsenite-induced cytotoxicity in DRG explants. *Free Radic. Biol. Med.* **44:** 1553–1561.
12. Chao, P.L. *et al.* 2007. N-acetylcysteine attenuates arsenite-induced oxidative injury in DRG explants. *Ann. N.Y. Acad. Sci.* **1122:** 276–288.
13. Lin, A.M.Y. *et al.* 2007. Endoplasmic reticulum stress is involved in arsenite-induced oxidative injury in rat brain. *Toxicol. Appl. Pharmacol.* **224:** 138–146.
14. Lin, A.M.Y. *et al.* 2007. Melatonin attenuates arsenite-induced apoptosis in rat brain: involvement of mitochondrial and ER pathways and aggregation of α-synuclein. *J. Pineal Res.* **43:** 163–171.
15. Zecca, L. *et al.* 2004. Iron, brain ageing and neurodegenerative disorders. *Nat. Rev. Neurosci.* **5:** 863–873.
16. Dexter, D.T. *et al.* 1989. Increased nigral iron content and alteration in other metal ions occurring in brain in Parkinson's disease. *J. Neurochem.* **52:** 1830–1836.
17. Floyd, R.A. & J.M. Carney. 1992. Free radicals damage to protein and DNA: mechanisms involved and relevant observation on brain undergoing oxidative stress. *Ann. Neurol.* **32:** S22–S27.
18. Mecocci, P. *et al.* 1993. Oxidative damage to mitochondrial DNA shows marked age-dependent increases in human brain. *Ann. Neurol.* **34:** 609–616.
19. Halliwell, B. & J.M. Gutteridge. 1984. Oxygen toxicity, oxygen radicals, transition metals and diseases. *J. Biochem.* **219:** 1–14.
20. Gotz, M.E. *et al.* 2004. The relevance of iron in the pathogenesis of Parkinson's disease. *Ann. N.Y. Acad. Sci.* **1012:** 193–208.
21. Lotharius, J. & P. Brundin. 2002. Impaired dopamine storage resulting from alpha-synuclein mutations may contribute to the pathogenesis of Parkinson's disease. *Hum. Mol. Genet.* **11:** 395–407.
22. Lin, A.M.Y. & L.T. Ho. 2000. Melatonin suppresses iron-induced neurodegeneration in rat brain. *Free Radic. Biol. Med.* **28:** 904–911.
23. Lin, A.M.Y. 2001. Coexistence of zinc and iron augmented oxidative injuries in the nigrostriatal dopaminergic system of SD rats. *Free Radic. Biol. Med.* **30:** 225–231.
24. Sengstock, G.J. *et al.* 1997. Intranigral iron infusion in the rat. Acute elevations in nigral lipid peroxidation and striatal dopaminergic markers with ensuing nigral degeneration. *Biol. Trace. Elem. Res.* **58:** 177–195.
25. Domingo, J.L. 2006. Aluminum and other metals in Alzheimer's disease: a review of potential therapy with chelating agents. *Alzheimers Dis.* **10:** 331–341.
26. Rodriguez, V.M. *et al.* 1998. Effects of oral exposure to mining waste on *in vivo* dopamine release from rat striatum. *Environ. Health Perspect.* **106:** 487–491.
27. Roth, J.A. & M.D. Garrick. 2003. Iron interactions and other biological reactions mediating the physiological and toxic actions of manganese. *Biochem Pharmacol.* **66:** 1–13.
28. Chandra, A.V. *et al.* 1981. Behavioral and neurochemical changes in rats simultaneously exposed to manganese and lead. *Arch. Toxicol.* **49:** 49–56.

29. Kalia, K., S.V. Chandra & P.N. Viswanathan. 1984. Effect of 54Mn and lead interaction on their binding with tissue proteins: *in vitro* studies. *Ind. Health* **22:** 207–218.
30. Mejia, J.J. *et al.* 1997. Effects of lead-arsenic combined exposure on central monoaminergic systems. *Neurotoxicol. Teratol.* **19:** 489–497.
31. Kikugawa, K. *et al.* 1989. Fluorescent and cross-linked proteins formed by free radical and aldehyde species generated during lipid peroxidation. *Adv. Exper. Med. Biol.* **266:** 345–356.
32. Paxinos, G. & C. Watson. 1986. *The Rat Brain in Stereotaxic Coordinates*. Academic Press. New York.
33. Chiueh, C.C. *et al.* 1983. 6-fluorocatecholamines as false adrenergic neurotransmitters. *J. Pharmacol. Exp. Ther.* **225:** 529–533.
34. Griffith, O.W. 1980. Determination of glutathione and glutathione disulfide using glutathione reductase and 2-vinylpyridine. *Anal. Biochem.* **106:** 207–212.
35. Sambrook, J., E.F. Fritch & T. Maniatis. Analysis and cloning of eukaryotic genomic DNA. In *Molecular Cloning*. Ford, N., C. Nolan & M. Ferguson, Eds.: 9.16–9.19. Cold Spring Harbor Laboratory Press. Cold Spring Harbor, NT.
36. Bernstam, L. & J. Nriagu. 2000. Molecular aspects of arsenic stress. *J. Toxicol. Environ. Health* **3:** 293–322.
37. Chattopadhyay, S. *et al.* 2002. Apoptosis and necrosis in developing brain cells due to arsenic toxicity and protection with antioxidants. *Toxicol. Lett.* **136:** 665–676.
38. Guidarelli, A. *et al.* 2005. Role of Bcl-2 in the arachidonate-mediated survival signaling preventing mitochondrial permeability transition-dependent U937 cell necrosis induced by peroxynitrite. *Free Radic. Biol. Med.* **39:** 1638–1649.
39. Chen, Y.C., S.Y. Lin-Shiau & J.K. Lin. 1998. Involvement of reactive oxygen species and caspase 3 activation in arsenite-induced apoptosis. *J. Cell. Physiol.* **177:** 324–333.
40. Garcia-Chavez, E. *et al.* 2003. Arsenite-induced formation of hydroxyl radical in the striatum of awake rats. *Brain Res.* **976:** 82–89.
41. Bau, D.T. *et al.* 2002. Oxidative DNA adducts and DNA-protein cross-links are the major DNA lesions induced by arsenite. *Environ. Health Persp.* **110:** 753–756.
42. Bernstam, L. & J. Nriagu. 2000. Molecular aspects of arsenic stress. *J. Toxicol. Environ. Health* **3:** 293–322.
43. Ramanathan, K. *et al.* 2005. Ascorbic acid and alpha-tocopherol as potent modulators of apoptosis on arsenic induced toxicity in rats. *Toxicol. Lett.* **156:** 297–306.
44. Lantz, R.C. *et al.* 1994. Effect of arsenic exposure on alveolar macrophage function. I. Effect of soluble As (III) and As (V). *Environ. Res.* **67:** 183–195.
45. Perry, T.L., D.V. Godin & A. Hansen. 1982. Parkinson's disease: a disorder due to nigral glutathione deficiency. *Neurosci. Lett.* **33:** 305–310.
46. Sofic, E. *et al.* 1992. Reduced and oxidized glutathione in the substantia nigra of patients with Parkinson's disease. *Neurosci. Lett.* **142:** 128–130.
47. de la Torre, M.R. *et al.* 1996. Human aging brain disorders: role of antioxidant enzymes. *Neurochem. Res.* **21:** 885–888.
48. Sakurai, T. *et al.* 2002. A major human arsenic metabolite, dimethylarsinic acid, requires reduced glutathione to induce apoptosis. *Chem. Res. Toxicol.* **15:** 629–637.
49. Yang, C.H. *et al.* 1999. Arsenic trioxide sensitivity is associated with low level of glutathione in cancer cells. *Br. J. Cancer* **81:** 796–799.
50. Lin, A.M.Y., C.F. Chen & L.T. Ho. 2002. Neuroprotective effect of intermittent hypoxia on iron-induced oxidative injury in rat brain. *Exp. Neurol.* **176:** 328–335.
51. Ahmad, S., K.T. Kitchin & W.R. Cullen. 2000. Arsenic species that cause release of iron from ferritin and generation of activated oxygen. *Arch. Biochem. Biophys.* **382:** 195–202.
52. Holtz, W.A. & K.L. O'Malley. 2003. Parkinsonian mimetics induce aspects of unfolded protein response in death of dopaminergic neurons. *J. Biol. Chem.* **278:** 19367–19377.
53. Imai, Y. *et al.* 2001. An unfolded putative transmembrane polypeptide, which can lead to endoplasmic reticulum stress, is a substrate of Parkin. *Cell* **105:** 891–902.
54. Vekrellis, K., H.J. Rideout & L. Stefanis. 2004. Neurobiology of alpha-synuclein. *Mol. Neurobiol.* **30:** 1–21.

Ann. N.Y. Acad. Sci. ISSN 0077-8923

ANNALS OF THE NEW YORK ACADEMY OF SCIENCES
Issue: *Neuroprotective Agents*

Isoflurane modulates neuronal excitability of the nucleus reticularis thalami *in vitro*

Pavle M. Joksovic[1] and Slobodan M. Todorovic[1,2,3]

Departments of [1]Anesthesiology and [2]Neuroscience and [3]Neuroscience Graduate Program, University of Virginia School of Medicine, Charlottesville, Virginia

Address for correspondence: Slobodan M. Todorovic, Department of Anesthesiology, University of Virginia Health System, Mail Box 800710, Charlottesville, VA 22908-0710. st9d@virginia.edu

The thalamus has a key function in processing sensory information, sleep, and cognition. We examined the effects of a common volatile anesthetic, isoflurane, on modulation of neuronal excitability in reticular thalamic nucleus (nRT) in intact brain slices from immature rats. In current-clamp recordings, isoflurane (300–600 μmol/L) consistently depolarized membrane potential, decreased input resistance, and inhibited both rebound burst firing and tonic spike firing modes of nRT neurons. The isoflurane-induced depolarization persisted not only in the presence of tetrodotoxin, but after replacement of Ca^{2+} with Ba^{2+} ions in external solution; it was abolished by partial replacement of extracellular Na^+ ions with N-methyl-D-glucamine. In voltage-clamp recordings, we found that isoflurane slowed recovery from inactivation of T-type Ca^{2+} current. Thus, at clinically relevant concentrations, isoflurane inhibits neuronal excitability of nRT neurons in developing brain via multiple ion channels. Inhibition of the neuronal excitability of thalamic cells may contribute to impairment of sensory information transfer in the thalamocortical network by general anesthetics. The findings may be important for understanding cellular mechanisms of anesthesia, such as loss of consciousness and potentially damaging consequences of general anesthetics on developing mammalian brains.

Keywords: thalamus; low-threshold-activated; isoflurane; calcium; sodium; reticular thalamic nucleus

Introduction

Recent studies implicate various thalamic nuclei in awareness and cognitive functions.[1–4] The rhythmicity of thalamocortical circuitry depends to a great extent on the ability of thalamic cells to burst in oscillatory patterns at hyperpolarized membrane potentials (burst firing) and to fire sustained-action potentials at depolarized membrane potentials (tonic firing).[2–4] It has been postulated that during tonic firing, which predominates during awake states, there is a faithful transfer of sensory information to cortical neurons; in contrast, during slow oscillations presented with burst firing pattern of these neurons, there is impairment of sensory transfer and transition to sleep states. A key element in rhythm generation within the thalamus is the GABAergic nucleus reticularis thalami (nRT), which is reciprocally connected to thalamocortical relay neurons and receives collateral excitatory connections from corticothalamic and thalamocortical fibers. *In vivo* extracellular recordings have shown that volatile general anesthetics depress the excitability of thalamic neurons, which, in turn, may underlie blockade of thalamocortical information transfer.[1] Thus, using whole-cell patch-clamp recordings in brain slices *in vitro*, we investigated the cellular excitability of nRT neurons in the presence of isoflurane (ISO), the prototypical volatile general anesthetic.

Materials and methods

In vitro tissue slice preparation

Experiments were done on transverse rat brain slices cut through the middle anterior portion of the nRT. We have detailed elsewhere the procedures for *in vitro* recording from intact nRT neurons in brain slices.[5,6] Sprague–Dawley rats were housed in a local animal facility in accordance with protocols approved by the University of Virginia Animal Use

doi: 10.1111/j.1749-6632.2009.05172.x

and Care Committee. Rats (age 7–14 days) of either sex were briefly anesthetized with ISO and decapitated. The brains were rapidly removed and placed in iced cold (4°C) cutting solution consisting, in mmol/L, of 2 $CaCl_2$, 260 sucrose, 26 $NaHCO_3$, 10 glucose, 3 KCl, 1.25 NaH_2PO_4, and 2 $MgCl_2$ equilibrated with a mixture of 95% O_2 and 5% CO_2. We glued a block of tissue containing the thalamus to the chuck of a vibrotome (model NVSL, WPI, Sarasota, FL) and cut 250–300 μm slices in a transverse plane. We incubated the slices in 36°C-oxygenated saline for 1 h before placing them in a recording chamber that had been superfused with external solution at a rate of 1.5 cc/min. The incubating solution consisted, in mmol/L, of 124 NaCl, 4 KCl, 26 $NaHCO_3$, 1.25 NaH_2PO_4, 2 $MgCl_2$, 10 glucose, and 2 $CaCl_2$ equilibrated with a mixture of 95% O_2 and 5% CO_2. Slices were maintained at room temperature in the recording chamber, where they remained viable for at least 1 h.

Recording procedures

The extracellular saline solution used for recording Ca^{2+} currents in whole-cell experiments consisted, in mmol/L, of 2 $CaCl_2$, 130 NaCl, 2.5 $MgCl_2$, 10 glucose, 26 $NaHCO_3$, 1.25 NaH_2PO_4, and 0.001 tetrodotoxin (TTX). This solution was equilibrated with a mixture of 95% O_2 and 5% CO_2 for at least 30 min, until its pH was 7.35–7.45. The extracellular solution for current-clamp experiments was the same as the incubating solution. However, for some current-clamp experiments, we replaced NaCl in the external solution with equimolar N-methyl-D-glucamine (NMDG) and 2 mmol/L $CaCl_2$ with 2 mmol/L $BaCl_2$; we then also included 1 μmol/L TTX in the external solution. To eliminate glutamatergic excitatory currents, most current-clamp recordings were done in the presence of 5 mol/L NBQX (2,3-dihydroxy-6-nitro-7-sulfamoyl-benzo [f]quinoxaline-2,3-dione) and 50 mol/L d-APV (2*R*-amino-5-phosphonovaleric acid; AP5) in the bath solution. To eliminate inhibitory synaptic currents, most current-clamp recordings were done in the presence of 20 μmol/L picrotoxin (a noncompetitive $GABA_A$ antagonist) in the bath solution.

To record T-currents in brain slices, we used an internal solution (solution 1) of, in mmol/L, 135–140 tetramethylammonium hydroxide (TMA-OH), 10 EGTA, 40 HEPES, and 2 $MgCl_2$ titrated to pH 7.15–7.25 with hydrofluoric acid (HF).[7] Recording electrodes for current-clamp studies contained, in mmol/L, KCl 130, $MgCl_2$ 5, EGTA 1, Na-HEPES 40, MgATP 2, and Na_3-GTP 0.1 (pH 7.2). For the data presented, membrane potential values were not corrected for the measured liquid junction potential of −10 mV in voltage-clamp experiments and −5 mV in current-clamp experiments. All recordings were obtained from thalamic neurons visualized with an infrared differential interference contrast camera (C2400; Hammamatsu, Hammamatsu City, Japan) on the Zeiss 2 FS Axioscope (Jena, Germany) with a 40X lens and patch-clamp pipette using a Sutter micromanipulator MP-285 (Sutter Instrument Co., Novato, CA).

Aliquots of anesthetic solution were prepared from saturated saline solution incubated with ISO (60 mL of saline with 40 mL of ISO in a closed 100 mL vial) for at least 24 h.[5–7] To quantify the actual anesthetic concentrations in solutions, we analyzed samples of saturated stock solutions and aliquots in a gas chromatograph calibrated with the appropriate anesthetic standards.[5–7] We found a loss of less than 10% if the solution was used within 30 min after preparation. Thus, all anesthetic solutions were used in our experiments within 30 min after preparation. Test solutions were maintained in all-glass syringes tightly sealed with parafilm punctured with a small escape hole for times when a whole cell was obtained and allowed anesthetic solution to fall by gravity.

Electrophysiological recordings

Recordings were made with standard whole-cell voltage and current-clamp techniques. Electrodes, which were fabricated from thin-walled microcapillary tubes (Drummond Scientific, Broomall, PA), had final resistances of 3–6 MΩ. We recorded membrane currents with an Axoclamp 200B patch-clamp amplifier (Molecular Devices, Foster City, CA). Voltage commands and digitization of membrane currents were done with Clampex 8.2 of the pClamp software package (Molecular Devices). Data were analyzed using Clampfit (Molecular Devices) and Origin 7.0 (OriginLab Corp., Northampton, MA). We filtered currents at 5–10 kHz.

Analysis of current

Statistical analysis was done using the Student *t* test, with statistical significance determined at $P < 0.05$.

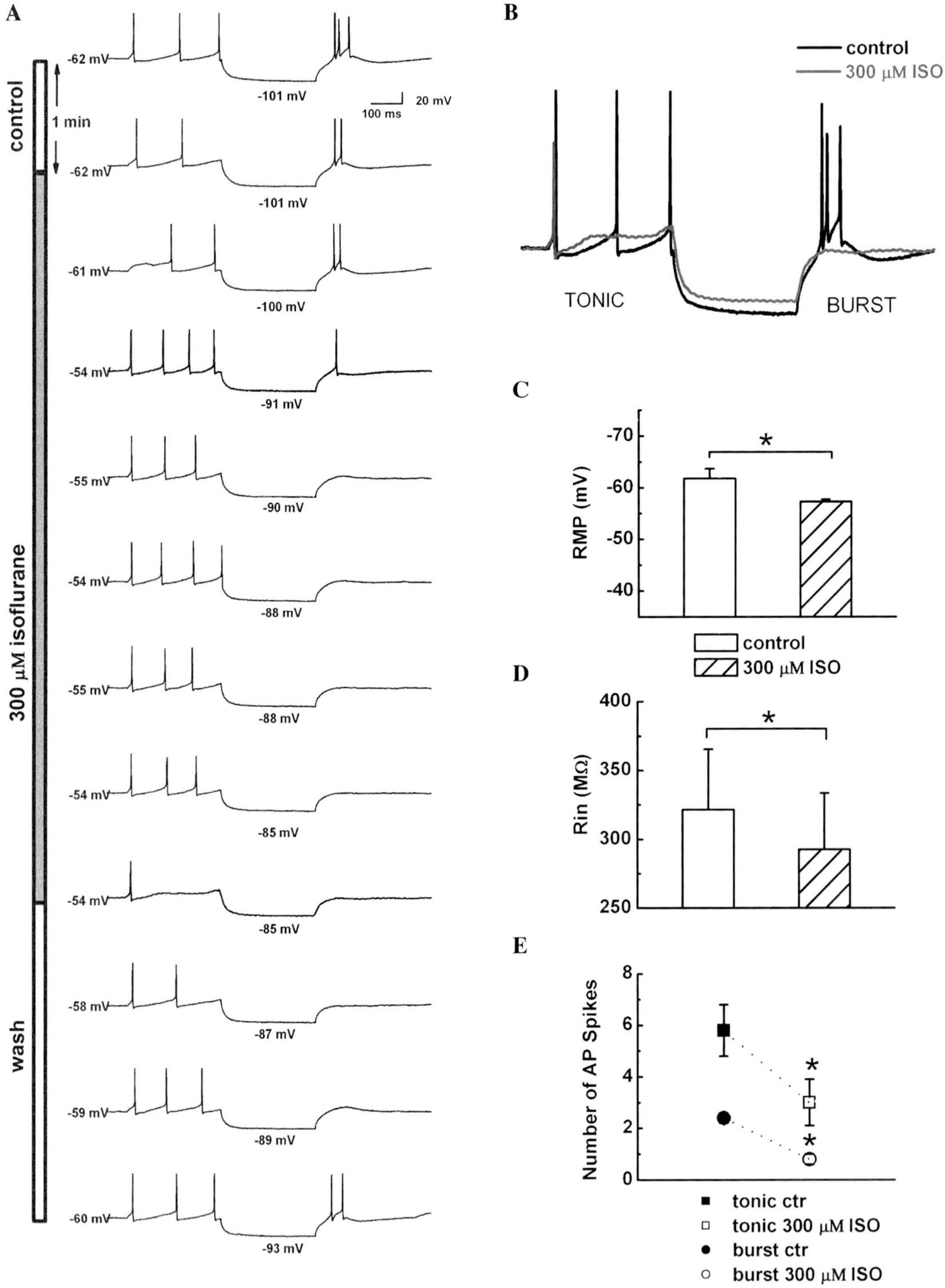

Figure 1. (A) This panel shows time course (*from the top to bottom*) in control conditions (*open bar*) during the application of 300 μmol/L ISO (*gray solid bar*) and after ISO wash (*open bar*) on (*from the left to the right*) resting

Input resistance (R_{in}) was determined from the slope of the peak voltage versus the current plot that resulted from injecting 80–200 ms-long current ranging from 100–500 pA.

Drugs and chemicals

TTX was purchased from Alomone Lab (Jerusalem, Israel). All other compounds were purchased from Sigma Chemical (St. Louis, MO). Drugs were delivered with a gravity-driven perfusion system. Manually controlled valves accomplished switching between solutions.

Results

Isoflurane modulates the cellular excitability of nRT neurons

To determine the effects of volatile anesthetics on sensory information transfer in the thalamocortical circuitry, we examined the effects of clinically relevant concentrations of ISO on spike firing of nRT cells in current-clamp experiments. In order to study both functional firing modes of these cells, we first injected a depolarizing current of 300-ms duration to evoke tonic firing of single action potentials (APs); we then injected a hyperpolarizing current of the same duration to asses membrane input resistance (R_{in}) and evoke rebound burst firing. As demonstrated by the time course of representative nRT shown in Figure 1A and the histogram in Figures 1C and D, bath applications of 300 μmol/L ISO reversibly depolarized resting membrane potential (RMP) in these cells for about 5 mV (average 4.6 ± 0.5 mV, $P < 0.001$, $n = 10$) and decreased R_{in} for about 10% (average 29 ± 6 MΩ, $P = 0.001$, $n = 10$). Bath applications of 600 μmol/L ISO further depolarized membranes for about 10 mV (average 9.6 ± 1.0 mV, $P < 0.01$, $n = 3$, data not shown). The traces in Figure 1B, which are normalized to baseline membrane potentials (black line), indicate that ISO at 300 μmol/L (gray line) decreased the initial number of APs in tonic mode from 3 to 1 and in burst mode from 3 to 0 with a concomitant decrease of about 10% in the amplitude of the hyperpolarizing pulse. In similar experiments from 10 nRT cells, we counted the number of APs in both tonic and burst firing mode, finding that ISO at 300 μmol/L significantly decreased spike firing in both by about 50% (Fig. 1E).

To examine probable ionic conductances involved in ISO-induced depolarization in nRT neurons, we did additional current-clamp experiments. When NaCl in the external solution was replaced with NMDG, ISO-induced depolarization was completely abolished ($n = 3$). Figure 2A shows a time course from representative nRT cells; application of NMDG hyperpolarized membranes for about 7 mV, while ISO applied with NMDG had little effect on membrane potential. However, inclusion of 1 μmol/L TTX in the external solution did not have a significant effect on ISO depolarization, suggesting the involvement of TTX-resistant Na^+ conductance ($n = 4$, data not shown). In two experiments, we replaced 2 mmol/L Ca^{2+} in the external solution with 2 mmol/L Ba^{2+}, which blocks many K^+ channels. As shown in Figure 2B, application of Ba^{2+}-containing external solution depolarized membranes for about 40 mV. Under these conditions, ISO further depolarized membranes by an additional 9 mV. These results suggest that resting Ba^{2+}-sensitive K^+ conductance is not sensitive to ISO, while resting TTX-resistant Na+ conductance in these cells is enhanced by ISO, which in turn depolarizes the neuronal membrane.

membrane potentials, tonic firing mode, R_{in}, and rebound burst firing. Note that ISO gradually and reversibly depolarized membranes from −62 mV to −54 mV; decreased R_{in}, as shown by the decrease in hyperpolarizing potential from −101 mV to −85 mV; and inhibited the number of action potentials during both tonic and burst firing. (**B**) This panel shows normalized traces from the control condition (*solid black line*) and at the end of ISO application (*solid gray line*) from the same cell as that shown in panel A. (C) Histograms indicate the average effects of ISO on RMP in 10 reticular thalamic nucleus (nRT) cells. (**D**) Histograms indicate the average effects of ISO on R_{in} in the same nRT cells as those shown in panel C. (**E**) Points indicate the average effects of ISO on control (ctr) number of action potential (AP) spikes in tonic (*squares*) and burst (*circles*) firing modes. In panels C–E, vertical lines indicates SEM and asterisks indicate significance $P < 0.05$.

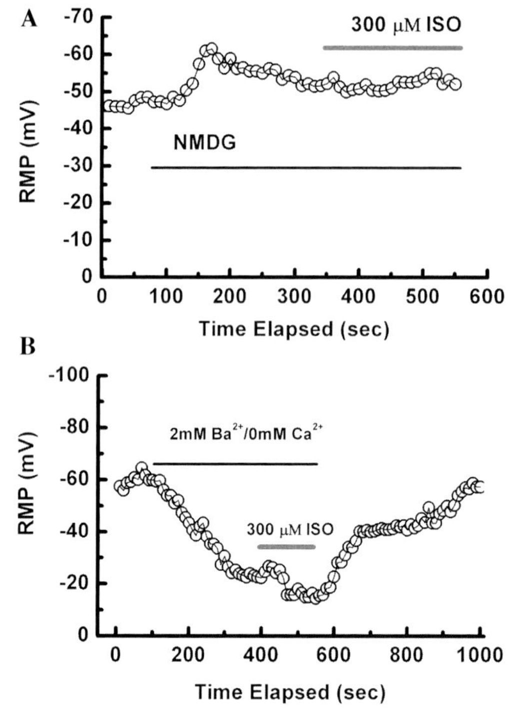

Figure 2. (A) Time course of the effects of N-methyl-D-glucamine (NMDG) and isoflurane (ISO) on resting membrane potential (RMP). Note that NMDG (black line) hyperpolarized this cell from −45 mV to −52 mV and subsequently co-applied ISO (*gray line*) had little effect. (B) Time course of the effects of 2 mmol/L Ba^{2+} and ISO on RMP in another reticular thalamic nucleus (nRT) cell. Note that the application of Ba^{2+} (*black line*) depolarized this cell from about −60 mV to about −20 mV; subsequently co-applied ISO (*gray line*) further depolarized the cell to resting membrane potential (RMP) of about −11 mV.

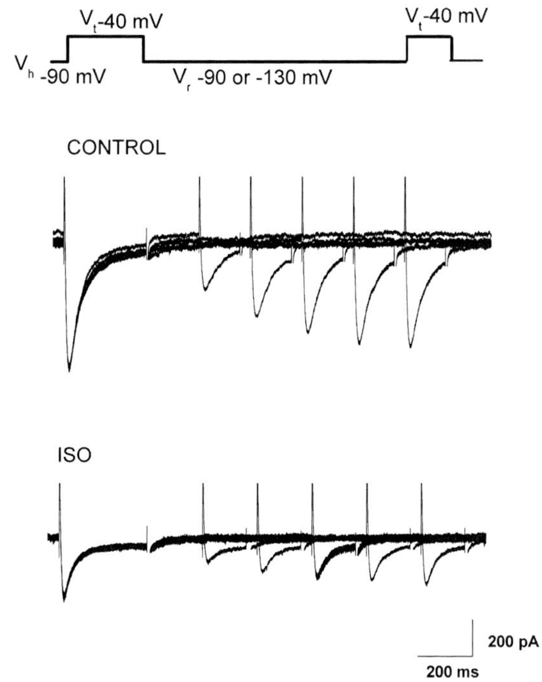

Figure 3. Paired-pulse protocol depicted on the top of this figure was used to study recovery from inactivation. Original traces show recovery from inactivation in control conditions (*middle panel*) and after bath application of 600 μmol/L isoflurane (ISO) (*bottom panel*) at −90 mV. In control conditions, T-current recovered to 86% of control after 1 s (last trace on the middle graph) while in the presence of ISO it recovered to 75% of control after same interval (last trace on bottom panel). Calibration bars pertain to both panels.

Isoflurane modulates recovery from inactivation of isolated T-currents in the nRT neurons

Because, in current-clamp recording, ISO inhibited rebound burst firing, we examined its effects on recovery from inactivation of T-currents, which is important in the generation of burst firing mode in these cells. Inactivation, a major biophysical property of voltage-gated Ca^{2+} channels, may differ substantially among distinct native T-channels.[8] The time- and voltage-dependent process of recovery from inactivation, which controls return of the availability of T-channels and underlying low-threshold calcium spikes (LTS) in the thalamus, is an important factor in determining the rate of repetitive low-threshold burst firing of APs in nRT neurons. By changing recovery from inactivation of T-currents or availability of T-channels at different potentials, anesthetics may influence burst firing of nRT neurons. Therefore, we investigated the influence of ISO on recovery from inactivation in 15 nRT cells.

For this purpose, we used a paired-pulse protocol in which a 300-ms step to −40 mV was used to inactivate most of the T-current. After a variable recovery interval (20 to 10,000 ms) at either −90 or −130 mV, a second step to −50 mV was used to determine the amount of T-current that had recovered from inactivation during the recovery period (Fig. 3). The percent recovery in the presence and

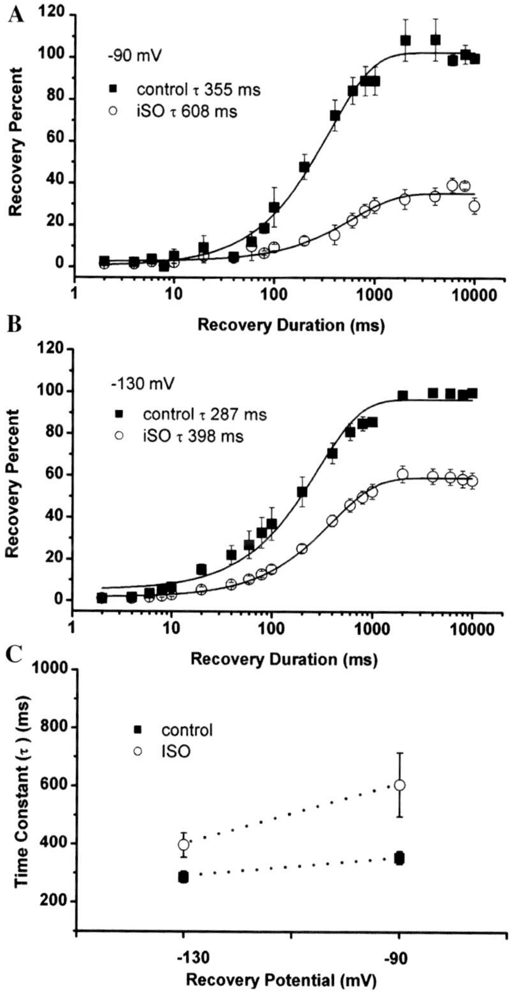

Figure 4. Percent recovery of peak inactivating T-current is plotted as a function of recovery duration at −90 mV (A) or −130 mV (B) in the absence (*filled squares*) and presence (*open circles*) of isoflurane (ISO). Symbols are average from 4–5 experiments, vertical lines are SEM, and solid lines are fitted by mono-exponential time course. (C) This graph shows differences between time constants in control conditions (*filled squares*) and after application of ISO (*open circles*) at recovery potentials of −90 and −130 mV from experiments depicted on plots A and B of this figure. Vertical lines indicate ± SEM of fitted values.

absence of 600 μmol/L ISO in the same cells ($n = 4$–5 for each protocol) was then plotted as a function of recovery duration at either 90 mV (Fig. 4A) or −130 mV (Fig. 4B). Recovery time courses with (open symbols) and without (filled symbols) ISO are reasonably well fitted with a single exponential function. Recovery from inactivation at −90 mV was slower in the presence of ISO by about 70%, with a time constant of 608 ± 110 ms with isoflurane as compared to 355 ± 22 ms in controls (Fig. 4A) and by about 38% at −130 mV (Fig. 4B, 287 ± 20 ms for controls and 398 ± 42 with ISO). Figure 4C summarizes the effects of ISO on recovery from inactivation of T-currents in nRT cells at membrane potentials of −90 and −130 mV. Overall, these results indicate relatively voltage-independent recovery from inactivation of T-currents under control conditions, but the effect of ISO was more prominent at −90 mV (Fig. 4C).

A characteristic of inactivation of T-currents in many native and recombinant systems is that recovery is influenced by the duration of the preceding inactivation step.[2] Our results confirm this; if a cell is held at −50 mV for 6 s before the recovery interval at potentials of −90 mV, recovery from inactivation is drastically slowed in comparison to that after a shorter inactivation pulse (from 355 ms to 855 ms, data not shown). However, the recovery time constant became even slower in the presence of ISO (855 ± 40 ms in control and 1150 ± 152 ms for isoflurane, a 34% difference; $n = 6$, data not shown). These findings indicate that ISO slows recovery from inactivation of T-currents regardless of the duration of the inactivating pulse.

Discussion

A major finding of this study is that ISO at a clinically relevant concentration *in vitro* at 300–600 μmol/L (corresponding roughly to 1–2 minimum alveolar concentration *in vivo*) profoundly inhibits neuronal excitability in nRT neurons in intact slices from the brains of young rats. This is manifested as depolarization of membrane potential accompanied by decreased R_{in}, decreased amplitude of rebound LTS, and diminished numbers of fast APs in both tonic and burst firing modes. ISO-induced depolarization of membrane potential was invariably associated with a decrease in R_{in}, which in turn indicates that this depolarization is mediated by the opening of some type of ion channels. Because we could completely abrogate this effect of ISO by partial replacement of Na^+ ions in external solution, it appears that TTX-resistant Na^+ conductance active at resting membrane potentials is increased by ISO, which in turn depolarized membranes.

We previously demonstrated that ISO inhibits isolated T-currents in these cells in voltage-dependent fashion.[6] Consistent with this is our present finding that ISO slowed recovery from inactivated states of T-currents, which in turn diminished the amplitude of LTS and underlying burst firing. Somewhat surprisingly, ISO depolarized nRT neurons but inhibited tonic firing of single APs. This could be attributed to several possible effects of ISO. First, a decrease in R_{in} may shunt APs generated by the injection of depolarizing current. Second, ISO-induced depolarization may enhance inactivation of voltage-gated Na^+ currents that control the generation of AP. Third, ISO may directly inhibit voltage-gated Na^+ currents.[9] This, to the best of our knowledge, is the first report of the effects of ISO on the excitability of rat nRT neurons. However, others have shown that ISO can inhibit the excitability of thalamic relay (TR) cells in rat brain slices.[10] Interestingly, given that ISO hyperpolarized TR cells by decreasing R_{in}, most likely as a consequence of the increase in background K^+ conductance, it seems that depolarization is a nucleus-specific effect of ISO.[10] However, despite the presumably different ionic mechanisms involved, the effect of ISO in both nRT and TR cells resulted in similar inhibition of tonic and burst firing modes.

Importantly, inhibition of neuronal excitability of nRT cells, together with previously reported inhibition in TR cells, may contribute to the impairment of sensory information transfer in the thalamocortical network by general anesthetics. Because the thalamus has a key function in the processing of sensory information, sleep, and cognition, our results indicate that the effects of ISO on multiple ion conductances involved in the electrogenesis of nRT cells may contribute to the clinical effects of general anesthetics. Extensive molecular and electrophysiological studies will be needed to identify the ion channels in nRT cells that mediate the effects of ISO on neuronal excitability.

Acknowledgments

This work was supported by NIH grant GM070726 to SMT.

Conflicts of interest

The authors declare no conflicts of interest.

References

1. Angel A. 1991. Adventures in anesthesia. *Exp. Physiol.* **76:** 1–38.
2. Llinas, R.R. *et al.* 1999. Thalamocortical dysrhythmia: a neurological and neuropsychiatric syndrome characterized by magnetoencephalography. *Proc. Natl. Acad. Sci. USA* **96:** 15222–15227.
3. McCormick, D.A. & T. Bal. 1997. Sleep and arousal: thalamocortical mechanisms. *Annu. Rev. Neurosci.* **20:** 185–215.
4. Steriade, M. 2005. Sleep, epilepsy and thalamic reticular inhibitory neurons. *Trends. Neurosci.* **28:** 317–324.
5. Joksovic, P.M. *et al.* 2005. Contrasting anesthetic sensitivities of T-type calcium channels of reticular thalamic neurons and recombinant CaV3.3 channels. *Br. J. Pharmacol.* **144:** 59–70.
6. Joksovic, P.M. *et al.* 2005. Different kinetic properties of two T-type Ca2+ currents of reticular thalamic neurons and their modulation by enflurane. *J. Physiol.* **566:** 125–142.
7. Todorovic, S.M. & C.J. Lingle. 1998. Pharmacological properties of T-type Ca2+ current in adult rat sensory neurons: effects of anticonvulsants and anesthetic agents. *J. Neurophysiol.* **79:** 240–252.
8. Huguenard, J.R. 1996. Low-threshold calcium currents in central nervous system neurons. *Annu. Rev. Physiol.* **58:** 329–358.
9. OuYang, W. & H.C. Hemmings, Jr. 2007. Isoform-selective effects of isoflurane on voltage-gated Na+ channels. *Anesthesiology* **107:** 91–98.
10. Ries, C.R. & E. Puil. 1999. Mechanism of anesthesia revealed by shunting actions of isoflurane on thalamocortical neurons. *J. Neurophysiol.* **81:** 1795–1801.

Ann. N.Y. Acad. Sci. ISSN 0077-8923

ANNALS OF THE NEW YORK ACADEMY OF SCIENCES
Issue: *Neuroprotective Agents*

Timing versus duration

Determinants of anesthesia-induced developmental apoptosis in the young mammalian brain

Sabina Rizzi,[1,2] Carlo Ori,[2] and Vesna Jevtovic-Todorovic[1]

[1]Department of Anesthesiology, University of Virginia, Charlottesville, Virginia. [2]Department of Anesthesiology and Pharmacology, University of Padova, Padova, Italy

Address for correspondence: Vesna Jevtovic-Todorovic, Department of Anesthesiology, University of Virginia Health System, PO Box 800710, Charlottesville, VA 22908. vj3w@virginia.edu

Rapidly accumulating evidence indicates that clinically used general anesthesia causes massive, widespread neuroapoptotic degeneration in the developing mammalian brain. Susceptibility to anesthesia-induced neurotoxicity has been documented in rats, mice, guinea pigs, primates, and in this study, piglets; in short, anesthesia-induced developmental neuroapoptosis is not species-dependent. Our findings with piglets, like those in other immature mammals, demonstrate that relatively short exposure to anesthesia is just as detrimental to species with long periods of synaptogenesis as it is to those with short periods of synaptogenesis. However, the highly reproducible findings in different species also indicate that the timing of exposure to anesthesia is critically important; that is, brain regions that are at the peak of synaptogenesis are most vulnerable even when the exposure to anesthesia is relatively brief. Because the peak of synaptogenesis is characterized by intense, highly programmed neuronal communication that is vital for the survival and proper function of immature neurons, we conclude that anesthesia causes severe disturbances in the fine equilibrium between excitatory and inhibitory neurotransmission in the developing mammalian brain, ultimately leading to neuronal redundancy and death.

Keywords: piglets; isoflurane; midazolam; nitrous oxide; fentanyl; synaptogenesis

Introduction

Rapidly accumulating evidence indicates that commonly used general anesthetics, administered alone or in clinically relevant cocktails during the early stages of mammalian brain development, cause severe, widespread neuronal degeneration.[1–5] Based on several mechanistic studies, it appears that anesthesia-induced neuronal damage is apoptotic and involves several pathways of caspase activation. The intrinsic mitochondria-dependent pathway appears to be activated first,[6,7] although others follow shortly. Activation of the extrinsic, death-receptor activated[6] and neurotrophic factor-activated (in particular, brain-derived neurotrophic factor)[5] pathways results in massive caspase-3 activation and DNA fragmentation.[3,6,7] At the ultrastructural level, the initial insult, detected mainly in the nucleus, is marked by clamping of the chromatin, followed by disruption of the nuclear membrane, intermixing of the cytoplasm and nucleoplasm, and the formation of apoptotic bodies.[3] Interestingly, despite massive neuronal demise, anesthesia-induced damage does not seem to result in significant gliosis.

A common finding in the animal studies done thus far is that the vulnerability of the immature mammalian brain to anesthesia-induced damage coincides with synaptogenesis.[1–4,6,8] Although synapse formation is the hallmark of this period, there are several other key elements. To make meaningful synapses and form functional circuitries, neurons have to migrate to their final destination, mature, and differentiate. This highly programmed series of events must occur in a specific order and in a highly homeostatic environment in which

doi: 10.1111/j.1749-6632.2009.05173.x

modulation of excitatory and the inhibitory neurotransmission is well balanced.[9] It has been proposed that general anesthetics, by creating an imbalance in excitatory and inhibitory neurotransmission, disturb the fine equilibrium and, if administered during the peak of synaptogenesis, can cause significant perturbation of normal synapse formation.[3,5,6] Neurons that do not form meaningful interneuronal connections are redundant and therefore die by apoptosis. (The apoptotic machinery in immature neurons is easily activated.) Interestingly, the processes of anesthesia-induced apoptotic activation and neuronal death are virtually the same as those that normally occur during early stages of synaptogenesis, the only difference between them being their magnitude. Normal neuronal pruning is highly controlled, its intensity varying during normal synaptogenesis but leading, ultimately, to the apoptotic death of a fairly low percentage of neurons (on average, approximately 1% with some regional variations).[1,4] In contrast, anesthesia-induced neuronal apoptosis results in the death of as many as 70-fold more neurons compared to age-matched controls.[3,4,6]

Duration of anesthesia versus duration of synaptogenesis

Initial studies of anesthesia-induced neuroapoptosis were done in rodents. Although the findings were both impressive and highly reproducible, they gave rise to the question of whether rodents are especially susceptible.[1–5,10] An even more important point was that the initial rodent studies begged the question of whether there is a direct correlation between the duration of anesthesia and the duration of synaptogenesis. For species with a relatively short span of synaptogenesis, anesthesia lasting several hours covers a substantial amount of time when proper communication between neurons is crucial. For example, the initial anesthesia neurotoxicity experiments dealt with mice and rats, in which synaptogenesis is 2–3 weeks long.[11] Thus, anesthesia protocols lasting for 6 to 7 h seem like a long exposure. Could exposure to anesthesia for this period be irrelevant to any kind of clinical setting, considering that human brain development spans a couple of years, including the last trimester of *in utero* and the first 2 or so years of postnatal life? (However, the argument could certainly be that prolonged, deep sedation in neonatal and pediatric intensive care units is often administered for days, thus exposing the human brain in the fragile early stages of its development to intense homeostatic unbalance.)

To address the correlation between the duration of synaptogenesis and anesthesia as potentially important determinants of the susceptibility to anesthesia-induced developmental neuroapoptosis, we and others have done studies using clinically relevant general anesthetics on species having relatively long durations of synaptogenesis: guinea pigs,[4] piglets, and primates.[8]

Guinea pigs

Synaptogenesis in guinea pigs lasts approximately 10 weeks[11] and, unlike synaptogenesis in humans, occurs mainly during the prenatal period. It starts early in pregnancy, reaches a peak between 35 and 40 days of gestation, and is virtually completed by the end of prenatal life (68–70 days).[12,13] We used three gestational ages and hence, three stages of brain growth: early (20 to 25 days *in utero*), peak (35 to 40 days *in utero*) and late (50+ days *in utero*). Examining anesthesia-induced neuroapoptosis, we found that the commonly used inhalational anesthetic isoflurane, alone or in combination with nitrous oxide and/or midazolam, administered for 4 h, induces severe and widespread apoptotic neurodegeneration in the guinea pig brain.[4] Moreover, when we quantified neuronal densities during the first week of postnatal life, when the brain is fully developed we discovered that most vulnerable brain regions, including the IV cortical layer of the occipital, retrosplenial, parietal, cingulated and piriformis cortices, as well as the amygdaloid nuclei, hippocampus, subiculum, and anterior thalamic nuclei showed significant decreases in neuronal densities as compared to those in both "true" controls (no anesthesia) and sham controls (treated with a continuous infusion of an intravenous narcotic, fentanyl, commonly used in pediatric patients). The overall anesthesia-induced decline in neuronal counts varied from 40%–50% as compared with controls.[4] Because the most prominent caspase-3 activation occurs between 35–40 days of gestational age, while the immature brain of older fetuses (50+ gestational days) were almost completely insensitive, we concluded that the peak of vulnerability coincided with the peak of synaptogenesis. Interestingly, fentanyl, which is commonly used in intensive care settings and, in some cases is infused for many hours, caused an increase in apoptotic damage as compared to the fetuses of mothers that were not anesthetized ("true" controls) although this increase was not significant compared to "true" controls. Furthermore, continuous infusion of fentanyl did not result in a permanent decrease in neuronal densities during later development.[4]

Piglets

Synaptogenesis in piglets lasts approximately 20 weeks[11] and, much like the process in humans, occurs both pre- and postnatally. Like guinea pigs, piglets are much larger than rat pups, which makes it technically feasible to obtain close control and continuous invasive and noninvasive monitoring of physiological parameters.

We used 5-day-old Yorkshire piglets for all experiments (average weight around 1700 g), because synaptogenesis in piglets reaches a plateau during the last 5 weeks of prenatal life and remains at that level during the first 5 weeks of postnatal life.[11] All efforts were made to minimize the number of animals used and their suffering. All experiments were approved by The Animal Use and Care Committee of the University of Virginia Health System and were conducted in accordance with the USA Public Health Service's Policy on Human Care and Use of Laboratory Animals. The animals were randomly designated as "true" control (no anesthesia, no monitoring); sham control (fentanyl given as an intravenous bolus at 30 μg/kg, followed by continuous infusion at 15 μg/kg/h for 4 h); and experimental (1 mg/kg of midazolam injected i.m., followed by 4 h of nitrous oxide at 75-vol% + isoflurane at 0.55-vol% + 24-vol% oxygen). For isoflurane, the minimum alveolar anesthetic concentration (MAC), which prevents purposeful movement in response to supramaximal noxious stimulation in 50% of subjects, is about 2.0-vol% in piglets.[14] Although the MAC for nitrous oxide anesthesia in piglets is not known, those for other mammals are between 104 and 180-vol%.[15,16]

We delivered nitrous oxide (N_2O) and oxygen (GTS, Allentown, PA) to piglets using a calibrated flowmeter. Isoflurane (Abbott Laboratories, Chicago, IL) was administered using an agent-specific vaporizer that delivered a set percentage of anesthetic. Midazolam (Sigma-Aldrich Chemical, St. Louis, MO) was dissolved in 10% dimethyl sulfoxide (DMSO) immediately before administration. For control experiments, 10% DMSO was used as a vehicle. Fentanyl, an intravenous narcotic, was purchased from Abbott Laboratories (Chicago, IL); rocuronium, an intravenous muscle relaxant, was purchased from Baxter Pharmaceutical Solutions, LLC (Bloomington, IN). These agents were delivered using a multichannel infusion pump (Harvard Apparatus, PHD 2000, Holliston, MA).

On the day of the experiment the anesthesia induction of sham and experimental animals was done using isoflurane as needed in ambient air (3 L of flow) delivered via nose cone. Each piglet was placed in the supine position and orotracheally intubated with a polyethylene tube (4 mm internal diameter). Artificial ventilation was immediately initiated with 25% oxygen/nitrogen and isoflurane (as needed while the invasive monitoring lines were placed), using 10–12 mL/kg tidal volume and 20–25 strokes per min delivered via SAR-830 ventilator (CWE, Ardmore, PA). The exhaled gases (e.g., oxygen, carbon dioxide, nitrous oxide, isoflurane) were continuously analyzed using the infrared analyzer (Datex Ultima, Chalfont, St. Giles, UK).

After the induction of general anesthesia, arterial and venous catheters (polyethylene, PE-50) were placed in the right femoral artery for continuous monitoring of blood pressure, heart rate and arterial blood gases, and in the left femoral vein for continuous infusion of intravenous lactate Ringer solution at 4 mL/kg/h. Femoral vascular access was chosen to avoid interference with blood flow to the brain. To facilitate artificial ventilation, piglets were paralyzed using continuous intravenous infusion of a muscle relaxant, rocuronium (15 nmol/kg/min)[17] after the placement of an intravenous line; the administration of rocuronium was discontinued 30 min before termination of the desired anesthesia protocol. After placement of the invasive lines, the animals were allowed 15–20 min to stabilize. The anesthesia protocol was then initiated and the minute ventilation was adjusted to maintain stable physiological parameters, which were continuously monitored for 4 h.

Monitoring of vital functions

The adequacy of ventilation and oxygenation was continuously monitored, first by analyzing the composition, in mmHg, of the exhaled end tidal oxygen (EtO_2 was kept around 22–23 mmHg) and carbon dioxide ($EtCO_2$) collected from the exhalation limb of the anesthesia breathing circuit. We also analyzed the composition of gases in the arterial blood (pH, partial pressure of oxygen, bicarbonate concentration, oxygen saturation, SaO_2 in %) (Nova Biomedical, Inc., Waltham, MA). Arterial blood pressure was continuously monitored using a 23Db blood pressure transducer referred to the mid-thoracic level. This was connected to the cannula inserted into the right femoral artery, which also allowed sampling of the arterial blood as needed. Systolic, diastolic, and mean arterial pressures were obtained using custom software in Pascal computer language and an Intel digital computer. Heart rate was derived from the pressure signal. The animal core temperature was continuously monitored with a rectal temperature probe and maintained using heating pads.

At the termination of an anesthesia protocol, piglets were kept normothermic and inspected continuously for 2 h after anesthesia. As soon as a regular breathing pattern, airway reflexes, and purposeful movements returned, the trachea was extubated. Animals were allowed to feed at will.

Histopathological studies

At 2 h after anesthesia treatment, piglets were deeply anesthetized and perfused with paraformaldehyde

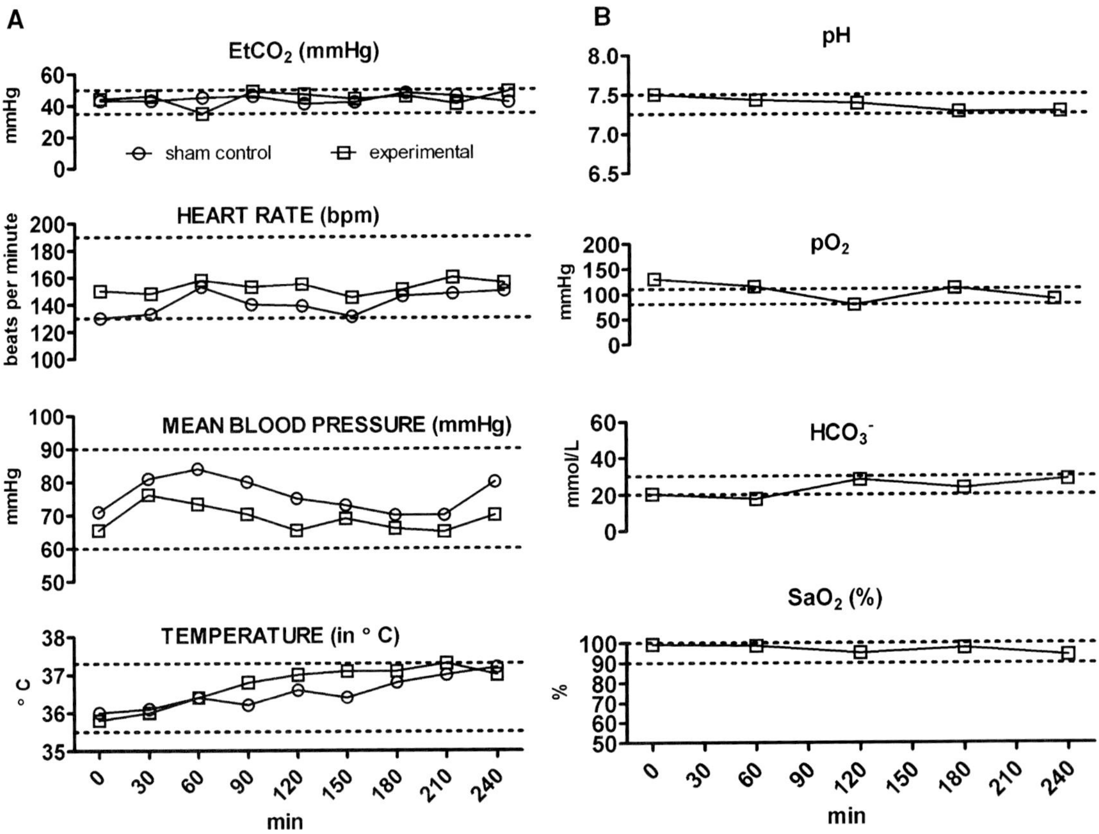

Figure 1. Anesthesia does not cause significant disturbances in vital signs (A), cardiorespiratory, or metabolic parameters (B) in 5-day-old piglets. Vital signs were monitored continuously and recorded every 30 min during anesthesia exposure (A). All measured parameters in experimental piglet (exposed to isoflurane, 0.55-vol%, + N_2O, 75-vol%, + midazolam, 1 mg/kg, i.m.) and sham control piglet (exposed to a continuous fentanyl infusion, 15 μg/kg/h) were within physiologically acceptable ranges (*dashed lines*).[23,24] Arterial blood gas analysis was done every hour during anesthesia exposure (B). All measured parameters in piglets (exposed to isoflurane, 0.55-vol%, + N_2O, 75-vol%, + midazolam, 1 mg/kg, i.m.) were within physiologically acceptable ranges (*dashed lines*).[23]

(4%) in cacodylate buffer (0.1%), pH 7.4, for histopathology studies of apoptosis. Caspase-3 immunochemical staining (ICC) was used because it is an excellent method for marking neurons in an early stage of apoptosis.[3,6,7] Brain tissue was sectioned into 50-μm-thick coronal sections, washed in 0.01 mol/L phosphate-buffered saline (PBS), quenched for 10 min in a solution of methanol containing 3% hydrogen peroxide, then incubated for 1 h in blocking solution (2% BSA/0.2% milk/0.1% triton X-100 in PBS). The tissue was incubated overnight in caspase-specific antibodies, such as rabbit anti-active caspase-3 antiserum, (D175, Cell Signaling Technology, Beverly, MA) diluted 1:1000 in blocking solution. After incubation with D175 primary antibody, sections were incubated for 1 h in secondary antibody (goat anti-rabbit 1:200 in blocking solution), then reacted in the dark with ABC reagents (standard Vectastain ABC Elite Kit, Vector Labs, Burlingame, CA). Sections were preincubated for 10 min in a filtered mixture containing 6 mL of 0.1 mol/L Tris buffer, 2 mg 3,3′-diaminobenzidine (DAB), and 400 mg imidazole, then for 15 min in 6 mL of the same DAB/imidazole/Tris mixture containing 3 μL H_2O_2.

Quantitative histology

To determine the density of caspase-3-positive neurons in a given brain region, we used the optical disector and fractionator method.[18] A counting frame (0.05 × 0.05 mm, disector height, 0.05 mm) and a high numerical aperture objective lens were used to visualize caspase-3-positive neurons. Unbiased sampling of each brain region was achieved by randomly selecting 10–12 viewing fields over which the counting frame was positioned for counting at different focal levels (Stereo Investigator System, MBF Bioscience, Burlington, VT).[3–7] The numerical density of caspase-3-stained neurons in any given region was expressed as the number of cells/mm³.

Statistical analyses

To identify anesthesia-induced pathomorphological changes, we assessed the stereological cell count data using ANOVA models that included a between-subject variable, such as treatment (experimental group, sham, and "true" controls). When ANOVAs with repeated measures were done, the Bonferroni correction or Tukey's test was used to help maintain prescribed alpha levels (e.g., 0.05). The data points are presented as mean ± SEM.

Findings

We used continuous monitoring of cardiovascular and respiratory functions to assure adequate tissue perfusion, as well as oxygenation and ventilation during anesthesia. Vital signs (Fig. 1A) and arterial blood gas values (Fig. 1B) were recorded. Figure 1A

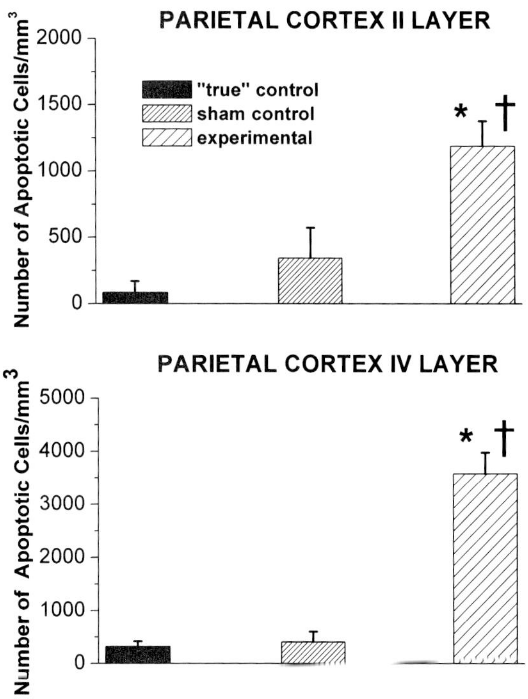

Figure 2. Anesthesia induces significant caspase-3 activation in the developing parietal cortex of 5-day-old piglets. In piglet brains, the sensitivity of the parietal cortices to general anesthesia is quantified as the number of caspase-3-positive cells/mm³ in layers II and IV. The density of caspase-3-positive neurons in "true" control was minimal in parietal cortical regions. In comparison, although a somewhat higher degree of caspase-3 labeling occurred in sham control (exposed to a continuous fentanyl infusion, 15 μg/kg/h), the difference was not statistically significant. The combination of isoflurane (0.55-vol%), N_2O (75 vol-%), and midazolam (1 mg/kg, i.m.) induced a significant increase in caspase-3 labeling as compared to labeling in both "true" and sham controls (*, $P < 0.05$, and †, $P < 0.05$, respectively in layer II; *, $P < 0.001$, and †, $P < 0.001$, respectively in layer IV) ($n = 1$ piglet per condition, $n = 5$ sections per brain region).

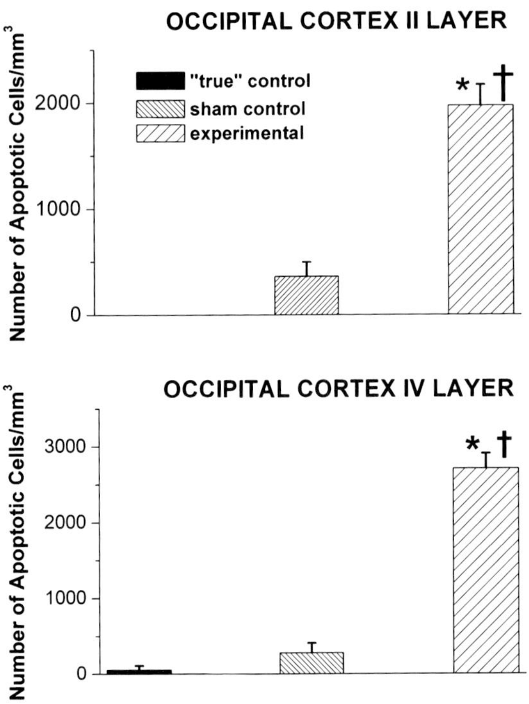

Figure 3. Anesthesia induces significant caspase-3 activation in the developing occipital cortex of 5-day-old piglets. The sensitivity of occipital cortices in piglet brains to general anesthesia is quantified as the number of caspase-3-positive cells/mm³ in layers II and IV. The density of caspase-3-positive neurons in "true" control was minimal in the parietal cortical regions. Although a somewhat higher degree of labeling occurred in sham control (exposed to continuous fentanyl infusion, 15 μg/kg/h), the difference from labeling in "true" control was not statistically significant. The combination of isoflurane (0.55-vol%), N_2O (75 vol-%), and midazolam (1 mg/kg, i.m.) caused a significant increase in caspase-3 labeling as compared to that in "true" and sham controls (*, $P < 0.001$, and †, $P < 0.001$, respectively) ($n = 1$ piglet per condition, $n = 4$–5 sections per brain region).

illustrates the results obtained from the experimental animal which, for anesthesia, was given a combination of midazolam, N_2O, and isoflurane, and sham control group which received a continuous infusion of fentanyl. Figure 1B illustrates the results obtained from the experimental animal only since this was the most toxic anesthesia regimen. All measured physiological parameters were within physiological ranges for piglets (indicated with dashed lines in each graph).

To determine the regional distribution and severity of anesthesia-induced neuroapoptosis caused by fentanyl and the anesthesia cocktail used, we have examined piglet brain regions stained with caspase-3 (Figs. 2–4). The developing parietal (Fig. 2) and occipital (Fig. 3) cortices (in particular, the II and IV cortical layers) were the most sensitive to anesthesia-induced damage. Even though the density of caspase-3-positive neurons in "true" control varied between the parietal and occipital cortices, the number of neurons undergoing apoptosis was small. A somewhat higher degree of apoptosis was detected in sham control (fentanyl-treated)[19] than in "true" control, although the difference was not statistically significant. The combination of three anesthetics (isoflurane, midazolam, and nitrous oxide) induced a statistically significant (on average 10- to 20-fold) increase in neuroapoptosis in both cortical regions—parietal and occipital—as compared to that in "true" controls (*, $P < 0.001$ except for parietal cortex-layer II where $P < 0.05$). Again in both cortical regions, this combination also induced a statistically significant (on average 5- to 7-fold) increase in neuroapoptosis as compared to

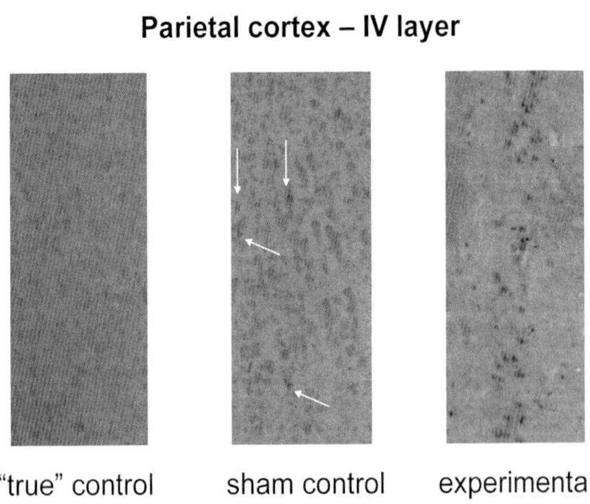

Figure 4. Anesthesia-induced caspase-3 activation in the IV layer of parietal cortex. Exposure of 5-day-old piglet to the triple anesthesia combination (isoflurane, 0.55-vol% + N_2O, 75-vol% + midazolam, 1 mg/kg, i.m.) caused significant caspase-3 activation. Only minimal caspase-3 labeling is shown in sham control (magnification, approximately 100x).

that in sham control (†, $P < 0.001$ except for parietal cortex-layer II where $P < 0.05$).

Figure 4 shows caspase-3 staining of the IV cortical layer of a parietal cortex not exposed to anesthesia (*left panel*, "true" control), one exposed to fentanyl anesthesia (*middle panel*, sham control), and one exposed to the triple anesthesia combination (*right panel*, experimental). In these scenes there was no caspase-3 labeling in "true" controls and minimal labeling in sham controls (marked with white arrows). However, substantial caspase-3 activation was seen in the experimental cortex.

Our piglet experiments indicate that isoflurane, a commonly used general anesthetic, administered in combination with nitrous oxide and midazolam, induces significant apoptotic neurodegeneration in the developing parietal and occipital cortices, specifically targeting the II and IV cortical layers. Although fentanyl, an intravenous narcotic, did not cause a significant increase in apoptotic damage in vulnerable brain regions, the observed caspase-3 activation was at least doubled compared to the amount in "true" control.

Although piglets have a brain-growth spurt that is twice as long as that in guinea pigs and 10 times longer than that in rats, piglets appear to be just as vulnerable as these species to anesthesia-induced developmental neuroapoptosis when exposed to only 4 hrs of general anesthesia.

Primates

Synaptogenesis in primates lasts for about 2 years and, as in humans, occurs both pre- and postnatally.[11] Therefore, primates, especially rhesus monkeys, in which brain development closely mimics that in humans, are good animal models for examining anesthesia-induced developmental neuroapoptosis. For the last several years, Slikker and colleagues[8] have been studying the neurotoxic effects of ketamine, an intravenous general anesthetic commonly used in the pediatric population. They have found that the developing brain of rhesus monkeys is highly sensitive to ketamine anesthesia administered during an early stage of synaptogenesis. For example, a continuous ketamine infusion that is required to achieve and maintain a surgical plane of anesthesia for 24 h causes in both the fetal rhesus brain cortex (122 days of gestation) and neonatal rhesus brain cortex (5 postnatal days) a significant increase in the number of caspase-3, Fluoro-Jade C, and silver-stain-positive cells when examined 6 h after the cessation of ketamine infusion.[8] Interestingly, like rodent and guinea pig brains, the rhesus brain at 35 postnatal days was insensitive to the same anesthesia treatment.[8]

Discussion

The timing, rather than the duration of anesthesia, determines the vulnerability of the developing brain to anesthesia-induced neuroapoptosis

Collectively, the animal studies published so far have confirmed that the duration of synaptogenesis is not a fundamental determinant of the severity of anesthesia-induced neuronal damage. This is true regardless of the duration of anesthesia exposure. For instance, anesthesia of fairly short duration, such as 4 h in guinea pigs or piglets and 24 h in primates, relative to the 10 and 20 weeks of synaptogenesis, respectively, in guinea pigs and piglets and the 2 years in primates, promotes significant activation of the apoptotic machinery in developing neurons.[5,8] Even in rats, despite the fact that histopathological signs of apoptosis could be captured after 6 h of anesthesia, the warning signs of activation of the apoptotic pathways (especially the intrinsic one) could be detected as early as within the first couple of hours of general anesthesia.[6] This indicates that, although the final stages of neuronal demise may take some time to evolve, the commitment to neuronal suicide occurs early during general anesthesia.

Guinea pig, piglet, and primate studies clearly confirm that, despite the maintenance of homeostasis and tight control of all vital parameters, significant neuronal apoptosis occurs in the immature brain. This suggests that general anesthetics rather than cardiovascular and respiratory abnormalities, such as hypoxia, hypercarbia, metabolic or respiratory acidosis, hypotension, or hypoglycemia, are the main culprit.[4,8]

The use of animal species in which brain development follows different schedules (e.g., pre- versus postnatal versus both pre- and postnatal) has enabled us to address the question of whether vulnerability to anesthesia neurotoxicity depends on when synaptogenesis occurs. The answer is that regardless of whether the peak of synaptogenesis occurs *in utero* or postnatally, the immature brain is at risk. Rodents, in which brain development occurs almost completely postnatally, were just as susceptible[1–3,5–7] as were guinea pigs,[4] in which brain development almost completely occurs postnatally, and just as susceptible as were piglets and primates,[8] in which brain development occurs both before and after birth.

So what seems to matter most when it comes to the vulnerability of the developing brain to anesthesia toxicity? Based on currently available data, the most important determinant appears to be the timing of the exposure to anesthesia relative to the time point in synaptogenesis. Specifically, brain regions that are at the peak of synaptogenesis are most vulnerable.[1,2,4,6,8] In all of the mammalian species studied, these are the brain regions that are most severely damaged, regardless of the duration or type of general anesthesia. The precise timing of regional brain development and the exact peak of synaptogenesis for each brain region has not been well established. Nevertheless, it is reasonable to propose that the region-specific vulnerability to general anesthesia demonstrated in the presently available studies is a consequence of the fact that these regions, at the time of anesthesia exposure, are at the peak of synaptogenesis. For example, when rat anterior thalamic nuclei and cerebral cortex are exposed at 7 days of age, they happen to be extremely susceptible[1,2,6]; when a piglet's thalamus is exposed at 5 days of age, it is not as sensitive (data not shown), but the cerebral cortex is very vulnerable. Although it was not conceived for that purpose, examination of anesthesia-induced neurodegenerative patterns during brain development could serve as a mapping tool to decipher the specific times when each brain region in different species is at the peak of synaptogenesis.

In conclusion, general anesthesia causes severe neurodegeneration in the mammalian developing brain. The main determinant of the severity of that neurodegeneration appears to be the timing, rather than the duration of the anesthesia exposure; brain regions are most sensitive at the peak of their synaptogenesis. This suggests that general anesthetics cause severe disturbance of the key elements of synaptogenesis by modulating the fine neurotransmitter balance and highly programmed neuronal communication[20] at the time when this communication is most vital for the survival and proper functioning of immature neurons. Indeed, anesthesia-induced activation of apoptotic neurodegeneration can lead to permanent harm, manifested as significant neuronal loss in susceptible brain regions[4,21] and behavioral impairments (e.g., cognitive deficits) later in life.[3,22]

Acknowledgments

This study was supported by the NIH/NICHD HD 44517 (to V.J-T.) and Harold Carron endowment (to V.J-T.). V.J-T. is an Established Investigator of the American Heart Association. The authors wish to thank Lisa Carter for technical assistance.

Conflicts of interest

The authors declare no conflicts of interest.

References

1. Ikonomidou, C., F. Bosch, M. Miksa, *et al.* 1999. Blockade of NMDA receptors and apoptotic neurodegeneration in the developing brain. *Science* **283:** 70–74.
2. Ikonomidou, C., P. Bittigau, M.J. Ishimaru, *et al.* 2000. Ethanol-induced apoptotic neurodegeneration and fetal alcohol syndrome. *Science* **287:** 1056–1060.
3. Jevtovic-Todorovic, V., R.E. Hartman, Y. Izumi, *et al.* 2003. Early exposure to common anesthetic agents causes widespread neurodegeneration in the developing rat brain and persistent learning deficits. *J. Neurosci.* **23:** 876–882.
4. Rizzi, S., L.B. Carter, C. Ori, *et al.* 2008. Clinical anesthesia causes permanent damage to the fetal guinea pig brain. *Brain Pathol.* **18:** 198–210.
5. Lu, L.X., J.H. Yon, L.B. Carter, *et al.* 2006. General anesthesia activates BDNF-dependent neuroapoptosis in the developing rat brain. *Apoptosis* **11:** 1603–1615.
6. Yon, J-H., J. Daniel-Johnson, L.B. Carter, *et al.* 2005. Anesthesia induces neuronal cell death in the developing rat brain via the intrinsic and extrinsic apoptotic pathways. *Neuroscience* **35:** 815–827.
7. Yon, J-H., L.B. Carter, R.J. Reiter, *et al.* 2006. Melatonin reduces the severity of anesthesia-induced apoptotic neurodegeneration in the developing rat brain. *Neurobiol. Dis.* **21:** 522–530.
8. Slikker, W., Jr., X. Zou, C.E. Hotchkiss, *et al.* 2007. Ketamine-induced neuronal cell death in the perinatal rhesus monkey. *Toxicol. Sci.* **98:** 145–158.
9. Yuan, J. & B.A. Yankner. 2000. Apoptosis in the nervous system. *Nature* **407:** 802–808.

10. Young, C., V. Jevtovic-Todorovic, Y.Q. Qin, *et al.* 2005. Potential of ketamine and midazolam, individually or in combination, to induce apoptotic neurodegeneration in the infant mouse brain. *Brit. J.Pharmacol.* **146:** 189–197.
11. Dobbing, J. & J. Sands. 1979. Comparative aspects of the brain growth spurt. *Early Hum. Dev.* **3:** 79–83.
12. Jones, D.G., M.M. Dittmer & L.C. Reading. 1974. Synaptogenesis in guinea-pig cerebral cortex: a glutaraldehyde-PTA study. *Brain Res.* **70:** 245–259.
13. Lennon, A.M., J. Francon, A. Fellous, *et al.* 1980. Rat, mouse, and guinea pig brain development and microtubule assembly. *J. Neurochem.* **35:** 804–813.
14. Satas, S., K. Haaland, M. Thoresen, *et al.* 1996. MAC for halothane and isoflurane during normothermia and hypothermia in the newborn piglet. *Acta Anaesthesiol. Scand.* **40:** 452–456.
15. Hornbein, T.F., E.I. Eger II, P.M. Winter, *et al.* 1982. The minimum alveolar concentration of nitrous oxide in man. *Anest. Analg.* **61:** 553–556.
16. Mahmoudi, N.W., D.J. Cole, H.M. Shapiro. 1989. Insufficient anesthetic potency of nitrous oxide in the rat. *Anesthesiology* **70:** 345–349.
17. Epemolu, O., A. Bom, F. Hope, *et al.* 2003. Reversal of neuromuscular blockade and simultaneous increase in plasma rocuronium concentration after the intravenous infusion of the novel reversal agent Org 25969. *Anesthesiology* **99:** 632–637.
18. West, M.J. 1999. Stereological methods for estimating the total number of neurons and synapses: issues of precision and bias. *TINS* **22:** 51–61.
19. Rajan, V., K.D.A. Beharry, P. Williams, *et al.* 1998. Pharmacodynamic effects and pharmacokinetic profile of continuous infusion fentanyl in newborn piglets. *Biol. Neonate* **74:** 39–47.
20. Lunardi, N., P. Joksovic, S.M. Todorovic, *et al.* 2008. General anesthetics cause structural and functional perturbations of the developing synapses in rat brain. Soc. Neurosci. Abst. Program 10.13.
21. Nikizad, H., J-H. Yon, L.B. Carter, *et al.* 2007. Early exposure to general anesthesia causes significant neuronal deletion in the developing rat brain. *Ann. N.Y. Acad. Sci.* **1122:** 69–82.
22. Fredriksson, A., T. Archer, H. Alm, *et al.* 2004. Neurofunctional deficits and potentiated apoptosis by neonatal NMDA antagonist administration. *Behav. Brain Res.* **153:** 367–376.
23. Chandler, C.J., B.Y. Ong & D.S. Sitar. 1989. Kinetic disposition of ethanol in the neonatal piglet and hemodynamic effects in the presence and absence of 4-methylpyrazole. *Toxicol. Appl. Pharmacol.* **99:** 185–192.
24. Chandler, C.J., B.Y. Ong & D.S. Sitar. 1990. Haemodynamic alterations in anaesthetized and acutely intoxicated newborn piglets. *Br. J. Pharmacol.* **101:** 227–231.

Ann. N.Y. Acad. Sci. ISSN 0077-8923

ANNALS OF THE NEW YORK ACADEMY OF SCIENCES
Issue: *Neuroprotective Agents*

Neuroprotective strategies in drug abuse-evoked encephalopathy

Ashraf Virmani,[1,2] Syed F. Ali,[3] and Zbigniew K. Binienda[4]

[1]Scientific & Medical Affairs, Sigma tau, Pomezia 00040, Italy. [2]European Mind & Metabolism Association (EMMA), London, UK and Rome, Italy. [3]Neurochemistry Laboratory and [4]Neurophysiology Laboratory, Division of Neurotoxicology, National Center for Toxicological Research, Food and Drug Administration, Jefferson, Arkansas

Address for correspondence: Prof. Ashraf Virmani, Sigma-tau, Via Pontina km 30,400, 00040 Pomezia (Roma) Italy. ashraf.virmani@sigma-tau.it

Encephalopathy is evidenced as an altered mental state with various neurological symptoms, such as memory and cognitive problems. The type of a substance-evoked encephalopathy will depend on the drug, substance, or combination being abused. The categories into which we could place the various abused substances could be tentatively divided into stimulants, amphetamines, hallucinogens, narcotics, inhalants, anesthetics, anabolic steroids, and antipsychotics/antidepressants. Other factors that may underlie encephalopathy, such as infectious agents, environmental, and other factors have also to be taken into account. Drugs of abuse can be highly toxic to the CNS following acute, but more so in chronic exposure, and can produce significant damage to other organs, such as the heart, lungs, liver, and kidneys. The damage to these organs may be at least partially reversible when drug abuse is stopped but CNS damage from repeated or prolonged abuse is often irreversible. The major pathways for the organ and CNS toxicity could be related to ischemic events as well as increased cell damage due to metabolic or mitochondrial dysfunction resulting in increased excitotoxicity, reduced energy production, and lowered antioxidant potential. These susceptibilities could be strengthened by the use of antioxidants to combat free radicals (e.g., vitamin E, lipoic acid); trying to improve energy generation by using mitochondriotropic/metabolic compounds (e.g., thiamine, coenzyme Q10, carnitine, riboflavin); by reducing excitotoxicity (e.g., glutamate antagonists) and other possible strategies, such as robust gene response, need to be investigated further. The drug-abuse-evoked encephalopathy still needs to be studied further to enable better preventative and protective strategies.

Keywords: leucoencephalopathy; nutrition; neurotoxicity; drug-abuse; cocaine; methamphetamine; alcohol; amphetamines

Introduction

Encephalopathy is usually evident as an altered mental state. Depending on the type and severity of encephalopathy, common neurological symptoms are progressive loss of memory and cognitive ability, subtle personality changes, inability to concentrate, lethargy, and progressive loss of consciousness.

The type of a substance-evoked encephalopathy will depend on the drug, substance, or combination being abused. In addition to the drug abuse, other factors, such as underlying pathologies, environmental, and nutritional factors or interactions with "legal" drugs, also have to be taken into account.

Neuroprotective strategies have to take this vulnerability into account both pre- and postnatally. Further, many cell types in the brain have different time and varying levels of sensitivity to damage. Drugs of abuse can be highly toxic to the CNS following acute, but more so in chronic exposure, and can produce significant damage to other organs, such as the heart, lungs, liver, and kidneys. The damage to these organs may be at least partially reversible when drug abuse is stopped but CNS damage from repeated or prolonged abuse is often irreversible. The spectrum of drug-induced neurotoxicity is constantly changing with the change in drug use culture, route and form of administration, changes in concentration, and types of impurities

doi: 10.1111/j.1749-6632.2009.05171.x

Table 1. Common risk factors affecting neuronal health

- Environmental toxins (PCB, dioxan, estrogens, 3-NPA, rotenone), alcohol, drugs
- Infectious disease (prions, virus, bacteria)
- Traumatic events (pregnancy complication, head injury)
- Brain tumor or increased intracranial pressure
- Brain ischemia
- Age (decreased anabolic hormone, state of health or disease)
- Nutritional deficiencies and intolerances
- Genetic vulnerability
- Poverty

and sources (transgenic plants or synthetic process of manufacturing) of the drug.

The pharmacological classification of drugs is most commonly based upon its effects on the CNS but also according to its legal status, depending in most cases upon its addiction potential. However, the abuse of drugs is not just limited to the illicit drugs, but also includes drugs obtained by legal prescription and even compounds available over-the-counter. The U.N.-affiliated International Narcotics Control Board (INCB Annual Report 2006) has reported that the abuse of prescription drugs has already outstripped traditional illegal drugs such as heroin, cocaine, and 3,4-methylenedioxymethamphetamine (Ecstasy, MDMA) in parts of Europe, Africa, and South Asia. The abuse of these legal drugs is done by using them in a manner and in quantities other than directed. In addition to their proper medicinal use, psychoactive drugs and stimulants are particularly subject to this type of abuse (Table 1). The most commonly abused psychoactive drugs are cocaine, amphetamines (methamphetamine; METH), MDMA and some inhalants, such as amyl or butyl nitrites. They are referred to by the slang term "uppers" and most used recreationally. Stimulants with significant mood-altering effects are usually strictly controlled and may be legally available only by prescription, such as amphetamine (Adderall), methylphenidate (Ritalin, Concerta), and METH (Desoxyn), or not at all in the case of MDMA. Therapeutically, amphetamine, methylphenidate, and METH are used in the treatment of attention deficit hyperactivity disorder (ADHD), narcolepsy, and life threatening obesity.[1]

Drug abuse is associated with significant health risks and it may also provoke encephalopathy. The possibility of triggering encephalopathy in an individual abusing illicit or legal chemical substance will depend on the level and type of substance being abused, the unique toxicity profile of that particular drug/substance or co-abuse of drugs, and the overall risk factor profile of that individual (both psychological and genetical).

Drug abuse in combination with other risk factors (e.g., nutritional deficiency, environmental toxins) may increase the potential for encephalopathy resulting from drug abuse (Table 2). Part of this risk profile will depend on the subject's physical and mental state, as well as his/her unique genetic susceptibility profile.

Further, as mentioned before, the drug-induced neurotoxicity will depend on abused drug amount, form, and level of impurities it contains. The major pathways for the organ and CNS toxicity could be related to increased risk of cell damage that would involve genetic, metabolic, or mitochondrial dysfunction resulting in increased excitotoxicity, reduced energy production, and lowered antioxidant potential (Fig. 1). These points of weakness can be strengthened by use of antioxidants to combat free radicals (e.g., vitamin E, lipoic acid); trying to improve energy generation by using mitochondriotropic/metabolic compounds (e.g., thiamine, coenzyme Q10, carnitine, riboflavin); by reducing excitotoxicity (e.g., glutamate antagonists); and other possible strategies.[2–5] However, drug-abuse-evoked encephalopathy still needs to be studied further to enable better preventative and protective strategies. The strategies presently available, in particular the nutritional approach, to protect drug-abusers from the metabolic syndrome and other diseases are discussed below.

Drug abuse and encephalopathy

Encephalopathy presents as an altered mental state with common neurological symptoms as mentioned above. Other neurological symptoms may include myoclonus, nystagmus, tremor, muscle atrophy and weakness, dementia, seizures, and loss of ability to swallow or speak.

Table 2. Commonly abused psychoactive drugs (modified from ref 5. Virmani *et al.*, 2007) ketamine* and PCP (phencyclidine)*

Drug category	Example
Stimulants	Cocaine
	Phenmetrazine (Preludin)
	Methcathinone
Amphetamines	Amphetamine
	Methamphetamine
	MDMA (Ecstasy, 3,4-Methylenedioxy-n-methylamphetamine)
	MDA (3,4-Methylenedioxy-amphetamine)
	Methylphenidate (Ritalin)
	Dextroamphetamine (Dexedrine)
	Phentermine (Duromine)
	Fenfluramine (Ponderax)
Hallucinogens	Lysergic acid diethylamide (LSD)
	Psilocybin
	Peyote (Mescaline)
	Igobaine
	Ketamine*
	PCP (Phencyclidine)*
	Bufotenin
Narcotics	Opium
	Morphine
	Heroin
	Codeine
	Hydromorphone
	Oxycodone (OxyContin)
	Hydrocodone (Vicodin)
	Meperidine (Demerol)
	Methadone
Inhalants	Butane
	Toulene
	Butyl nitrite
	Amyl nitrite
Anesthetic	Ketamine
	Gamma hydroxybutrate (GHB)
	PCP (phencyclidine)
	Nitrous oxide
Anabolic steroids	Methandrostenolone (Dianabol)
	Nandrolone (Deca-Durabolin)
Antipsychotics/antidepressants	Quetiapine
	Bupropion
Depressants	Barbiturates/benzodiazepines
	Methaqualone (Mandrax)
	Flunitrazepam (Rohypnol)
	Glutethimide
	Chloral hydrate (Equithesin)

*Hallucinogens as well as anesthetic use.

The type of substance-evoked encephalopathy will depend on the drug, substance, or combination being abused. Other factors that may underlie encephalopathy, such as infectious agent (bacteria, virus, or prion), environmental agents, brain tumor, or increased intracranial pressure, prolonged exposure to toxic elements (solvents, alcohol, smoke, radiation, paints, industrial chemicals, heavy metals), chronic progressive trauma, poor nutrition, or lack of oxygen or blood flow to the brain, in addition to "legal" drugs also have to be taken into account.[6]

Critical windows of CNS vulnerability to these agents occur both pre- and postnatally. The many cell types in the brain have different times and varying levels of sensitivity to damage.

Drugs of abuse can be highly toxic to the CNS following acute, but more so in chronic exposure, and can produce significant damage to other organs, such as the heart, lungs, liver, and kidneys. The damage to these organs may be at least partially reversible when drug abuse is stopped but CNS damage from repeated or prolonged abuse is often irreversible.

Further the drug abuse is known to affect the nutritional status by adversely affecting both the mind and the body. The role of drug abuse as a risk factor in provoking the disease pathogenesis known as the metabolic syndrome is still not well studied. Thus drug abuse is generally associated with significantly higher health risks.[3,4] Although amphetamines are popular and considered safe by abusers, a variety of adverse effects have been associated with their use, such as the serotonin syndrome, hepatotoxicity, neurotoxicity, and psychopathology.[7] Treatment with antipsychotics has been associated with increased risk of developing diabetes and ketoacidosis.[8–10] The role of drug abuse in disease pathogenesis is well studied for alcohol abuse[11] but not for other drugs of abuse. Further research is needed in this field. The increased health risk due to drug abuse could be related to increased susceptibility to organ damage, for example, alcohol abuse is associated with liver injury. The drug abuse in combination with other risk factors, such as nutritional deficiency, may increase cell damage by triggering neurotoxicity processes within the cells.[3,12,13]

Categories of abused substances

Substances often abused include nicotine (tobacco), caffeine (coffee, tea, cola), and ephedrine (in anti-allergy mixtures) (See Table 1). The categories

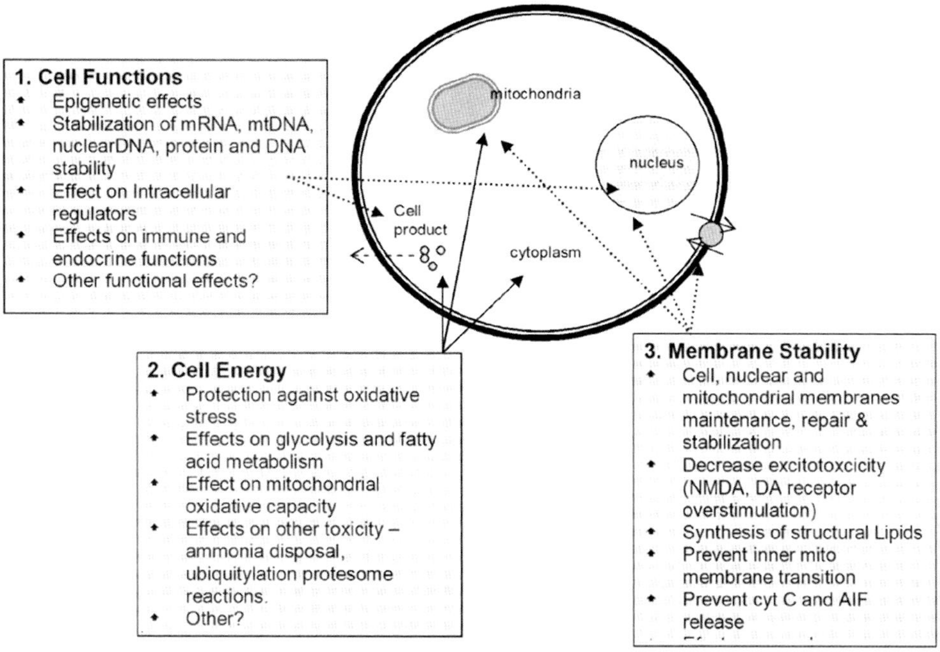

Figure 1. Some neuroprotective targets in the cell.

into which we could place the various abused substances could be tentatively divided into stimulants, amphetamines, hallucinogens, narcotics, inhalants, anesthetics, anabolic steroids, and antipsychotics/antidepressants.

However, there are certain compounds that do not fall into these categories, such as the depressant which can still be used as drugs of abuse. Thus, certain depressant drugs may inhibit certain functions of the CNS but their effects may manifest as euphoria, relaxation, and disinhibition. This is also true for the other drug abuse categories (cannabinoid, hallucinogens, narcotic, alcohol, inhalants, anesthetic, anabolic steroids, and antipsychotics) these may not necessarily make a person feel depressed or tranquilized but may lead to hyperexcitation and euphoria. This is the case for alcohol, barbiturates (Seconal, Tuinal, and Amytal), benzodiazepines (Rohypnol), cannabis, gamma-hydroxybutrate (GHB), opiates (heroin, morphine, codeine, methadone, and pethidine), as well as some solvents and inhalants.

Another factor in categorizing the substances of drug abuse is that the biological and psychological outcome is difficult to predict because how a particular drug will affect a particular subject will vary greatly, depending on the physical and psychological state of the abuser. In the case of hallucinogens, it is not only an abuser's perception that is distorted, but there are physiological drug effects on the body leading to dilation of pupils, loss of appetite, increased activity, excessive talking or laughing, a sense of emotional and psychological euphoria and well-being, jaw clenching, sweating, panic, paranoia, loss of contact with reality, irrational or bizarre behavior, stomach cramps, and nausea.

Factors underlying encephalopathy

As mentioned above, several factors probably play a role in the pathogenesis of encephalopathy due to drug abuse:

- Direct toxic action of the drug and its metabolites
- Toxic action of contaminants found with the drugs/substances being abused
- Indirect toxicity due to damage of other organs (e.g., liver, kidney, lungs, heart)
- Malnutrition
- Anoxia, ischemia, vasculitis due to cardiovascular damage or increased seizures
- Genetic susceptibility

The exact role of drugs in the pathogenesis of encephalopathy is not clear but each compound has its own specific toxicity profile that can either affect the brain directly or indirectly via damaging effects on other body systems, especially hepatic, renal, gastrointestinal, and cardiovascular.

Drug abuse is associated with significant health risk, for example, cardiac (angina pectoris, myocardial infarction, and sudden cardiac death) and cerebrovascular pathology is higher among cocaine users.[14,15]

In combination with the psychopathological effects of drugs, potential negative drug-drug interaction, the risk of nutritional imbalances and higher rates of diabetic complications, there is also a higher risk of the metabolic syndrome.[3,4]

Genetic susceptibility

Another factor that is beginning to be recognized by advances in genomics research is the role genetic susceptibility plays in the development of the encephalopathy. An individual's genetic patrimony, which includes ethnicity and gender, might also influence susceptibility to the stimulant-abuse-evoked increase in risk of encephalopathy. Because the stimulant efficacy, as well its potential toxicity, depend on the cellular metabolism and machinery, any genetic polymorphism may have a positive or negative influence depending on how metabolism/excretion/action of the stimulant is affected by single or multiple genes or by changes in gene expression.[16] The damage, as well as the severity of liver damage, following alcohol abuse is linked to a specific gene profile.[17] This is probably true also for stimulant-evoked damage. Despite the above indications and the cellular toxicity risk associated with stimulate abuse, more studies are needed in this area to establish a definite link of genetic susceptibility and drug abuse with encephalopathy.

Each drug of abuse has a unique toxicity profile

Encephalopathy resulting from drug abuse depends on the activity profile of each compound or combination of compounds in many cases in which the subject abuses more than one type of drug. The stimulants may mask some of the effects of depressant drugs, such as alcohol, benzodiazepines, and barbiturates. On their own, the effects of stimulants manifest as increased wakefulness, increased physical activity, decreased appetite, increased respiration, high fever, euphoria, irritability, insomnia, confusion, tremors, convulsions, anxiety, paranoia, and aggressiveness. These collateral effects, especially seizures, may in themselves lead to brain damage. Thus, high fever and convulsions may prove to be fatal per se and long-term abuse of stimulants may result in permanent brain damage.[18]

The region of brain affected will often depend on specific distribution of the drug, that is, certain inhalants, cocaine, and amphetamines concentrate in specific areas of the brain associated with the reward and pleasure.[19] Some problems with drugs are caused by the fact that users mix drugs which have different effects and may combine to increase the relative health risk. The same is true for the drug metabolites and other toxic contaminants that may be present with the abused drug.

Drug abuse is associated with a variety of neurological complications. The use of certain recreational drugs shows a marked temporal association with the onset of both hemorrhagic and ischemic strokes.[20] Delayed onset of stroke has also been observed.[21]

These risk factors, in combination with malnutrition, can affect cellular expression, intermediary metabolism, and inflammation, and therefore directly and indirectly influence susceptibility. Thus, the encephalopathies resulting are typical of region affected and toxicity profile of the stimulant drug abused.

Direct toxic actions of abused drugs

Research in animal experiments, as well as on various neuronal cell types in culture, suggests that most drugs of abuse, such as stimulants like cocaine and amphetamines, have direct toxic action upon the CNS. In the case of the stimulants, at least part of their toxicity has been linked to the increase in extracellular levels of catecholamines, especially dopamine. It is the release of dopamine (DA) and formation of its metabolites that is thought to cause the augmentation of reactive oxygen species (ROS). In a recent *in vitro* model, METH toxicity in a clonal DA producing cell line (CATHa) was shown to involve DA, because DA release and DA synthesis inhibitors both attenuated METH toxicity.[22,23] There is evidence that brain injury observed after amphetamine and METH administration is provoked by an increase in free radical formation and mitochondrial damage, which leads to a failure of cellular energy metabolism followed by a secondary excitotoxicity as discussed further below.[24–28] The other possibility is that METH may initially cause mitochondrial dysfunction that later leads to excessive DA release. Attenuation of this type of stimulant-evoked excitotoxicity by various agents, for example, anti-convulsant, mitochondriotropic, antioxidant and anti-inflammatory agents may play a role in the future prevention and treatment of stimulant-evoked encephalopathy.

Cocaine abuse and encephalopathy

The chemical substance, benzoylmethylecgonine, is also referred to as cocaine (crack, freebase rocks, rock) is derived from the leaves of *Erythroxylon coca*. It is highly addictive and gives a feeling of exhilaration and euphoria when sniffed, smoked, or injected. Its use during pregnancy could cause birth defects as well as mental development problems.

Cocaine has a range of toxicities affecting not only the CNS but also various other body systems.[29] In general, death and even toxicity is not always related to the dosage or blood levels, although most deaths occur after prolonged drug use possibly due to accumulation of toxic metabolites and damaging actions.[30] Cocaine ranks first in total encounters, major medical complications, and drug-related deaths.[31]

Cocaine is fat soluble and freely crosses the blood-brain barrier and has sympathomimetic actions on the limbic system. In the CNS, the primary neurotoxic action of cocaine may manifest as encephalopathy and the secondary actions include compromised blood flow (stroke, ischemia), cerebral vasculitis, and vasospasm.[32,33] Neurological complications include seizure, intracerebral hemorrhage, and brain injury due to hyperthermia and/or seizures, and headache. Rupture of aneurysms and arteriovenous malformations have been detected in up to half of the patients with hemorrhagic stroke due to cocaine abuse. Cocaine abuse may also trigger cerebral inflammatory vascular changes leading to encephalopathy.[34] Encephalopathy related to cocaine induced hypertension has also been described.[35] Cocaine-induced seizures are a severe manifestation of toxicity unlike the withdrawal-evoked seizures of alcohol abuse. Movement disorders and cerebral atrophy correlating with the duration of abuse have been described. These alterations in nigrostriatal dopamine function are thought to cause the extrapyramidal motor dysfunction, including dystonic reactions, bradykinesia, akinesia, akathisia, pseudoparkinsonism, and catalepsy.[36]

Cocaine induced toxic encephalopathy presents with neurobehavioral and MRI changes. Cocaine has been shown to cause irreversible changes in the cerebral white matter.[37,38] Toxic leucoencephalopathy has been described for both intravenous and inhalative abuse of cocaine. Even asymptomatic cocaine abusers have been found to have significant white matter lesions on MRI.

The underlying mechanism of cocaine neurotoxicity is not clear but is thought to be related to increased ischemic insults and changes in brain metabolism. This is shown by *in vivo* magnetic resonance studies in which cocaine dependence is associated with T2 signal hyperintensities and metabolite abnormalities in cerebral white matter.

There are records of perfusion defects in nearly 70% of cocaine abusers which tend to persist up to 6 months despite abstinence.[39]

In animal models, chronic exposure to cocaine also induces structural and functional changes in the nucleus accumbens that are presumably mediated by altered gene expression, that is, decreased myelin-related transcripts and decreased myelin basic protein (MBP).[40]

Cocaine-evoked metabolic compromise and damage is probably also affected by its combination with other drugs/stimulants. Toxic encephalopathy induced by cocaine, especially in simultaneous intoxication with amphetamine, morphine, and heroine is associated with an increase in lactate as well as changes in N-acetylaspartate/creatine ratios (NAA/Cr),[33,37,41,42] suggesting conversion of aerobic metabolism to anaerobic energy production, but whether this is due to mitochondrial impairment secondary to hypoxia, due to macrophage invasion, or due to direct consequence of cocaine-induced neuroaxonal toxicity remains unknown.[33,43]

The effects of cocaine can be augmented with concomitant alcohol use because concomitant use of alcohol and cocaine results in the *in vivo* formation of ethylbenzoylecgonine (cocaethylene) with far greater toxicity than cocaine.

Treatment strategies against cocaine neurotoxicity are not yet well defined but may be amenable to neuroprotection.[44,45] A strategy whereby the cocaine related risk factors, such as metabolic dysfunction with reduced energy and increased ROS and inflammation, may be tackled, should be implemented.[3,28] For example, the antioxidant compound selenium has been shown to protect against cocaine-induced myocardial oxidative stress.[46] Animal experiments also suggest cocaine-induced hepatotoxic neurobehavioral and biochemical changes can be ameliorated by the mixed opioid agonist-antagonist buprenorphine.[47,48] Protection against cocaine and combined cocaine-ethanol toxicities by a partial inverse agonist of benzodiazepine receptors Ro 15-4513 has also been shown in mice.[49,80] Other strategies such as liver detoxification and prevention of renal failure have also been proposed.[50,51]

Amphetamines abuse and encephalopathy

In terms of drug categories, the drugs classified as amphetamines are amphetamine (Adderal), methamphetamine (Desoxyn, speed, crystal), 3,4-methylenedioxyamphetamine (MDA), 3,4-methylenedioxymethamphetamine (MDMA, Ecstasy) as well as methylphenidate (Ritalin), phentermine (Duromine), and fenfluramine (Ponderax) (Table 1). Amphetamines are widely abused, addictive, legally and illegally available drugs. Amphetamines are usually taken by mouth but can be snorted, smoked, or injected. These stimulants generally increase alertness, attention, and enhance physical performance. Symptoms opposite to the drug's effects occur when an amphetamine is suddenly discontinued. The stimulant action of amphetamines is linked to their chemical structures, which are similar to the monoamine neurotransmitters, such as norepinephrine and dopamine. The increase in dopamine is associated with a sense of euphoria that can accompany the use of these drugs. Due to the sympathomimetic actions they also increase heart rate, constrict blood vessels causing an increase in blood pressure, as well as increasing blood glucose, and open up the pathways of the respiratory system. Thus, amphetamines generally affect the cardiovascular and neurological systems.[15] A recent study in rats combined Fluoro-Jade C staining of degenerating terminals prelabeled with axonally transported Fluoro-Ruby to unequivocally demonstrate terminal degeneration of dopaminergic terminals and axons in the caudate-putamen following d-amphetamine exposure.[52]

Some of the adverse actions of the amphetamines are linked to the increase of blood pressure which can cause burst blood vessels and may in rare cases, lead to paralysis and coma.[53]

Another mechanism could be the direct amphetamine toxicity because some people suffer a bad or toxic reaction to even low doses of amphetamines. Further, due to tolerance higher and higher doses are taken and these high doses and associated adverse reactions to the drug can lead to brain damage or could even be fatal due to the increased risk of convulsions, coma, and brain hemorrhage. Regular, heavy use of amphetamines is associated with hallucinations, paranoia, mental illness, and brain damage. Widely abused amphetamine drugs belong to a large family of phenethylamines, which include MDMA, MDA, and METH, affect brain metabolism by inducing cortical hypometabolism and cerebellar hypermetabolism.[54] Part of their action on brain cells is due to the stimulant action, but part could be related to the inherent toxicity of these substances.[55] Each has its own particular toxicity profile and thus potential to induce encephalopathy.[4,56]

Methamphetamine-evoked encephalopathy. METH (speed) is a powerful stimulant of abuse with potent addictive and neurotoxic properties with its own unique toxicity profile. In the short term, METH use causes increases in heart rate, blood pressure, temperature, and rate of breathing, constriction of blood vessels, and cardiac arrhythmia. Prolonged METH use is associated with stroke, cardiac valve sclerosis, decreases in lung function, pulmonary hypertension, reduced cognition and mental health.[57,58] These adverse effects are related in part to its cardiac toxicity, immunosuppressive effects, and its detrimental effects on oral health. In the brain it causes loss of dopaminergic and serotonergic terminals, possibly by increasing excitotoxicity, and mitochondrial dysfunction.[55,59,60] The increased risk of stroke from the abuse of METH can lead to irreversible damage to the brain. METH, like other drugs of abuse, affects cellular energy requirements and, in particular, glucose metabolism, but metabolism of amino acids and fatty acids may also be affected. PET scans show that glucose metabolism is 14% higher in the whole brain in abusers compared to non-abusers.[61] Protracted abstinence may reverse some of the METH-induced alterations in brain function but many deficits persist.

The possibility that METH may induce encephalopathy has not been reported per se but METH abuse has been linked to long-term brain cell damage. In recently abstinent METH dependent subjects, electroencephalography revealed EEG abnormalities, increased EEG power in the delta and theta bands that were consistent with a generalized encephalopathy.[62] Prenatal METH exposure has been linked to CNS injury. Echoencephalographic study found cranial abnormalities in 35.1% of the drug-exposed infants.[63] The abnormalities in the drug-exposed infants suggested intraventricular hemorrhage, as well as echodensities associated with necrosis and cavitary lesions mainly in the basal ganglion, frontal lobes, and posterior fossa.

METH abusers suffer cognitive deficits correlated with the changes in the limbic and paralimbic cortices, reduced hippocampal volume, and abnormal metabolic activity. MRI showed striatal damage in a group of METH abusers who had abused METH for periods ranging from 4 to 15 years.[64] Part of the toxic effect of METH is also attributed to its pro-inflammatory action because the co-administration of nonsteroidal anti-inflammatory drugs (NSAIDs) with METH significantly attenuates striatal dopamine terminal degeneration and microgliosis.[65]

Chronic exposure to METH in laboratory animals has been shown to cause degeneration in dopaminergic and serotonergic nerve terminals[66] as well as cell bodies in distinct brain regions, such as the somatosensory cortex,[67] the frontal cortex, the hippocampus,[68] and thalamus.[69]

Some of the damage to the CNS that is observed following amphetamine and METH administration is known to be linked to increased formation of free radicals. This increase could be, in part, related to mitochondrial dysfunction and/or cause damage to the mitochondria, thereby leading to a failure of cellular energy metabolism and an increase in secondary excitotoxicity.[60,70] In a study to examine the neurotoxic actions of METH in the brains of children exposed to METH *in utero*, the toxic actions were linked to abnormality in energy metabolism using MRI as localized 1H-MRS.[71]

Antioxidants, such as selenium, as well as other agents, such as carnitines and neuropeptide Y, have been reported to protect against the METH toxicity in the CNS.[72,73]

The protective effects against METH neurotoxicity have been shown by NSAIDs' inhibitory activity on METH-evoked inflammation, possibly via effects on cytokines and nitric oxides, or their suppressive action against microglia activation. Other agents that prevent microglial activation, such as MK801 and dextromethorphan, have also been shown to protect against METH-induced neurotoxicity.[74]

3,4-Methylenedioxymethamphetamine-evoked encephalopathy. A brain stimulant, MDMA (ecstasy), is just one of a large family of phenethylamines, including MDA, N-ethyl-3,4-methylenedioxyamphetamine (MDEA), and N-methyl-1-(1,3-benzodioxol-5-yl)-2-butanamine (MDBD), all of which are abused. Fake "ecstasy" is widely sold as a mixture of drugs, such as ketamine and ephedrine, which have their own toxicity problems. MDMA users report that it causes a sense of euphoria, followed by a feeling of calm. MDMA-induced hyperthermia combined with strenuous exercise could lead to brain hyperthermia that often may be fatal.[75] MDMA overdose is associated with high blood pressure, faintness, panic attacks, and in severe cases, a loss of consciousness and seizures. Prolonged use may cause disseminated intravascular coagulation, brain edema, rhabdomyolysis, acute renal and hepatic failure, cardiac arrhythmia, and neurotoxicity.[76] Research on long-time users suggests it may cause brain damage and mental illness.[77]

MDMA use may be associated with a drug-induced neuropathological state and it has been reported to cause toxic leukoencephalopathy.[78] MDMA-induced cell and nerve terminal degeneration has been shown.[79] This neurotoxic action could be partly related to long-lasting effects of MDMA on glucose metabolism in the human brain because it reduces glucose metabolism globally in the brain but mainly in striatum and amygdala.[80]

Methcathinone-evoked encephalopathy. Methcathinone (ephedron) is a stimulant drug, a structural analogue of cathinone and methamphetamine, commonly made by the oxidation of ephedrine. Methcathinone has effects similar to

METH and its adverse events are similar to cocaine, because it induces hypertension and tachycardia. It affects the catecholaminergic systems in the CNS and its abuse potential is similar to that of the amphetamines.

Recent studies have recently described cases of "ephedron" encephalopathy.[81,82] Clinical signs of brain lesions appeared 3–14 (mean 6.8 $\pm$ 4.9) months after the beginning of the regular drug intake.[81] In the acute stage of the disease, most patients suffered from a combination of extrapyramidal disorders (Parkinsonism, muscular dystonia, tremor, myoclonia) with pronounced postural instability, pseudobulbar syndrome, autonomic, and cognitive and affective personality abnormalities. These studies suggested that the main mechanism underlying the "ephedron encephalopathy" development were related to the manganese accumulation in the brain and this triggered secondary pathogenetic mechanisms, such as mitochondrial dysfunction, oxidative stress, etc. Treatment strategies relied in reducing manganese by induction courses of calcium and sodium EDTA that accelerates manganese excretion.

Hallucinogens abuse and encephalopathy

Hallucinogens have been used since ancient times but became popular in the 1960s. The most common hallucinogens are d-lysergic acid (LSD), phencyclidine (PCP, angel dust), igobaine, ketamine, mescaline, peyote, and psilocybin (mushrooms).[83] In addition, there are other fungi and medicinal herbs which are rich in hallucinogenic substances and which are sometimes abused. With larger doses there is a risk of convulsions, coma, heart failure, and death. PCP and ketamine can cause respiratory depression, heart rate abnormalities, and a withdrawal syndrome. The mushrooms have a lower hallucinogenic effect but greater physical effects, such as increased heart rate and blood pressure. Almost all can give rise to neurotoxic symptoms but it is the possibility of poisoning mainly due to other contaminants that can give rise to encephalopathy and late dystonia.[84] The hallucinogen psilocybin has been tentatively linked with multifocal cerebral demyelination.[83]

Lysergic acid diethylamide-evoked encephalopathy. LSD distorts perception and with effects varying according to the dosage, situation, and mood. The effects of LSD are primarily exerted in the serotonergic systems of the raphe nuclei and locus ceruleus. LSD has been reported to potentiate the neurotoxic action of MDMA in animal experiments.[85] In these experiments the MDMA-induced neurotoxicity was dose dependently increased by LSD and attenuated by 5-HT2A/2C receptor antagonist MDL 11,939.

LSD and other sympathomimetic drugs, such as cocaine, amphetamines, and PCP, can also provoke a hypertensive crisis, which, if untreated, can cause hypertensive encephalopathy. In treating this condition agents with few or no CNS side effects (avoid clonidine hydrochloride (Catapres), methyldopa (Aldomet), and reserpine) and decreased cerebral blood flow (avoid Diazoxide) are recommended, for example, nitroprusside. The last one, despite its effects on intracranial pressure, is advocated as the agent of choice for treatment of hypertensive encephalopathy.[86] Other stimulant agents that may provoke hypertensive encephalopathy include ephedrine and caffeine alkaloids.[87]

Narcotics abuse and encephalopathy

The class of narcotics includes opioids, heroin, morphine, and meperidine.[88] Heroin is the diacetyl derivative of morphine which can be smoked, swallowed, sniffed (chasing the dragon), or injected. Pregnant women who use heroin risk giving birth to small babies who may be addicted to heroin and suffer withdrawal symptoms. Symptoms of an overdose include rapid heartbeat, heart failure, shortness of breath, unconsciousness, and coma. Treatment is with naloxone, which counteracts the effects of heroin, morphine, and other opiates because it targets the same receptors in the CNS. Medical consequences of chronic heroin injection use include collapsed veins and infections. It is also associated with liver, lung, and kidney disease. Some additives in street heroin do not readily dissolve and clog blood vessels affecting the lungs, liver, kidneys, or brain.

The most common neurological complication with heroin abuse in the hospital is coma due to overdose. Other cerebral complications of narcotic overdose include delirium, delayed postanoxic encephalopathy, stroke, involuntary movement disorder, as well as peripheral nerve lesions, and muscle disorders. Neuropathologically, there can be brain edema, myelin damage, astrocytic clasmatodendrosis, globus pallidus cysts, and reduced neuronal populations. The dose pattern associated with the most neurological disturbances is heroin abuse for more than 6 months in dosages more than 0.4 g per day.[89] Diagnosis of heroin related neurological complication should bear in mind temporal relationship to the use, other drugs, or diseases that could mimic the condition should be excluded.

Heroin-evoked encephalopathy. Many cases of spongiform leukoencephalopathy in heroin addicts have been reported and MR imaging and CT appear to be essential for making this diagnosis because clinical history is often unreliable and findings at physical examination are nonspecific.[90] Intravenous heroin abuse provokes hypoxic-ischemic leukoencephalopathy[91] and the inhalation of "heroin" pyrolysate, generated by heating the drug on aluminum foil, induces toxic leukoencephalopathy revealed by the MRI that corresponds to spongiform changes in white matter and the degeneration of multivacuolar oligodendrocytes.[92]

Inhalation of the vapors can result in the relatively rare toxic spongiform leukoencephalopathy with patients progressing through three defined clinical stages with one-quarter reaching the terminal stage, which invariably leads to death.[92] Imaging studies indicate a lipophilic toxin-induced demyelinating process, mainly involving the central motor system, as the most likely cause of heroin leukoencephalopathy.[90] MR findings of spongiform leukoencephalopathy secondary to chasing heroin can progress despite apparent abstinence of the drug suggesting the MR changes may represent an evolving injury.[43] Ryan and colleagues did MR spectroscopy in these type of subjects which showed increased lactic acid and myoinositol, decreased N-acetyl aspartate and creatine, normal to slightly decreased choline, and normal lipid peak. They suggested that the encephalopathy could be due to impaired energy metabolism at the cellular level. This was further substantiated in another study in which a patient with near fatal toxic leucoencephalopathy after inhalation of heated heroin where clinical recovery and reversible white matter changes were observed following antioxidant therapy with ubiquinone (Coenzyme Q10).[93] Coenzyme Q10 is necessary for the proper function of the mitochondrial respiratory chain and is also a strong antioxidant. It has been shown to have neuroprotective activity in many different models of neurotoxicity.[12] Other metabolic cofactors may also be affected in drug abuse.[3] A recent study reported that heroin pyrolysate inhalation was associated with tetrahydrobiopterin (BH4) deficiency.[94] This study showed that the patient suffered from temporary Parkinsonism and this was probably related to altered dopamine metabolism due to a reversible deficiency of BH4. These aspects of metabolic dysfunction are discussed further below.

Methadone-evoked encephalopathy. There was a case report on encephalopathy associated with the synthetic opioid, methadone. Methadone is used clinically in the treatment of opioid addiction. However, methadone can have neurotoxic consequences as in the case of the 3-year-old boy who ingested methadone accidentally.[95] The accidental exposure to methadone resulted in a coma with acute obstructive hydrocephalus caused by cerebellar edema and supratentorial lesions. On this occasion, the patient was successfully treated with methylprednisolone and cerebrospinal fluid external drainage.

Inhalants abuse and encephalopathy

There are inexpensive and readily available carbon-based products that are abused to produce a "high" when inhaled. These include butane, toluene, butyl nitrite, and amyl nitrite found in common products, such as aerosols, adhesives, cigarette lighters, paints, petrol, etc. Acute symptoms include loss of muscle control, slurred speech, drowsiness, hallucinations, or loss of consciousness. The volatile solvents are rapidly absorbed via the lungs and rapidly reach the brain. The fumes replace oxygen in the lungs and can cause suffocation and heart failure. In the long term, they are toxic to the cells in the liver, kidneys, and brain.

Solvent-evoked encephalopathy. Heavy solvent use over years can cause brain damage. There are many published cases of the inhalation of butane and toluene resulting in a prolonged semiconscious state with encephalopathic symptoms.[96] The toxicological properties of butane are probably related to asphyxia, replacement of oxygen by butane, which probably leads to anoxic damage to heart and CNS.[96]

However, solvents also possess other toxic properties per se. Both butane and toluene cause damage to the white matter damaging myelin in both the central and peripheral nervous system with severity of damage being correlated with the duration of abuse.[97] The neurological symptoms reflect these neurotoxic actions of inhalant abuse and depend on parts of brain that are damaged.[97] White matter hyperintensities in cerebrum, brain stem, and cerebellum on T2-weighted images have been reported following toluene abuse.[98] In some patients, toluene abuse also results in more diffuse white matter change linked to brain atrophy, including hippocampal and cerebral atrophy and thinning of the corpus callosum.[99] Abnormalities in the substantia nigra and the red nucleus have also been reported.[97] Encephalopathies resulting from other solvents have also been described, such as paint thinner,[100] and petrol.[101]

Anesthetics abuse and encephalopathy

Encephalopathy's resulting from PCP (see Hallucinogens), anesthetic gas, and nitrous oxide have been reported before.[102]

Ketamine and GHB may cause brain damage[103,104] but specific encephalopathies have not been described. Ketamine is a powerful anesthetic used mainly in farm animals. Ketamine can cause loss of consciousness, vomiting, and death.

GHB is both a sedative and a steroid, formerly sold in many health food stores to promote bodybuilding. Now illegal, GHB usually comes as a liquid, pill, or powder. GHB induces sleep, which in combination with other drugs, particularly alcohol, may result in coma or death. GHB is often used as a "date rape" drug because it is difficult to detect in a drink. Coma and seizures can occur following abuse of GHB. GHB and two of its precursors, gamma butyrolactone (GBL) and 1,4 butanediol (BD), have been involved in poisonings, overdoses, date rapes, and deaths.

Nitrous oxide is a gas used for anesthesia in dental surgery. Sometimes called "laughing gas," nitrous oxide produces immediate loss of motor control and a floating sense of disconnected perceptions. Extended use can cause brain damage, long-lasting numbness in the feet and hands, and sometimes, suffocation.

Other designer drugs abuse and encephalopathy

There are already growing numbers of so-called designer drugs, produced in laboratories, similar to other compounds. An example is the synthetic opiate Fentanyl, which is 80–100 times more powerful than heroin. Fentanyl acts very fast (1–4 min and lasts 30–90 min). Another synthetic opiate is meperidine. There are also dozens of synthetic amphetamines. All designer drugs will work by targeting known pleasure mechanisms in the brain, looking to maximize pleasure and minimize side effects. The potential neurotoxicity of these new designer drugs and possible role in triggering encephalopathy has to be studied further.

Role of mitochondrial dysfunction

Mechanisms involving cellular energy failure and mitochondrial dysfunction have been implicated in alcohol encephalopathy as well as other neurodegenerative diseases. Metabolism plays a major part in various forms and development of encephalopathies. There are two major types of metabolic encephalopathy, related to deficiency in glucose, oxygen, or metabolic cofactors, and those due to peripheral organ dysfunction. In substance abuse-evoked encephalopathy, metabolic disturbances also play a major role in the pathogenesis.

Most of the cellular energy derives from oxidation of carbohydrates and fatty acids in the mitochondria via the Krebs cycle and the respiratory chain. The toxicity profile of the drugs of abuse (and their metabolites) is probably related to mitochondrial dysfunction, either directly via effects on respiratory processes or indirectly via nutritional and oxygen deficiencies. Mitochondrial dysfunction is known to underlie many forms of encephalopathy, for example, mitochondrial myopathy, encephalopathy, lactic acidosis, and stroke-like episodes (MELAS). For example, mutation of the mitochondrial DNA (mtDNA) G13513A, encoding the ND5 subunit of respiratory chain complex I causes mitochondrial encephalopathy with lactic acidosis.[105] Because mitochondria contain their own machinery for nucleoside and nucleotide metabolism and have physically separate nucleotide pools, compounds interfering with intracellular substrates pools, that is, deoxynucleosides triphosphate precursors imbalance, can also provoke partial depletion of mtDNA and encephalopathy.[106,107] Thus, as a strategy against the drug abuse-evoked encephalopathy the mitochondria are a prime target. Indeed, as discussed below, supplementation with mitochondrial respiratory chain cofactor, coenzyme Q10 has been shown to ameliorate recovery following heroin-evoked encephalopathy.[93] Other metabolic cofactors may also be affected in drug abuse.[12,13] Thus, heroin pyrolysate inhalation may also be associated with BH4 deficiency.[94]

Present and future protective strategies against encephalopathy

It is important for clinicians, as well as the drug abusers, to be aware of the potential neurological damage caused by psychoactive drugs. Clinicians need to assess type, frequency, as well as the dosage of drug and type that has been abused. Impurities of the drug, risky administration techniques, and the use of mixtures of various drugs, especially in combination with alcohol should also be assessed. Reliable laboratory procedures for detection of psychoactive drugs are now widely available. However, to assess encephalopathy the imaging techniques, especially MRI, are the most reliable in the detection of complications associated with drug abuse.[108] The MR spectra may also be used to assess the effectiveness of various treatment strategies.[62]

Stopping the drug/substance abuse

To reduce the possibility of the irreversible brain damage in drug abusing individuals, the first strategy would be to stop (or wean off) the subject from the drug/substance abuse. The treatment strategy should make an effort to prevent but also to educate about the dangers of the habit. Addicts would need to be helped in breaking the habit even if it would mean in some instances substituting the habit with other less harmful drugs, for example, naloxone or methadone in combination with psychoeducation, family interventions, and cognitive therapy. Research also suggests other potential therapeutic strategies for the treatment against specific abused drugs during the critical withdrawal phase. Previous work with repeated administration of amphetamine in rats has shown that amphetamine withdrawal produces decreased motivation to work for a non-drug reward, and this withdrawal is reversed by administration of a dopamine partial agonist. Repeated systemic treatment with the dopamine partial agonist terguride, the full dopamine agonist ropinirole and acetyl-L-carnitine, a compound with a potential antidepressant effect, during methamphetamine withdrawal restored responding for the sweet solution, suggesting that these drugs may represent potential therapeutic strategies for the treatment of methamphetamine addiction during the withdrawal phase.[109] These compounds could be useful in combination with behavior modification programs in reducing the risk factors triggering the drug abuse habit and associated encephalopathy.

Developing better neuroprotective strategies

Secondly, or better, concomitantly, a neuroprotective strategy has to be employed to prevent further damage and possibly reverse damage that has already occurred. The metabolic derangements caused by the inherent toxicity of the abused drugs as well as the consequences, such as increased toxins due to organ damage, should also be tackled.[109] Toward this aim, new strategies to restore normal metabolism, prevent nutritional deficiencies, and use of potential neuroprotective compounds needs to be investigated further.[4,5,110]

Correcting nutritional deficiency may be an important strategy in preventing the drug abuse-evoked damage because drug abuse may cause nutritional insufficiencies. Many alcoholics are malnourished, because alcohol prevents the body from properly absorbing, digesting, and using nutrients.[111] Alcohol abuse is linked with marked steatosis and liver injury and malnutrition is common and is associated with vitamin (B1, B2, B6, B12, C, K, A, and D) and mineral deficiencies (selenium, zinc, magnesium, iron, and phosphorus).[111] Thiamine (B1) deficiency in alcoholics causes neurological damage leading to the Wernicke/Korsakoff syndrome. Wernicke's encephalopathy (WE) is a neurological emergency which presents with symptoms of confusion, ophthalmoplegia, and ataxia. Mechanisms involving cellular energy failure and mitochondrial dysfunction have been implicated in this syndrome.[2]

Dietary supplementation may provide a means to reduce the risk of drug-evoked neurotoxicity. Thus, encephalopathy may be triggered by initial cellular injury from oxidation damage, where antioxidant supplements would be protective. As mentioned before, dietary supplements may also combat the neurotoxic actions of drugs of abuse directly.[3,4,12] Coenzyme Q10 reduces the neurotoxicity of cocaine and METH[13,112] and L-carnitine reduces the toxicity of METH.[72]

Supplementation with L-carnitine also alleviates alcohol-induced liver damage, possibly by reducing hepatic concentrations of thiobarbituric acid reactive substances, an indicator of lipid peroxidation.[113] In animal experiments, supplementation with creatine has been reported to protect against the dopamine depleting effects of neurotoxic doses of METH.[114] Rats fed with 1% creatine in a normal diet had greater striatal dopamine after one week of METH treatment. Indices of oxidative damage were reduced in the creatine fed compared to the animals on normal diet.[114]

Another potential strategy being examined by us and other groups is the potential of epigenetic modulation in reducing the risk of developing the drug abuse-evoked encephalopathy. The genetic vulnerability may be amenable to modulation in an appositive manner by nutritional and dietary supplements to reduce the potential damage.

Conclusion

Major pathways for CNS neurotoxicity could be related to increased risk of cell damage that would involve genomic, metabolic, and mitochondrial dysfunction resulting in increased excitotoxicity, reduced energy production, and lowered antioxidant potential. In particular, the role of mitochondrial dysfunction in provoking drug abuse generated neurotoxicity is noteworthy.

The drug-abuse-evoked encephalopathy still needs to be studied further to enable better preventative and protective strategies. While treatment of the neurological complication may not be sufficient enough in restoring the quality of life, neuroprotective as well as social and rehabilitative care may be more effective.

Acknowledgments

The authors thank Mr. Latif Suleman Kara and Mr. Aziz Ahmed Juma for their help.

Conflicts of interest

The authors declare no conflicts of interest.

References

1. Greenhill, L.L. 2006. The science of stimulant abuse. *Pediatr. Ann.* **35:** 552–556.
2. Desjardins, P. & R.F. Butterworth. 2005. Role of mitochondrial dysfunction and oxidative stress in the pathogenesis of selective neuronal loss in Wernicke's encephalopathy. *Mol. Neurobiol.* **31:** 17–26.
3. Virmani, A., Z. Binienda, S. Ali, *et al.* 2006. Links between nutrition, drug abuse, and the metabolic syndrome. *Ann. N.Y. Acad. Sci.* **1074:** 303–314.
4. Virmani, A., Z. Binienda, S. Ali, *et al.* 2007. Metabolic syndrome in drug abuse. *Ann. N.Y. Acad. Sci.* **1122:** 50–68.
5. Virmani, A., L.C. Schmued, F. Gaetani, *et al.* 2007. Encephalopathies related to abuse of psychoactive drugs. In *Drug Related Encephalopathies.* 227–260. Nova Science Inc. New York.
6. Richter, R.W., Ed. 1975. Clinicopharmacological aspects of mind altering and addictive drugs. In *Medical Aspects of Drug Abuse.* 1–78. Harper & Row. New York.
7. Maurer, H.H. 2004. Chemistry, pharmacology, toxicology, and hepatic metabolism of designer drugs of the amphetamine (ecstasy), piperazine, and pyrrolidinophenone types: a synopsis. *Ther. Drug Monit.* **26:** 127–131.
8. Henderson, D.C. *et al.* 2000. Clozapine, diabetes mellitus, weight gain, and lipid abnormalities: a five-year naturalistic study. *Am. J. Psych.* **157:** 975–981.
9. Timar, O., F. Sestier & E. Levy. 2000. Metabolic syndrome X: a review. *Can. J. Cardiol.* **16:** 779–789.
10. Kohen, D. 2004. Diabetes mellitus and schizophrenia: historical perspective. *Br. J. Psych. Suppl.* **47:** S64–S66.
11. Albano, E. 2006. Alcohol, oxidative stress and free radical damage. *Proc. Nutr. Soc.* **65:** 278–290.
12. Virmani, A., F. Gaetani & Z. Binienda. 2005. Effects of metabolic modifiers such as carnitines, coenzyme Q10 and PUFAs against different forms of neurotoxic insults: metabolic inhibitors, MPTP, and methamphetamine. *Ann. N.Y. Acad. Sci.* **1053:** 183–191.
13. Virmani, A. *et al.* 2006. Coenzyme Q10 and the metabolic approach to neuroprotection. *Agro Food Industry Hi-tech* **17:** 20–22.
14. Karch, S.B. 2005. Cocaine cardiovascular toxicity. *South Med. J.* **98:** 794–799.
15. Darke, S., S. Kaye & J. Duflou. 2006. Comparative cardiac pathology among deaths due to cocaine toxicity, opioid toxicity and non-drug-related causes. *Addiction* **101:** 1771–1777.

16. Dodd, P.R. *et al.* 2004. Genes and gene expression in the brain of the alcoholic. *Addict. Behav.* **29:** 1295–1309.
17. Day, C.P. 2006. Genes or environment to determine alcoholic liver disease and non-alcoholic fatty liver disease. *Liver Int.* **26:** 1021–1028.
18. NIDA Infofacts. Crack and Cocaine http://www.nida.nih.gov/pdf/infofacts/Cocaine06.pdf.
19. Volkow, N. D., J.S. Fowler & G.J. Wang. 2003. The addicted human brain: insights from imaging studies. *J. Clin. Invest.* **111:** 1444–1451.
20. Brust, J.C. 2002. Neurologic complications of substance abuse. *J. Acquir. Immune. Defic. Syndr.* **31:** S29–S34.
21. Neiman, J., H.M. Haapaniemi, M. Hillbom. 2000. Neurological complications of drug abuse: pathophysiological mechanisms. *Eur. J. Neurol.* **7:** 595–606.
22. Fornai, F. *et al.* 2001. Dose-dependent protective effects of apomorphine against methamphetamine-induced nigrostriatal damage. *Brain Res.* **898:** 27–35.
23. Choi, H.J. *et al.* 2002. Methamphetamine-induced apoptosis in a CNS-derived catecholaminergic cell line. *Mol. Cells* **13:** 221–227.
24. Yamamoto, B.K. & W. Zhu. 1998. The effects of methamphetamine on the production of free radicals and oxidative stress. *J. Pharmacol. Exp. Ther.* **287:** 107–114.
25. Stephans, S.E. *et al.* 1998. Substrates of energy metabolism attenuate methamphetamine-induced neurotoxicity in striatum. *J. Neurochem.* **71:** 613–621.
26. Imam, S.Z. & S.F. Ali. 2000. Selenium, an antioxidant, attenuates methamphetamine-induced dopaminergic toxicity and peroxynitrite generation. *Brain Res.* **855:** 186–191.
27. Imam, S.Z. & S.F. Ali. 2001. Aging increases the susceptibility to methamphetamine-induced dopaminergic neurotoxicity in rats: correlation with peroxynitrite production and hyperthermia. *J. Neurochem.* **78:** 952–959.
28. Virmani, A. & Z. Binienda. 2004. Role of carnitine esters in brain neuropathology. *Mol. Aspects Med.* **25:** 533–549.
29. Benowitz, N.L. 1992. How toxic is cocaine? *Ciba Found Symp.* **166:** 125–143.
30. Karch, S.B. 2005. Cocaine cardiovascular toxicity. *South Med. J.* **98:** 794–799.
31. Treadwell, S.D. & T.G. Robinson. 2007. Cocaine use and stroke. *Postgrad. Med. J.* **83:** 389–394.
32. Brown, E. *et al.* 1992. CNS complications of cocaine abuse: prevalence, pathophysiology, and neuroradiology. *AJR Am. J. Roentgenol.* **159:** 137–147.
33. Kondziella, D., E.R. Danielsen, P. Arlien-Soborg. 2007. Fatal encephalopathy after an isolated overdose of cocaine. *J. Neurol. Neurosurg. Psychiatry* **78:** 437–438.
34. Diez-Tejedor, E. *et al.* 1998. Encephalopathy and biopsy-proven cerebrovascular inflammatory changes in a cocaine abuser. *Eur. J. Neurol.* **5:** 103–107.
35. Grewal, R.P. & B.L. Miller 1991. Cocaine induced hypertensive encephalopathy. *Acta Neurol. (Napoli)* **13:** 279–281.
36. Ruttenber, A.J. *et al.* 1997. Fatal excited delirium following cocaine use: epidemiologic findings provide new evidence for mechanisms of cocaine toxicity. *J. Forensic Sci.* **42:** 25–31.
37. Maschke, M. *et al.*1999. Toxic leukoencephalopathy after intravenous consumption of heroin and cocaine with unexpected clinical recovery. *J. Neurol.* **246:** 850–851.
38. De Roock, S. *et al.* 2007. Extensive pallidal and white matter injury following cocaine overdose. *Intensive Care Med.* **33:** 2030–2031.
39. Volkow, N.D. *et al.* 1988. Cerebral blood flow in chronic cocaine users: a study with positron emission tomography. *Br. J. Psychiatry* **152:** 641–648.
40. Albertson, D.N. *et al.* 2004. Gene expression profile of the nucleus accumbens of human cocaine abusers: evidence for dysregulation of myelin. *J. Neurochem.* **88:** 1211–1219.
41. Gottfried, J.A. *et al.* 1997. Delayed posthypoxic demyelination. Association with arylsulfatase A deficiency and lactic acidosis on protein MR spectroscopy. *Neurology* **49:** 1400–1404.
42. Vella, S. *et al.* 2003. Acute leukoencephalopathy after inhalation of a single dose of heroin. *Neuropediatrics* **34:** 100–104.
43. Ryan, A. *et al.* 2005. Fatal toxic leukoencephalopathy: clinical, radiological, and necropsy findings in two patients. *J. Neurol. Neurosurg. Psychiatry* **76:** 1014–1016.
44. Herning, R.I. *et al.* 1997. Cocaine dependence: a clinical syndrome requiring neuroprotection. *Ann. N.Y. Acad. Sci.* **825:** 328–331.
45. Johnson, B.A. *et al.* 2001. Treatment advances for cocaine-induced ischemic stroke: focus on dihydropyridine-class calcium channel antagonists. *Am. J. Psychiatry* **158:** 1191–1198.
46. Kim, H. *et al.* 2000. Selenium deficiency potentiates methamphetamine-induced nigral neuronal loss: comparison with MPTP model. *Brain Res.* **17:** 247–252.
47. Hayase, T. *et al.* 2000. Relationship between cocaine-induced hepatotoxic neurobehavioral & biochemical

changes in mice: the antidotal effects of buprenorphine. *Life Sci.* **67:** 45–52.

48. Hayase, T. *et al.* 2004. Microarray profile analysis of toxic cocaine-induced alterations in the expression of mouse brain gene sequences: a possible 'protective' effect of buprenorphine. *J. Appl. Toxicol.* **24:** 15–20.
49. Hayase, T., Y. Yamamoto & K. Yamamoto. 1997. Protection against cocaine and combined cocaine-ethanol toxicities in mice by imidazobenzodiazepine Ro 15-4513. *Toxicology* **117:** 171–182.
50. Wholey, M.H., E. Ogasawara & M.H. Ramadan. 1990. Acute rhabdomyolysis associated with cocaine intoxication: a case report. *Hawaii Med. J.* **49:** 386–387.
51. Kramer, L. *et al.* 2003. Successful treatment of refractory cerebral oedema in ecstasy/cocaine-induced fulminant hepatic failure using a new high-efficacy liver detoxification device (FPSA-Prometheus). *Wien Klin. Wochenschr.* **115:** 599–603.
52. Bowyer, J.F. & L.C. Schmued. 2006. Fluoro-Ruby labeling prior to an amphetamine neurotoxic insult shows a definitive massive loss of dopaminergic terminals and axons in the caudate-putamen. *Brain Res.* **1075:** 236–239.
53. White, S.R. 2002. Amphetamine toxicity. *Semin. Respir. Crit. Care Med.* **23:** 27–36.
54. Gouzoulis-Mayfrank, E. *et al.* 1999. Neurometabolic effects of psilocybin, 3,4-methylenedioxyethylamphetamine (MDE) and d-methamphetamine in healthy volunteers. A double-blind, placebo-controlled PET study with [^{18}F]FDG. *Neuropsychopharmacol.* **20:** 565–581.
55. Quinton, M.S. & B.K. Yamamoto. 2006. Causes and consequences of methamphetamine and MDMA toxicity. *AAPS J.* **8:** E337–E347.
56. Filley, C.M. & B.K. Kleinschmidt-DeMasters. 2001. Toxic leukoencephalopathy. *N. Engl. J. Med.* **345:** 425–432.
57. Welder, A.A. 1992. A primary culture system of postnatal rat heart cells for the study of cocaine and methamphetamine toxicity. *Toxicol. Lett.* **60:** 183–196.
58. Varner, K.J. *et al.* 2002. Cardiovascular responses elicited by the "binge" administration of methamphetamine. *J. Pharmacol. Exp. Ther.* **301:** 152–159.
59. Cadet, J.L., S. Jayanthi & X. Deng. 2003. Speed kills: cellular and molecular bases of methamphetamine-induced nerve terminal degeneration and neuronal apoptosis. *FASEB J.* **17:** 1775–1788.
60. Riddle, E.L., A.E. Fleckenstein & G.R. Hanson. 2006. Mechanisms of methamphetamine-induced dopaminergic neurotoxicity. *AAPS J.* **8:** E413–E418.
61. London, E.D. *et al.* 2004. Mood disturbances and regional cerebral metabolic abnormalities in recently abstinent methamphetamine abusers. *Arch. Gen. Psych.* **61:** 73–84.
62. London, E.D. *et al.* 1999. Brain imaging studies of cocaine abuse: implications for medication development. *Crit. Rev. Neurobiol.* **13:** 227–242.
63. Dixon, S.D. & R. Bejar. 1989. Echoencephalographic findings in neonates associated with maternal cocaine and methamphetamine use: incidence and clinical correlates. *J. Pediatr.* **115:** 770–778.
64. Chang, L. *et al.* 2005. Enlarged striatum in abstinent methamphetamine abusers: a possible compensatory response. *Biol. Psychiatry* **57:** 967–974.
65. Asanuma, M. *et al.* 2003. Methamphetamine-induced neurotoxicity in mouse brain is attenuated by ketoprofen, a non-steroidal anti-inflammatory drug. *Neurosci. Lett.* **352:** 13–16.
66. Seiden, L.S., M.W. Fischman, & C.R. Schuster. 1976. Long-term methamphetamine induces changes in brain catecholamines in tolerant rhesus monkeys. *Drug Alcohol Depend.* **1:** 215–219.
67. Commins, D.L. & L.S. Seiden. 1986. Alpha-methyltyrosine blocks methylamphetamine-induced degeneration in the rat somatosensory cortex. *Brain Res.* **365:** 15–20.
68. Ryan, L.J. *et al.* 1990. Histological and ultrastructural evidence that D-amphetamine causes degeneration in neostriatum and frontal cortex of rats. *Brain Res.* **518:** 67–77.
69. Schmued, L.C. & J.F. Bowyer. 1997. Methamphetamine exposure can produce neuronal degeneration in mouse hippocampal remnants. *Brain Res.* **759:** 135–140.
70. Pubill, D. *et al.* 2005. Free radical production induced by methamphetamine in rat striatal synaptosomes. *Toxicol. Appl. Pharmacol.* **204:** 57–68.
71. Smith, L.M. *et al.* 2001. Brain proton magnetic resonance spectroscopy in children exposed to methamphetamine in utero. *Neurology* **57:** 255–260.
72. Virmani, A. *et al.* 2003. Possible mechanism for the neuroprotective effects of L-carnitine on methamphetamine-evoked neurotoxicity. *Ann. N.Y. Acad. Sci.* **993:** 197–207.
73. Thiriet, N. *et al.* 2005. Neuropeptide Y protects against methamphetamine-induced neuronal apoptosis in the mouse striatum. *J. Neurosci.* **25:** 5273–5279.
74. Thomas, D.M. & D.M. Kuhn. 2005. MK-801 and dextromethorphan block microglial activation and protect against methamphetamine-induced neurotoxicity. *Brain Res.* **1050:** 190–198.

75. Freedman, R.R., C.E. Johanson & M.E. Tancer. 2005. Thermoregulatory effects of 3,4-methylenedioxymethamphetamine (MDMA) in humans. *Psychopharmacology* **183:** 248–256.
76. Caballero, F. *et al.* 2002. Ecstasy-induced brain death and acute hepatocellular failure: multiorgan donor and liver transplantation. *Transplantation* **74:** 532–537.
77. Herning, R.I. *et al.* 2005. Neuropsychiatric alterations in MDMA users: preliminary findings. *Ann. N.Y. Acad. Sci.* **1053:** 20–27.
78. Bertram, M. *et al.* 1999. Toxic leukoencephalopathy following "ecstasy" ingestion. *J. Neurol.* **246:** 617–618.
79. Jensen, K.F. *et al.* 1993. Mapping toxicant-induced nervous system damage with a cupric silver stain: a quantitative analysis of neural degeneration induced by 3,4-methylenedioxymethamphetamine. *NIDA Res. Monogr.* **136:** 133–149.
80. Buchert, R. *et al.* 2001. Long-term effects of 'ecstasy' abuse on the human brain studied by FDG PET. *Nucl. Med. Commun.* **22:** 889–897.
81. Levin, O.S. 2005. "Ephedron" encephalopathy. *Zh. Nevrol. Psikhiatr Im. S. S. Korsakova* **105:** 12–20.
82. Ismailova, T.F., N.V. Fedorova & L.M. Savchenko. 2005. The treatment of patients with toxic encephalopathy caused by using surrogate psychoactive manganese-containing compounds. *Zh. Nevrol. Psikhiatr. Im. S. S. Korsakova* **105:** 18–21.
83. Spengos, K., A. Schwartz, & M. Hennerici. Multifocal cerebral demyelination after magic mushroom abuse. *J. Neurol.* **247:** 224–225.
84. Carod Artal, F.J. 2003. Neurological syndromes associated with the ingestion of plants and fungi with a toxic component (II). Hallucinogenic fungi and plants, mycotoxins and medicinal herbs. *Rev. Neurol.* **36:** 951–960.
85. Armstrong, B.D. *et al.* 2004. Potentiation of (DL)-3,4-methylenedioxymethamphetamine (MDMA)-induced toxicity by the serotonin 2A receptior partial agonist d-lysergic acid diethylamide (LSD), and the protection of same by the serotonin 2A/2C receptor antagonist MDL 11,939. *Neurosci. Res. Commun.* **35:** 83–95.
86. Gifford, R.W., Jr. 1991. Management of hypertensive crises. *JAMA* **266:** 829–835.
87. Berman, J.A. *et al.* 2006. Complicated hypertension related to the abuse of ephedrine and caffeine alkaloids. *J. Addict. Dis.* **25:** 45–48.
88. Brecher, E.M. 1972. The narcotics: opium, morphine, heroin, methadone, and others; alcohol, the barbiturates, the tranquilizers, and other sedatives and hypnotics; coca leaves, cocaine, the amphetamines, "speed" and cocaine again; LSD and LSD-like drugs. In *Licit and Illicit Drugs*. E.M. Brecher, et al., Eds.: 101, 76. Little, Brown. Boston.
89. Gekht, A.B. *et al.* 2003. Neurological disturbances in heroin addicts in acute withdrawal and early postabstinence periods. *Zh. Nevrol. Psikhiatr. Im. S. S. Korsakova* **103:** 9–15.
90. Chang, Y.J., C.H. Tsai & C.J. Chen. 1997. Leukoencephalopathy after inhalation of heroin vapor. *J. Formos Med. Assoc.* **96:** 758–760.
91. Keogh, C.F. *et al.* 2003. Neuroimaging features of heroin inhalation toxicity: "chasing the dragon". *Am. J. Roentgenol.* **180:** 847–850.
92. Hagel, J. *et al.* 2005. "Chasing the dragon"—imaging of heroin inhalation leukoencephalopathy. *Can. Assoc. Radiol. J.* **56:** 199–203.
93. Gacouin, A. *et al.* 2003. Reversible spongiform leucoencephalopathy after inhalation of heated heroin. *Intensive Care Med.* **29:** 1012–1015.
94. Heales, S., F. Crawley & P. Rudge. 2004. Reversible Parkinsonism following heroin pyrolysate inhalation is associated with tetrahydrobiopterin deficiency. *Mov. Disord.* **19:** 1248–1251.
95. Anselmo, M. *et al.* 2006. Methadone intoxication in a child: toxic encephalopathy? *J. Child Neuro.* **21:** 618–620.
96. Doring, G. *et al.* 2002. Butane abuse associated encephalopathy. *Klin. Padiatr.* **214:** 295–298.
97. Kile, S.J. *et al.* 2006. Bithalamic lesions of butane encephalopathy. *Pediatr. Neurol.* **35:** 439–441.
98. Yamanouchi, N. *et al.* 1995. White matter changes caused by chronic solvent abuse. *AJNR Am. J. Neuroradiol.* **16:** 1643–1649.
99. Borne, J. *et al.* 2005. Neuroimaging in drug and substance abuse part II: opioids and solvents. *Top Magn. Reson. Imaging* **16:** 239–245.
100. Ohnuma, A., I. Kimura & S. Saso. 1995. MRI in chronic paint-thinner intoxication. *Neuroradiology* **37:** 445–446.
101. Cairney, S. *et al.* 2005. Neurological and cognitive recovery following abstinence from petrol sniffing. *Neuropsychopharmacology* **30:** 1019–1027.
102. Shulman, R.M., T.J. Geraghty & M. Tadros. 1996. A case of unusual substance abuse causing myeloneuropathy. *Hum. Reprod.* **11:** 566–567.
103. Jansen, K.L. & R. Darracot-Cankovic. 2001. The nonmedical use of ketamine, part two: a review of problem use and dependence. *J. Psychoactive Drugs* **33:** 151–158.
104. Drasbek, K.R., J. Christensen & K. Jensen. 2006. Gamma-hydroxybutyrate—a drug of abuse. *Acta Neurol. Scand.* **114:** 145–156.

105. Wang, S.B. *et al.* 2008. Mutation of mitochondrial DNA G13513A presenting with Leigh syndrome, Wolff-Parkinson-White syndrome and cardiomyopathy. *Pediatr. Neonatol.* **49:** 145–149.

106. López, L.C. *et al.* 2009. Unbalanced deoxynucleotide pools cause mitochondrial DNA instability in thymidine phosphorylase deficient mice. *Hum. Mol. Genet.* 18: 714–722.

107. Martí, R. *et al.* 2003. Alteration of nucleotide metabolism: a new mechanism for mitochondrial disorders. *Clin. Chem. Lab. Med.* **41:** 845–851.

108. Hoefer, M.E. *et al.* 2006. Effects of terguride, ropinirole, and acetyl-L-carnitine on methamphetamine withdrawal in the rat. *Pharmacol. Biochem. Behav.* **83:** 403–409.

109. Kunze, K. 2002. Metabolic encephalopathies. *J. Neurol.* **249:** 1150–1159.

110. Virmani, M.A. *et al.* 1995. Protective actions of L-carnitine and acetyl-L-carnitine on the neurotoxicity evoked by mitochondrial uncoupling or inhibitors. *Pharmacol. Res.* **32:** 383–389.

111. Leevy, C.M. & S.A. Moroianu. 2005. Nutritional aspects of alcoholic liver disease. *Clin. Liver Dis.* **9:** 67–81.

112. Klongpanichapak, S. *et al.* 2006. Attenuation of cocaine and methamphetamine neurotoxicity by coenzyme Q10. *Neurochem. Res.* **31:** 303–311.

113. Bykov, I., H. Jarvelainen & K. Lindros. 2003. L-carnitine alleviates alcohol-induced liver damage in rats: role of tumor necrosis factor-alpha. *Alcohol Alcohol.* **38:** 400–406.

114. Cass, W.A., M.P. Smith & L.E. Peters. 2005. Protection against the dopamine depleting effects of neurotoxic doses of methamphetamine. ISN/ESN Satellite Meeting, Abst. # 11: 39.

Ann. N.Y. Acad. Sci. ISSN 0077-8923

ANNALS OF THE NEW YORK ACADEMY OF SCIENCES
Issue: *Neuroprotective Agents*

Statins and neuroprotection

A prescription to move the field forward

W. Gibson Wood,[1] Gunter P. Eckert,[2] Urule Igbavboa,[1] and Walter E. Müller[2]

[1]Department of Pharmacology, University of Minnesota, Geriatric Research Education and Clinical Center, VA Medical Center, Minneapolis, Minnesota. [2]Department of Pharmacology, Biocenter Niederursel, University of Frankfurt, Frankfurt, Germany

Address for correspondence: W. Gibson Wood, PhD, Department of Pharmacology, University of Minnesota, 6-120 Jackson Hall, 321 Church St., Minneapolis, MN 55455. woodx002@umn.edu

There is growing interest in the use of statins, HMG-CoA reductase inhibitors, for treating specific neurodegenerative diseases (e.g., cerebrovascular disease, Parkinson's disease, Alzheimer's disease, multiple sclerosis) and possibly traumatic brain injury. Neither is there a consensus on the efficacy of statins in treating the aforementioned diseases nor are the mechanisms of the purported statin-induced neuroprotection well-understood. Part of the support for statin-induced neuroprotection comes from studies using animal models and cell culture. Important information has resulted from that work but there continues to be a lack of progress on basic issues pertaining to statins and brain that impedes advancement in understanding how statins alter brain function. For example, there are scant data on the pharmacokinetics of lipophilic and hydrophilic statins in brain, statin-induced neuroprotection versus cell death, and statins and brain isoprenoids. The purpose of this mini-review will be to examine those aforementioned issues and to identify directions of future research.

Keywords: Alzheimer's disease; cerebrovascular disease; cholesterol; HMG-CoA reductase; isoprenoids; neurodegeneration; neuroprotection; statins; stroke

Introduction

Statins are universally recognized for their effectiveness in reducing serum cholesterol levels and reducing the morbidity and mortality associated with coronary heart disease.[1,2] What has not received as much attention, but is a topic of emerging interest, is the efficacy of statins in the prevention or treatment of certain neurodegenerative diseases, for example, cerebrovascular disease,[3] Parkinson's disease,[4] Alzheimer's disease,[5] and multiple sclerosis.[6] A recent report also indicates that statins may be effective in treating traumatic brain injury.[7] There have been several recent and excellent reviews on statins and neuroprotection.[5,8–12] Many of those reviews have covered clinical and experimental data both pro and con concerning the use of statins in neurodegenerative diseases. In this review, our intention is not to reexamine that body of data. Instead, the focus of this review will be on specific issues pertaining to statin use in animal and cell culture studies and recommendations to move the field forward. The issues which will be examined are: (1) the pharmacokinetics of lipophilic and hydrophilic statins in brain; (2) statin-induced neuroprotection versus cell death; and (3) statins and brain isoprenoids.

Pharmacokinetics of lipophilic and hydrophilic statins in brain

There have been no comprehensive studies published on the uptake, distribution and metabolism of statins in brain. A small number of studies have provided some data on statin levels in brain. One study of 12 human subjects found that lovastatin acid but not pravastatin was detected in the cerebrospinal fluid following a 5 day drug treatment and it was concluded that pravastatin did not pass the blood-brain barrier.[13] The conclusion that pravastatin did not pass the blood-brain barrier is tempered by the

doi: 10.1111/j.1749-6632.2009.05359.x

detection limit of the GC/MS method used in that study and the elimination half-life of pravastatin. The detection limit of the statins was 0.5 ng/mL. Lovastatin acid, which has a partition coefficient of 1.51 as compared with pravastatin with a partition coefficient of −0.47,[14] showed a peak drug level of 1.3 ng/mL in cerebral spinal fluid (CSF) 2.5 h following drug administration. Certainly, based on the differences in the partition coefficients of the two statins, it would be expected that higher levels of lovastatin acid would be detected than pravastatin but the level of lovastatin acid detected was near the detection limit of the assay. The GC/MS assay method may not have had the sensitivity to detect pravastatin. Further impeding pravastatin detection, is that the elimination half-life of pravastatin in serum has been reported to be 1.8 h[15] and the first determination of pravastatin in CSF was 1 h after drug administration. In the same study, it was also observed that there was a 30% reduction in lovastatin acid levels between 2.5 and 4.0 h following drug administration. The elimination half-life of lovastatin in serum is approximately 3 h.[15] It has not been determined if statins are metabolized in the central nervous system (CNS). Alternatively, the reduction in lovastatin acid might be due to active transport out of the CNS which could involve brain acid transporters and is discussed later in this section. Transport of statins into brain was determined in another study using the uptake of radiolabeled statins and an *in situ* rat brain perfusion technique.[16] Permeability of statins into brain was strongly associated with drug lipophilicity and pravastatin permeability was similar to sucrose and it was concluded that pravastatin did not cross the blood-brain barrier.[16] Uptake time points were 10, 20, and 30 s which may have been too early following drug administration. In the same study, it was shown that pravastatin partitions through brain capillary endothelial cells over a 10 min incubation period *in vitro*, albeit at a slower rate as compared with simvastatin and lovastatin.

Two recent studies report unequivocally that pravastatin can be detected in brain.[17,18] As part of a study on statins and brain gene expression in mice, we quantified statin levels in brain and found that simvastatin, lovastatin, and pravastatin could be detected in cerebral cortex of mice administered the drugs *in vivo*.[17] Initially, we determined simvastatin, lovastatin, and pravastatin levels in the cerebral cortex of mice who received statins for 21 days. Mice were sacrificed 24 h after the last statin administration, cerebral cortex dissected and statin levels were determined by LC-MS/MS. Relatively low levels of simvastatin and lovastatin lactones were detected but pravastatin was not detected in the cerebral cortex 24 h after the last drug administration. The low levels of simvastatin and lovastatin and the absence of pravastatin at 24 h were puzzling because of the significant effects of all three statins on brain gene expression. To begin to examine the possibility that statins did not accumulate in brain, we examined statin levels in mice given a single administration and then sacrificed at 1, 3, and 6 h following drug administration. Simvastatin, lovastatin, and pravastatin were all detected in the cerebral cortex. Not surprisingly, brain levels of the three statins reflected their lipophilicity with simvastatin levels > lovastatin levels > pravastatin levels. The maximum average concentration of pravastatin in the cerebral cortex was 100 pmol/g and these levels are above the reported 50% inhibitory concentration (IC50) on membrane bound HMG-CoA reductase. Between 1 and 6 h there was a large reduction in statin levels and is similar to the reduction in lovastatin levels in the CSF study[13] discussed earlier in this review. Statins in brain would appear to be rapidly eliminated but the mechanism for the reduction has not been determined. Since those initial findings on statin levels in brain, a second paper reported levels of simvastatin and pravastatin in mouse brain homogenates after a 3 day drug treatment.[18]

A general conclusion of the four studies discussed above is that lipophilic statins can easily cross the blood-brain barrier. Consensus is not observed as to whether hydrophilic statins, such as pravastatin, can enter the brain. The two studies[13,16] which concluded that pravastatin did not cross the blood-brain barrier may have been limited with respect to assay sensitivity and the sampling times. On the other hand, the two studies[17,18] which found that pravastatin could be detected in brain used high drug concentrations (100 mg/kg and 200 mg/kg per body weight) and sensitive LC-MS/MS methods to quantify drug levels at pmol concentrations. Membrane partitioning of pravastatin and probably other statins administered as acids, such as atorvastatin most likely does not explain how a statin acid enters the brain. However, pravastatin has been shown to be transported into cells by organic anionic transporters (OATs) and these transporters are expressed in brain.[19–21] Another transporter that shuttles statin acids into cells is the monocarboxylic acid transporter.[22] Uptake of lovastatin and simvastatin lactones occurs by simple diffusion but the acid form of the two statins is taken up by means of a transport mechanism for monocarboxylic acid in bovine brain capillary endothelial cells.[22] We found that simvastatin, lovastatin, and pravastatin significantly increased expression of the gene that encodes the monocarboxylic acid transporter in brain tissue of mice chronically administered those drugs.[17] An additional mechanism which could potentially facilitate movement of statins into brain is statin lactonization. Atorvastatin acid as well as simvastatin acid can undergo lactonization and thus could increase the availability of the lactone forms, particularly atorvastatin, which then could cross the blood-brain barrier.[23] While atorvastatin is administered as an acid it undergoes lactonization *in vivo*.[23] Serum levels of atorvastatin lactone and acid were comparable in human subjects.[24] The partition coefficients of atorvastatin lactone (4.2) and simvastatin lactone (4.4)[14] are quite similar and it is predicted that atorvastatin lactone would indeed cross the blood-brain barrier.

CSF and brain levels of statins showed a marked decline within a few hours after drug administration. It is not known if statins are metabolized in brain. Simvastatin, atorvastatin, and lovastatin are substrates for CYP3A4, which is the primary CYP isoform involved in the metabolism of those drugs,[15] and this enzyme is present in rodent brain.[25] There are no published data on whether statins induce CYP3A4 in brain. Pravastatin is not metabolized by CYP3A4 and it is eliminated mostly unchanged.[15] A different mechanism which could contribute to the elimination of statins from brain is the transporter P-glycoprotein (P-gp). Previous studies have shown that P-gp is involved in the excretion, absorption, and distribution of hydrophobic and amphipathic drugs.[26] Statins are substrates for P-gp and this transporter may play a role in statin efflux from cells.[27,28] P-gp is a major component of the blood-brain barrier[29] and it is located in different brain cell types including neurons.[28] P-gp could act as a transporter both at the blood-brain barrier and neuronal cells.

Statin-induced neuroprotection versus cell death

In studies using animal models and various cell types, statins have been shown to provide protection to various types of insults, for example, *N*-methyl-D-aspartate (NMDA) and glutamate,[30,31] amyloid beta-protein,[32] oxygen glucose deprivation,[33,34] sodium nitroprusside,[35] and bone morphogenetic protein.[36] However, there are data indicating that statins can have toxic effects on brain neural cells, for example, Refs. 37–42. In general, what distinguishes the studies on protective effects of statins versus toxic effects are the drug concentrations used in the different studies. Most studies reporting neuroprotection have used statin concentrations ranging between 100 nM and 1 μM although it was reported that rosuvastatin at a concentration of 5 μM reduced toxicity of oxygen-glucose deprivation in rat primary cortical neurons.[34] Effects of rosuvastatin alone on cell viability were not reported in that study. Statin-induced reductions in cell viability have typically used drug concentrations ranging, for example, between 2 μM and 300 μM. An exception is a recent study which found that simvastatin at a concentration of 0.1 μM and 1 μM induced cell death in a mouse cerebellar slice culture preparation.[43] Several issues are raised by this interesting study. One possibility is that statin effects differ in cerebellar tissue as compared to other brain areas. Cholesterol abundance is less in mouse synaptic plasma membrane of the cerebellum as compared with membranes of the cerebral cortex and hippocampus.[44] Statin-induced reduction of cholesterol may have more pronounced effects in brain regions where cholesterol levels are lower relative to other brain regions. Also, there are no available data on comparisons between effects of statins on brain slices from postnatal mice versus primary neurons from embryonic mice which may have an influence of the actions of statins. A prudent observation is that the use of high statin concentrations in neural cells is unwarranted unless the goal is to induce cell dysfunction and death.

Even though statins are shown to be associated with neuroprotection both *in vitro* and *in vivo*, the issue of drug concentration should also be considered with respect to statin dosage used when treating human patients. We have shown that chronic administration of simvastatin (50 mg/kg/day for

21 days) in mice and guinea pigs[17,35] increased gene expression and protein levels of Bcl-2, the major anti-apoptotic gene/protein member of the Bcl-2 family. Both lovastatin (20 mg/kg/day i.p. for 14 days) and atorvastatin (20 mg/kg/day orally for 7 or 21 days) administered to rats reduced the pro-inflammatory calcitonin gene-related peptide and substance P in the dorsal root ganglion.[36] The statin concentrations used in those three studies are noticeably higher than doses taken by human subjects, which generally range between 5 and 80 mg tablet per day.[45] The human dosage is not based on body weight. If statins were prescribed for human patients based on body weight, a 70 kg human male would be taking approximately 0.07/mg/kg/day to 1.14/mg/kg/day, which is far less than statin concentrations used in animal studies. The issue of statin concentration also applies to the *in vitro* studies where relatively low drug concentrations (0.1 to 1 μM) were employed. Brain statin concentrations were found to be at the pmol level in brain tissue of mice administered different statins[17,18] and those *in vivo* levels are distinctly lower than the statin concentrations used in studies of neuroprotection in neural cells. It is worth noting that there are no data on intracellular statin concentrations of drug treated cells and is further evidence of the lack of basic data on statins.

Statins and brain isoprenoids

The mevalonate pathway produces several biologically active molecules which play an important role in cell function. One of those molecules is cholesterol, which has certainly garnered intensive study. Upstream of cholesterol in that pathway are two isoprenoids farnesyl pyrophosphate (FPP) and geranylgeranyl pyrophosphate (GGPP) which are receiving increasing attention both with respect to normal function and their potential contributions to pathophysiology associated with coronary heart disease, cancer, and neurodegenerative diseases.[46–49] Until recently, the protective effects of statins in coronary heart disease were largely attributable to a reduction in cholesterol levels but there is emerging evidence that the reduction of isoprenoid levels specifically FPP and GGPP may also be important in preventing cardiovascular disease by reducing the abundance of prenylated proteins.[46] FPP and GGPP belong to a group of isoprenoids which include, for example, ubiquinone and dolichol. FPP is a C_{15} isoprenoid, which is the key branch point in the synthesis of ubiquinone, dolichol, and GGPP, as well as cholesterol. In addition to its critical role in synthesis, FPP posttranslationally prenylates by farnesyl transferase the small GTPases such as H-ras, Rheb, and other proteins containing a cysteine in the C-terminal CaaX box (C = cysteine, a = aliphatic amino acid and X = C-terminal amino acid).[50,51] FPP is a substrate for geranylgeranyl pyrophosphate synthase resulting in the production of GGPP, a 20-carbon lipid as compared with the 15-carbon FPP. Whereas FPP prenylates proteins containing a cystine of the CaaX box of the C terminal, GGPP on the other hand prenylates proteins containing a C-terminal leucine residue by geranylgeranyl prenyltranferase-1 (GGTase-1), such as the Rho family of GTPase and Rac-1. These and other prenylated proteins are integral components of complex signaling networks and control diverse cellular activities including intracellular vesicle transport, cell adhesion, endocytosis, cytoskeletal organization, receptor signaling, cell cycle progression, and gene expression.[51]

It has been suggested that the neuroprotective effects of statins may be due in part to a reduction in FPP and/or GGPP levels which in turn lessens the abundance of prenylated proteins and which may or may not be cholesterol independent.[5,9,48] To rule out the contribution of statin-induced lowering of cholesterol levels, one approach is to incubate cells with a squalene synthase inhibitor which prevents the production of squalene and subsequently cholesterol. The reasoning is that reducing cholesterol levels by non-statin intervention leaves FPP and GGPP levels unaffected. If reducing cholesterol levels by squalene synthase inhibition has the same effect, such as increasing protein A as did a statin, then the conclusion is that the effects are cholesterol-dependent. On the other hand, if there is no change in the effect of non-statin cholesterol reduction on protein A then the conclusion is that such effects may be mediated by statin-induced reduction of FPP or GGPP. To test those possibilities, two different approaches can be used: (1) incubating cells with exogenous FPP or GGPP in the presence of a statin; or (2) incubating cells with specific inhibitors of FPP and GGPP transferases involved in protein prenylation. If the addition of FPP or GGPP reduces effects of the statin on protein A, then one interpretation is that the statin effects are due to a reduction of FPP or GGPP levels but that has never been directly tested in brain, that is, FPP and GGPP levels determined. There are no *in vivo* or *in vitro* data on effects of statins on FPP and GGPP levels in brain. In the example of using an inhibitor of one of the transferases, if effects on response A are similar to the statin effects, then the conclusion is that statin-induced reduction of FPP or GGPP and not cholesterol is the underlying mechanism.

In practice, the manipulation of FPP, GGPP, and cholesterol levels as described above seems a workable approach to tease out the contributions of the different mevalonate-derived lipids acted upon by statins. We and other groups have used such an approach[32,52,53] but it is problematic for several different reasons. In a typical experiment, μmol amounts or greater of FPP or GGPP are incubated with cells. Recent studies of mouse brain[54] and human brain[55] have demonstrated that levels of FPP and GGPP are in the pmol to nmol range and that GGPP abundance is markedly higher than FPP. Until those two studies, data on brain FPP and GGPP levels had not been determined and thus the rationale was not clear for incubating cells with μmol amounts of FPP and GGPP. In view of the finding that brain GGPP levels were several fold higher than FPP levels, adding μmol amounts of FPP to cells could possibly have confounding effects on regulation within the HMG-CoA reductase pathway. An example of unexpected consequences when perturbing a member of the HMG-CoA reductase pathway is a study which reported that cells treated with the squalene synthase inhibitor, zaragozic acid, showed over a 250-fold increase in FPP levels but only a 4-fold increase in GGPP levels in the mouse fibroblast cell line NIH3T3.[56] The reasoning for reducing cholesterol levels by means that do not reduce FPP and GGPP levels allows one to determine if effects of statins are due to only cholesterol reduction. However, the key observation that zaragozic acid treatment of cells has such a remarkable impact on FPP levels belies the notion that only cholesterol levels are altered by such treatment. That experiment was a relatively uncomplicated experiment in design but the fact that FPP and GGPP levels were quantified provided major insight into FPP and GGPP homeostasis and such insight is lacking in understanding isoprenoid regulation in brain and underscores the need for more research. To date, there are no published data effects of statins *in vivo* or *in vitro* on brain FPP and GGPP levels.

Conclusions

Statins may be efficacious in preventing and treating certain neurodegenerative diseases and support is based in part on animal and cell culture studies. Further progress in understanding the mechanisms of statin-induced neuroprotection are hampered by a lack of fundamental data on actions of statins in the CNS. Three major topics which need to be addressed are the pharmacokinetics of lipophilic and hydrophilic statins in brain, cell protection versus cell death and regulation of brain isoprenoids. Table 1 summarizes suggested directions of research under each of the three topics. There is inadequate knowledge on each of these topics which we suggest has in some instances resulted in erroneous conclusions. For example, the notion that hydrophilic statins do not cross the blood-brain barrier is not supported by the limited data available. Basic studies are needed on statin transport in and out of brain as well as whether metabolism of statins occurs in the CNS. The issue of statin-induced cell protection versus cell death may simply be explainable by drug concentration but this issue requires further investigation. Regulation of brain FPP and GGPP

Table 1. Statins in brain: recommendations for future research

Pharmacokinetics	Protection versus cell death	FPP and GGPP
Active transport of statins in and out of brain	Role of statin concentration *in vivo* and *in vitro*	Statin effects on brain FPP and GGPP levels
Brain metabolism of statins	Human therapeutic drug doses versus experimental doses	Regulation of FPP and GGPP in brain
Statin lactonization	Brain region/cell specific effects	FPP used for cholesterol or GGPP

FPP: farnesyl pyrophosphate; GGPP: geranylgeranyl pyrophosphate.

are not understood. It is assumed that FPP and GGPP levels are reduced in brains of animals and neural cells treated with statins but there are no reported data. What is instructive is that the two recent studies reporting brain levels of FPP and GGPP in mice and humans found that GGPP was in greater abundance than FPP and isoprenoid levels were in the range of pmol to nmol. From a practical standpoint, those data have relevance to the procedure of examining effects of statins by adding back μmol amounts of FPP and/or GGPP in neural cells. Statins may be neuroprotective but efforts toward understanding the potential mechanisms will be enhanced by advancements in the CNS pharmacokinetics and pharmacodynamics of statins.

Note added in proof

After acceptance of this manuscript, we (Eckert *et al.*, Neurobiology of Disease, 2009, 35, 251–257) reported that FPP and GGPP levels were significantly elevated in brain tissue of Alzheimer's disease (AD) patients compared with control subjects but that cholesterol levels were unchanged. FPP synthase gene expression was significantly elevated in the AD brain however gene expression of HMG-CoA reductase did not differ between the two groups. These results indicate a disease-specific targeting of isoprenoid regulation independent of HMG-CoA reductase. In the same study, additional support for the hypothesis of selective disruption of FPP and GGPP homeostasis in AD, we showed for the first time that statin induced inhibition of HMG-CoA reductase *in vivo* significantly reduced FPP, GGPP, and cholesterol abundance in mice with the greatest effect on the isoprenoids. Impaired regulation of FPP and GGPP in AD could impact on protein prenylation and certainly contribute to AD neuropathophysiology.

Acknowledgment

This work was supported in part by grants from the National Institutes of Health AG-23524, AG-18357, Department of Veterans Affairs, Hanna Bragard-Apfel Foundation, and Alzheimer Forschung Initiative.

Conflicts of interest

The authors declare no conflicts of interest.

References

1. Tobert, J.A. 2003. Lovastatin and beyond: the history of the HMG-CoA reductase inhibitors. *Nat. Rev.* **2:** 517–526.
2. Law, M.R. *et al.* 2003. Quantifying effect of statins on low density lipoprotein cholesterol, ischaemic heart disease, and stroke: systematic review and meta-analysis. *Br. Med. J.* **326:** 1–7.
3. Nassief, A. & J.D. Marsh. 2008. Statin therapy for stroke prevention. *Stroke* **39:** 1042–1048.
4. Wahner, A.D. *et al.* 2008. Statin use and the risk of Parkinson disease. *Neurology* **70:** 1418–1422.
5. Eckert, G.P. *et al.* 2005. Statins: drugs for Alzheimer's disease? *J. Neural Transm.* **112:** 1057–1071.
6. Neuhaus, O. & H.P. Hartung. 2007. Evaluation of atorvastatin and simvastatin for treatment of multiple sclerosis. *Expert. Rev. Neurother.* **7:** 547–556.
7. Tapia-Perez, J.H. *et al.* 2008. Effect of rosuvastatin on amnesia and disorientation after traumatic brain injury (NCT003229758). *J. Neurotrauma.* **25:** 1011–1017.
8. Stepien, K. *et al.* 2005. Neuroprotective properties of statins. *Pharmacol. Rep.* **57:** 561–569.
9. Eckert, G.P. *et al.* 2007. Cholesterol-lowering drugs and Alzheimer's disease. *Future Lipidol.* **2:** 423–432.
10. Tapia-Perez, H. *et al.* 2007. Statins and brain protection mechanisms. *Revista de Neurologia* **45:** 359–364.
11. Farooqui, A.A. *et al.* 2007. Comparison of biochemical effects of statins and fish oil in brain: the battle of the titans. *Brain Res. Rev.* **56:** 443–471.
12. Orr, J.D. 2008. Statins in the spectrum of neurologic disease. *Curr. Atheroscler. Rep.* **10:** 11–18.
13. Botti, R.E. *et al.* 1991. Concentrations of pravastatin and lovastatin in cerebrospinal fluid in healthy subjects. *Clin. Neuropharmacol.* **14:** 256–261.
14. Ishigami, M. *et al.* 2001. A comparison of the effects of 3-hydroxy-3-methylglutaryl-coenzyme A (HMG-CoA) reductase inhibitors on the CYP3A4-dependent oxidation of mexazolam *in vitro*. *Drug Metab. Dispos.* **29:** 282–288.
15. Schachter, M. 2004. Chemical, pharmacokinetic and pharmacodynamic properties of statins: an update. *Fund Clin. Pharmacol.* **19:** 117–125.
16. Saheki, A. *et al.* 1994. *In vivo* and *in vitro* blood-brain barrier transport of 3-hydroxy-3-methylglutaryl coenzyme A (HMG-CoA) reductase inhibitors. *Pharm. Res.* **11:** 305–311.
17. Johnson-Anuna, L.N. *et al.* 2005. Chronic administration of statins alters multiple gene expression patterns in mouse cerebral cortex. *J. Pharmacol. Exp. Ther.* **312:** 786–793.

18. Thelen, K.M. *et al.* 2006. Brain cholesterol synthesis in mice is affected by high dose of simvastatin but not of pravastatin. *J. Pharmacol. Exp. Ther.* **316:** 1146–1152.
19. Hasegawa, M. *et al.* 2003. Contribution of organic anion transporters to the renal uptake of anionic compounds and nucleoside derivatives. *J. Pharmacol. Exp. Ther.* **305:** 1087–1097.
20. Takeda, M. *et al.* 2004. Evidence for a role of human organic anion transporters in the muscular side effects of HMG-CoA reductase inhibitors. *Eur. J. Pharmacol.* **483:** 133–138.
21. Kusuhara, H. *et al.* 1999. Molecular cloning and characterization of a new multispecific organic anion transporter from rat brain. *J. Biol. Chem.* **274:** 13675–13680.
22. Tsuji, A. *et al.* 1993. Transport mechanism of 3-hydroxy-3-methylglutaryl coenzyme A reductase inhibitors at the blood-brain barrier. *J. Pharmacol. Exp. Ther.* **267:** 1085–1090.
23. Jacobsen, W. *et al.* 2000. Lactonization is the critical first step in the disposition of the 3-hydroxy-3-methylglutaryl-CoA reductase inhibitor atorvastatin. *Drug Metab. Dispos.* **28:** 1369–1378.
24. Kantola, T. *et al.* 1998. Effect of itraconazole on the pharmacokinetics of atorvastatin. *Clin. Pharmacol. Ther.* **64:** 58–65.
25. Pai, H.V. *et al.* 2002. Differential metabolism of alprazolam by liver and brain c (P4503A) to pharmacologically active metabolite. *Pharmacogenomics* **2:** 243–258.
26. Schinkel, A.H. 1997. The physiological function of drug-transporting P-glycoproteins. *Semin. Cancer Biol.* **8:** 161–170.
27. Bogman, K. *et al.* 2001. HMG CoA reductase inhibitors and P-glycoprotein modulation. *Br. J. Pharmacol.* **132:** 1183–1192.
28. Hirrlinger, J. *et al.* 2002. Expression of mRNAs of multidrug resistance proteins (Mrps) in cultured rat astrocytes, oligodendrocytes, microglial cells and neurons. *J. Neurochem.* **82:** 716–729.
29. Sun, H. *et al.* 2003. Drug efflux transporters in the CNS. *Adv. Drug Deliv. Rev.* **55:** 83–105.
30. Zacco, A. *et al.* 2003. 3-Hydroxy-3-methylglutaryl coenzyme A reductase inhibitors protect cortical neurons from excitotoxicity. *J. Neurosci.* **23:** 11104–11111.
31. Bösel, J. *et al.* 2005. Neuroprotective effects of atorvastatin against glutamate-induced excitotoxicity in primary cortical neurones. *J. Neurochem.* **92:** 1386–1398.
32. Johnson-Anuna, L.N. *et al.* 2007. Simvastatin protects neurons from cytotoxicity by up-regulating Bcl-2 mRNA and protein. *J. Neurochem.* **101:** 77–86.
33. Lim, J.H. *et al.* 2006. Simvastatin prevents oxygen and glucose deprivation/reoxygenation-induced death of cortical neurons by reducing the production and toxicity of 4-hydroxy-2E-nonenal. *J. Neurochem.* **97:** 140–150.
34. Domoki, F. *et al.* 2009. Rosuvastatin induces delayed preconditioning against oxygen-glucose deprivation in cultured cortical neurons. *Am. J. Physiol. Cell Physiol.* **296:** C97–C105.
35. Franke, C. *et al.* 2007. Bcl-2 upregulation and neuroprotection in guinea pig brain following chronic simvastatin treatment. *Neurobiol. Dis.* **25:** 438–445.
36. Bucelli, R.C. *et al.* 2008. Statins decrease expression of the proinflammatory neuropeptides calcitonin gene-related peptide and substance P in sensory neurons. *J. Pharmacol. Exp. Ther.* **324:** 1172–1180.
37. Michikawa, M. & K.Yanagisawa. 1999. Inhibition of cholesterol production but not of nonsterol isoprenoid products induces neuronal cell death. *J. Neurochem.* **72:** 2278–2285.
38. Tanaka, T. *et al.* 2000. Geranylgeranyl-pyrophosphate, an isoprenoid of mevalonate cascade, is a critical compound for rat primary cultured cortical neurons to protect the cell death induced by 3-hydroxy-3-methylglutaryl-CoA reductase inhibition. *J. Neurosci.* **20:** 2852–2859.
39. Schulz, J.G. *et al.* 2004. HMG-CoA reductase inhibition causes neurite loss by interfering with geranylgeranylpyrophosphate synthesis. *J. Neurochem.* **89:** 24–32.
40. Jiang, Z. *et al.* 2004. Lovastatin-induced up-regulation of the BH3-only protein, Bim, and cell death in glioblastoma cells. *J. Neurochem.* **89:** 168–178.
41. März, P. *et al.* 2007. Statins induce differentiation and cell death in neurons and astroglia. *Glia* **55:** 1–12.
42. Klopfleisch, S. *et al.* 2008. Negative impact of statins on oligodendrocytes and myelin formation *in vitro* and *in vivo*. *J. Neurosci.* **28:** 13609–13614.
43. Xiang, Z. & S.A. Reeves. 2009. Simvastatin induces cells death in a mouse cerebellar slice culture (CSC) model of developmental myelination. *Exp. Neurol.* **215:** 41–47.
44. Chochina, S.V. *et al.* 2001. Amyloid β-peptide$_{1-40}$ increases neuronal membrane fluidity: role of cholesterol and brain region. *J. Lipid Res.* **42:** 1292–1297.
45. Solomon, K.R. & M.R. Freeman. 2008. Do the cholesterol-lowering properties of statins affect cancer risk? *Trends Endocrinol. Metab.* **19:** 113–121.
46. Liao, J.K. & U. Laufs. 2004. Pleiotropic effects of statins. *Annu. Rev. Pharmacol. Toxicol.* **45:** 89–118.

47. Swanson, K.M. & R.J. Hohl. 2006. Anti-cancer therapy: targeting the mevalonate pathway. *Curr. Cancer Drug Targets* **6:** 15–37.
48. Cole, S.L. & R. Vassar. 2006. Isoprenoids and Alzheimer's disease: a complex relationship. *Neurobiol. Dis.* **22:** 209–222.
49. Wood, W.G. *et al.* 2007. Cholesterol—a Janus faced molecule in the central nervous system. In *Handbook of Neurochemistry and Molecular Neurobiology-Neural Membranes and Transport*. A Lajtha & M.E.A. Reith, Eds.: 151–170. Springer. New York.
50. Basso, A.D. *et al.* 2006. Farnesyl transferase inhibitors. *J. Lipid Res.* **47:** 15–31.
51. Mc Taggart, S.J. 2006. Isoprenylated proteins. *Cell Mol. Life Sci.* **63:** 255–267.
52. Cole, S.L. 2005. Statins cause intracellular accumulation of amyloid precursor protein. β-secretase-cleaved fragments, and amyloid β-peptide via an isoprenoid-dependent mechanism. *J. Biol. Chem.* **280:** 18755–18770.
53. Ostrowski, S.M. *et al.* 2007. Statins reduce amyloid-β production through inhibition of protein isoprenylation. *J. Biol. Chem.* **282:** 26832–26844.
54. Tong, H. *et al.* 2008. Quantitative determination of farnesyl and geranylgeranyl diphosphate levels in mammalian tissue. *Anal. Biochem.* **378:** 138–143.
55. Hooff, G.P. *et al.* 2008. Isoprenoid quantitation in human brain tissue: a validated HPLC-fluorescence detection method for endogenous farnesyl- (FPP) and geranylgeranylpyrophosphate (GGPP). *Anal. Bioanal. Chem.* **392:** 673–680.
56. Tong, H. *et al.* 2005. Simultaneous determination of farnesyl and geranylgeranyl pyrophosphate levels in cultured cells. *Anal. Biochem.* **336:** 51–59.

Ann. N.Y. Acad. Sci. ISSN 0077-8923

ANNALS OF THE NEW YORK ACADEMY OF SCIENCES
Issue: *Neuroprotective Agents*

Neuroprotective effects of *Lepidium meyenii* (Maca)

Alejandro Pino-Figueroa, Diane Nguyen, and Timothy J. Maher

Department of Pharmaceutical Sciences, Massachusetts College of Pharmacy and Health Sciences, Boston, Massachusetts

Address for correspondence: Alejandro Pino-Figueroa, Department of Pharmaceutical Sciences, Massachusetts College of Pharmacy and Health Sciences, 179 Longwood Avenue, Boston, MA 02115. alejandro.pino@my.mcphs.edu

The neuroprotective activity of the plant *Lepidium meyenii* (Maca) was studied in two experimental models: *in vitro* and *in vivo*. Crayfish neurons were pretreated with vehicle or the pentane extract from Maca, subjected to H_2O_2, and their viability determined microscopically and chemically. A significant concentration-neuroprotective effect relationship was demonstrated. The pentane extract was then administered intravenously to rats prior to and following middle cerebral artery occlusion. While infarct volumes were decreased for the lower dose, higher doses increased infarct volumes compared to controls. These results suggest a potential application of Maca as a neuroprotectant.

Keywords: Maca; *Lepidium*; crayfish neurons; cerebral ischemia

Introduction

Much interest has focused on the prevention and treatment of neurodegenerative diseases and stroke,[1,2] but challenges relating to the complexity of the central nervous system (CNS) and neuronal death have been difficult to overcome.[3–9] One focus of the search for effective new drugs has been on complementary and alternative medicines. Medicinal plants have the great advantage that they have followed an indirect clinical trial during centuries of traditional use and usually many of the adverse effects and toxicities are known. In addition, they have been an important source of chemical compounds used as drugs or to model the synthesis of new drugs. Naturally occurring compounds also have the advantage of having been developed in living organisms during evolution to protect and improve the organism's survivability. Facing the complexity of neurodegeneration,[9,10] natural based drugs may be good candidates to target oxidative stress, stabilization of membranes, inactivation of enzymes, inhibition of apoptosis, or inhibition of inflammation so as to inhibit or decrease the cellular death and neuronal injury observed in focal ischemic stroke and many neurodegenerative diseases.

The Peruvian plant, *Lepidium meyenii* (Maca), was probably domesticated between the years 4000–1200 BC as indicated by primitive Maca cultivars that have been found in archeological sites in Peru.[11] Knowledge of this plant and its medicinal properties has been transferred from generation to generation and continues today.[12] The root (hypocotyls) of Maca can be baked or eaten after decoction, but typically is dried and stored for years before its consumption.[13] Thereafter, Maca has been traditionally used as a food and an essential folk medicine;[14] its tremendous value has led many Peruvians to regard Maca as a fundamental component of their diet and medicinal treatments.[15] Used to enhance sexual behavior in men and women, fertility, energy, and reduce stress and menopausal symptoms,[13] it is also recommended in traditional medicine as effective in cancer prevention and treatment, anemia, gastritis, high blood pressure, and depression.[12,16] While several studies have already been conducted to examine Maca as a potential treatment in various disorders, pharmacological studies are still needed to determine and better characterize the properties attributed to this plant.

Chemical studies have demonstrated that the hypocotyls of the plant contain various compounds: alkaloids (macaridine, lepidilin A, lepidilin B, lepidine, tetrahydro-β-carbolines, and others),[17–19] glucosinolates (glucotropaeolin, glucoalyssin, glucobrassicanapin, glucobrassicin, and others),[19–21] aromatic isothiocyanates (benzylisothiocyanate, 4-methoxybenzylisothiocyanate, and others),[19]

doi: 10.1111/j.1749-6632.2009.05174.x

steroids (brassicasterol, ergostadienol, and others),[22] benzylated amides (macamides),[18,23–25] and acyclic polyunsaturated oxoacids (macaenes).[19,23] Most likely other compounds will be discovered in the future. The aerial parts of the plant contain essential oils mainly constituted by phenylacetonitrile, benzaldehyde, and 3-methoxyphenylacetonitrile.[26]

The published pharmacological results of Maca investigations provide information about the effect of the whole hypocotyls or its crude extract administered orally, especially regarding the fertility enhancer and pro-aphrodisiac effects in mice,[27,28] rats,[29–37] and humans,[38–40] and the preventive effect on the UV-induced skin damage.[41] Other results demonstrate the antistress,[42] antiosteoporosis,[43] and prostate size reduction effects in mice and rats.[44,45] Recent studies have demonstrated the effect on learning and depression in ovariectomized mice,[46] on memory impairment induced by scopolamine[47] and ovariectomy in mice.[48] Clinical studies have also demonstrated the effect of the dried powdered hypocotyls on serotonin-selective reuptake inhibitor (SSRI)-induced sexual dysfunction[49] and on postmenopausal psychological signs.[50] *In vitro* studies have demonstrated antioxidant and antiapoptotic activity in macrophages,[51] absence of toxicity to rat hepatocytes[52] and also the lack of direct androgenic effects in prostatic cancer cells.[53] One study reported estrogenic effects as increasing proliferation of human breast cancer cells (MCF-7).[52] Most of the studies in animals did not report toxicity,[13] however preliminary toxicological assessments in humans have shown that 90 days consumption of 0.6 g/day of dried hypocotyl powder leads to significant increases in diastolic blood pressure and plasma aminotransferase (AST).[54] Overall, there still is a need for additional pharmacological studies to demonstrate other properties attributed to this plant and answer questions remaining about the efficacy, doses, mechanisms of action, responsible compounds, biopharmaceutical properties, safety, toxicity, adverse effects, and possible clinical applications of the plant, preparations, or its isolated compounds.

The goal of this study was to determine the possible neuroprotective properties of the lipophilic compounds from *Lepidium meyenii* tested *in vitro* in cell culture, and *in vivo* in rats subjected to focal ischemic stroke. The lipophilic nature of some of the constituents of Maca could facilitate their passage through the blood-brain barrier and act within the CNS. Some constituents present in Maca have reported activity in the CNS.[55–57] Standardized extracts could act along with endogenous compounds, or mimic endogenous compounds with demonstrated neuroprotective efficacy, or block neurodegenerative processes.[58] Maca could be a neuroprotective agent alone or act synergistically with other agents to prevent neurodegeneration and/or reduce cell death in stroke and other neurodegenerative diseases.

Materials and methods

Plant material and extract preparations

Dried hypocotyls of *Lepidium meyenii*, procured from Arequipa, Peru, were botanically identified at the faculty of Pharmacy and Biochemistry of the Catholic University of Arequipa, and then were chemically identified at the Massachusetts College of Pharmacy and Health Sciences (MCPHS) and the University of Mississippi. The dried hypocotyls (750 g) were comminuted into a powder and extracted with 3 L of methanol (HPLC grade, Pharmco-AAPER, Brookfield, CT) for a period of 48 h. The methanol extract was then filtered, concentrated in a rotary-evaporator to 1 L and mixed with an equal volume of distilled water, underwent a liquid–liquid continuous re-extraction with n-pentane 98% (Sigma-Aldrich, St. Louis, MO) for 24 h, after which time it was dried in a rotary-evaporator and the residue was kept under refrigeration. The yield of the pentane extract was 0.68%.

In all of the *in vitro* experiments, the pentane fraction was dissolved in 10% DMSO (Sigma-Aldrich) in phosphate-buffered saline (PBS, Mediatech, Manassas, VA). For the *in vivo* study, the pentane extract was redissolved in methanol with six times its weight of poly-vinyl-pirrolidone (PVP) 30 K (GAF Chemicals Corporation, Wayne, NJ), the solution was dried in a rotary evaporator until constant weight and the residue dissolved in sterile water before administration.

Cells and culture media

In this study we used *Orconectes limosus* (crayfish) neuronal cells, OLGA-PH-J/92 (ATCC, Manassas, VA). This cell line exhibits certain transformation features, such as anchorage independence and loss of contact inhibition. Its stable growth characteristics and morphology from the primary culture throughout higher passages may suggest that the cells are neuronal stem cells (ATCC product description).

The crayfish neuronal cells were cultured in minimum essential medium (MEM, Sigma-Aldrich) supplemented with sodium bicarbonate (2.2 g/L, Sigma-Aldrich), HEPES (9.52 g/L, Sigma-Aldrich), sodium pyruvate (0.11 g/L, Sigma-Aldrich), and 10% fetal bovine serum (ATCC). The pH of the supplemented base media was then adjusted to 6.8.[59]

In vitro neuroprotection assay

The cells were cultured in T-flasks at 27° C until 80% confluent growth. The medium was removed from the flask, a scraper was used to detach the cells, and the cells were suspended in supplemented MEM. The cell suspension underwent total cell counting with trypan blue dye using a hemocytometer to determine the number of viable cells per μL to ensure a seeding density of 1×10^5 cells per well. MEM was subsequently added to yield a total volume of 180 μL per well. Twenty-four h after the cell seeding the wells were pretreated with 20 μL of the pentane extract solutions or vehicle. The final concentrations of pentane extract assayed were 0.1, 0.3, 1, 3, 10, and 30 μg/mL. Five replicates were performed for every assay. Three h later, 20 μL of 0.001 mol/L hydrogen peroxide (H_2O_2, Sigma-Aldrich), as a neurotoxic agent,[60] or vehicle, were added to the wells. Microscopic morphology of the cells was observed and photographed 18 h later.

Cell viability assay for concentration-effect correlation

Cell viability was measured using a colorimetric method for the determination of cells in proliferation, with tetrazolium compound 3-(4,5-dimethylthiazol-2-yl)-5-(3-carboxymethoxyphenyl)-2-(4-sulphophenyl)-2H-tetrazolium salt (MTS, Promega, Madison, WI), which is bioreduced by cells into a formazan blue product that is soluble in the cell culture medium. Ten μL of MTS reagent was added to wells 3 h after the H_2O_2 treatment and an absorbance measurement was performed on well plates using a 96-well plate reader at a wavelength of 490 nm, after an incubation period of 24 h. Estimation of the viable cells is possible as the absorbance of the blue color is directly proportional to the number of metabolically active cells. The neuroprotective effect is estimated as the percentage of absorbance increase compared with the absorbance in the wells treated only with H_2O_2 (maximal damage), 0% of neuroprotection. The absorbance in the wells treated only with vehicle (no damage) was considered as 100% of neuroprotection.

Animals

Thirty-six (36) adult male Sprague–Dawley rats (300–350 g) from Charles River Laboratories (Wilmington, MA) were housed under standard conditions of ambient temperature (74 ± 3°F), relative humidity (55 ± 15%), and 12:12 h light:dark cycles, five days before the study and were divided into four groups of nine animals each. Food and water were available *ad libitum*. All experimental animal protocols were reviewed and approved by the Institutional Animal Care and Use Committee (IACUC).

Development of focal infarction

Animals were anesthetized with i.p. chloral hydrate (Sigma-Aldrich) 400 mg/kg. The common carotid arteries were isolated via a ventral midline cervical incision and both arteries were eventually ligated for one h. Then, a 1.5 cm scalp incision was made at the midpoint between the right eye and the right ear. The temporalis muscle was separated and retracted to expose the zygoma and squamosal bone. A hole was made with a dental drill 1 mm rostal to the anterior junction of the zygoma and squamosal bone. Bone and dura mater were carefully pierced to expose the middle cerebral artery. The artery was occluded with a bipolar coagulator (Radionics, LabX, Riverview, FL). The craniotomy was cleaned and the temporalis muscle and overlying skin were allowed to fall back and were sutured separately. After one h the common carotid arteries were reperfused and the ventral incision cleaned and sutured.[61]

Treatment

The four groups of animals received a double tail vein injection, the first when anesthetized before surgery (30 min prior to stroke), and the second when the common carotid arteries were reperfused at the end of surgery (one h after stroke). One group of animals (Control) was treated with aqueous PVP solution and the other three groups (Maca) were treated with the pentane extract at doses of 3, 10, and 30 mg/kg per injection.

Infarct volume evaluation

Twenty-four h after the treatment, the animals were deeply anesthetized with i.p. chloral hydrate and decapitated. The brains were extracted and kept in a cold saline solution under refrigeration for 15 min. Brains were sliced and treated with 2% triphenyltetrazolium-chloride (TTC, Sigma-Aldrich) solution for 30 min and kept in the dark. The stained slices were transferred to 10% formalin buffered solution (Sigma-Aldrich), for photographs after 24 h. Infarct volumes, measured using the Image J program, were expressed as percentages relatives to the total tissue in the brain hemisphere.

Statistical analysis

Data were analyzed for statistical significance and results are presented as mean ± SEM. Homogeneity of variances was assessed using the ANOVA. A P-value less than 0.05 was considered significant. If the P-value in the ANOVA test was significant, post hoc Bonferroni testing was performed when indicated. The concentration-effect relationship was analyzed by linear regression.

Results

Crayfish neurons neuroprotective assay

Following pretreatment of crayfish neurons with pentane extract solutions or vehicle, and treated with H_2O_2, differences in cell appearance could be microscopically detected as shown in Figures 1A to D. As compared to the dendritic shape and dense concentration of untreated cells, Figure 1A, and the spherical shape and sparse concentration of cells subjected to H_2O_2 (negative control), Figure 1B, cells treated with different concentrations of the pentane fraction exhibited varying cell shapes and densities. Cells treated with 30 μg/mL pentane extract displayed healthier dendritic cell shapes than cells treated with 3 μg/mL pentane extract as shown in Figures 1C and D. Linear regression analysis of the six concentrations of pentane extract demonstrated a significant concentration effect ($P \leq 0.03$ and $r = +0.85$). Figure 2 shows the percentages of neuroprotection as calculated from the absorbances of the MTS-treated wells after the experiments with the various pentane extract solutions (0.1 to 30 μg/mL) and H_2O_2 in the crayfish neurons. Results indicate that the effective concentration 50% (EC_{50}) to be approximately 2.8 μg/mL.

In vivo neuroprotective assay

The effect of the pentane extract was also evaluated in rats subjected to focal ischemic stroke. The results show statistically significant differences for the three doses (3, 10, 30 mg/kg) as shown in Figure 3. The control group showed an overall percentage of ischemic tissue of 23 ± 1.5 and the dose of 3 mg/kg was the only dose showing significant neuroprotective effects (13.5 ± 2.2%; $P \leq 0.002$). Doses of 10 and 30 mg/kg actually showed a significant increase in brain damage. The neuroprotective effect of the 3 mg/kg dose on the brain of a representative animal compared to a control brain is shown in Figures 4A and B. The colorless area represents the ischemic or dead tissue.

Discussion

Several studies have found Maca extracts to produce different pharmacological effects in animals and humans. Lipophilic extracts, which concentrate most of the active constituents found in the hypocotyls of *Lepidium meyenii*, have demonstrated to be the most pharmacologically interesting.[31] Because traditional claims and preliminary studies have supported the suggestion that the pentane extract of the Maca root could act as a neuroprotective agent, this study was developed to demonstrate the possible neuroprotective properties of the pentane extract from Maca by both *in vitro* and *in vivo* models, attempting to demonstrate and associate cellular and organic protection.[62]

The *in vitro* model using crayfish neurons subjected to oxidative stress with H_2O_2 allowed for the evaluation of the protective effect of the pentane extract.[60] Oxidative stress, defined as a disturbance in pro-oxidant-antioxidant balance, has been implicated in several neurodegenerative diseases characterized by cell death. Although reactive oxygen species (ROS), such as H_2O_2, are produced by normal metabolic processes, overproduction may result in oxidative-stress injuries that damage the integrity of cell function causing subsequent death by either necrosis or apoptosis.[10] Under optimal conditions in cell culture, without oxidative stressors,

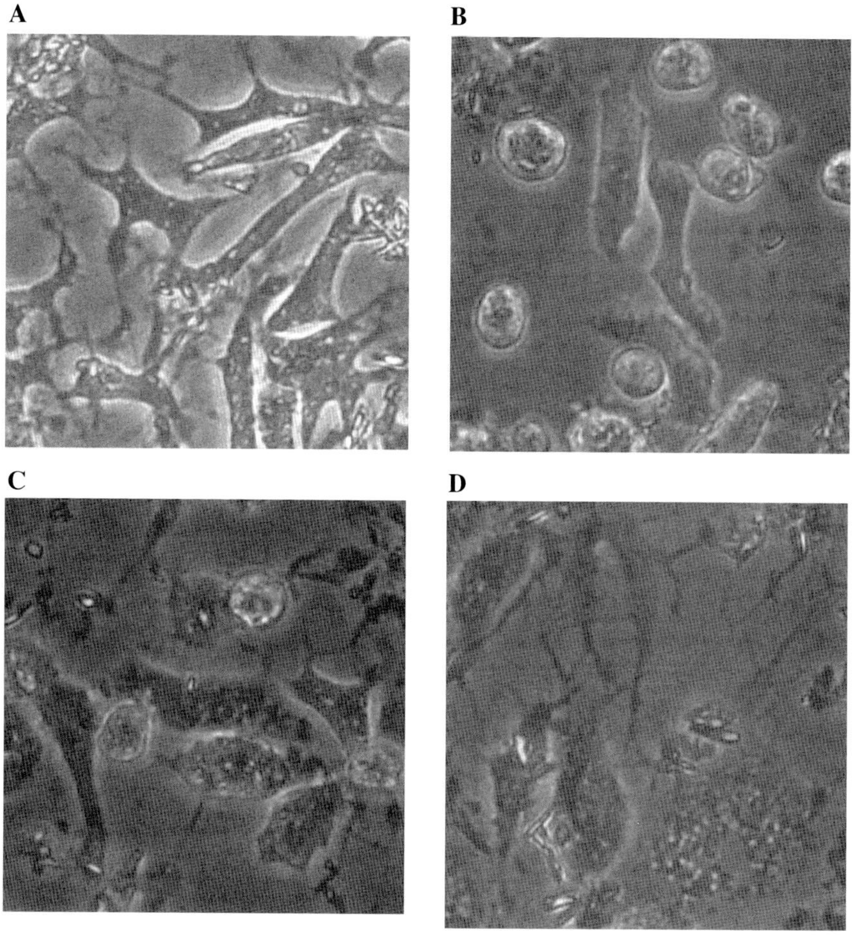

Figure 1. (A) *In vitro* model of neuroprotection with crayfish neurons. Control crayfish neurons without treatment. (B) Crayfish neurons treated with H_2O_2 0.001 mol/L. (C) Crayfish neurons pretreated with 3 μg/mL of pentane extract of *Lepidium meyenii* (Maca) and treated 3 h later with H_2O_2 (0.001 mol/L). (D) Crayfish neurons pretreated with 30 μg/mL of pentane extract of *Lepidium meyenii* (Maca) and treated 3 h later with H_2O_2 (0.001 mol/L).

the crayfish neurons assume appropriate dendritic shapes, extending and forming synapses with their surrounding neurons.[59,63] When oxidative stressors are applied these neurons lose their dendrites and transform into spherical shapes, suggesting a reversion to an undifferentiated state. Microscopic evaluations and cellular viability assays revealed a reduction in H_2O_2-induced stress in cells treated with the pentane extract. Cells treated with 30 μg/mL of the pentane fraction displayed more appropriate dendritic cell shapes and greater cell density compared to those treated with 3 μg/mL. Moreover, the cell viability assay demonstrated a significant linear correlation between the concentration of the pentane extract and the percentage of neuroprotection, ranging from 6.7% for the 0.1 μg/mL to 87.9% for the 30 μg/mL pentane extract.

The reduction of H_2O_2-induced cell oxidative stress *in vitro* by the pentane extract of *Lepidium meyenii* demonstrated in this preliminary study on crayfish neurons support the suggestion that this natural product has potential neuroprotective properties. Several possible mechanisms including the direct scavenging of ROS, stabilizing cell membranes to prevent lipid peroxidation, alleviating the damage by increasing the intracellular defensive mechanisms, or the inhibition or blockade of the biochemical cascades leading to cell death could be operating. Future studies are required to demonstrate the mechanisms involved and the

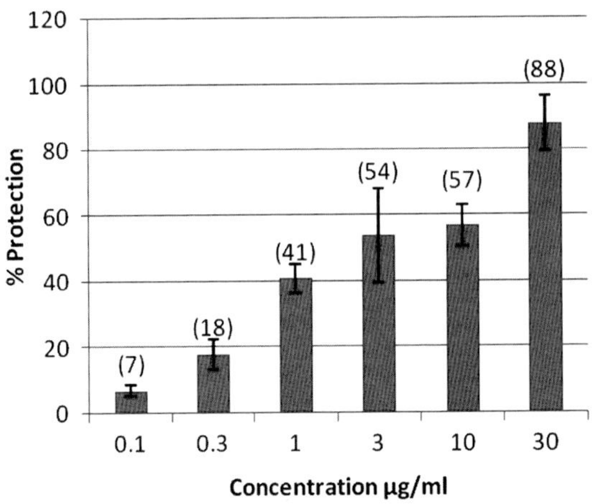

Figure 2. Concentration-effect of pentane extract of *Lepidium meyenii* (Maca) on % neuroprotection in crayfish neurons subjected to oxidative damage. Neurons were pretreated with the pentane extract and 3 h later 0.001 mol/L H_2O_2 was added. Bars represent the mean ± SEM, values in parentheses represent the mean.

participation of specific chemical entities. The techniques and comprehensive method developed to test neuroprotection on cells sets a foundation for future studies involving these and other neural cells and procedures.[64]

The effect of the pentane extract *in vivo* was then assessed in rats subjected to focal ischemic stroke. Occlusion of the middle cerebral artery (MCAO) in the rat is technically feasible and its histological consequences are consistent under controlled experimental conditions.[64] Improvement of the method includes 1 h transient occlusion of the common carotid arteries. Drugs demonstrating reduction of the infarct size in experimental stroke are considered potential neuroprotective candidates for the treatment of stroke and neurodegenerative diseases. In this study, 3 mg/kg of the pentane extract administered intravenously 30 min prior and 1 h after the onset of stroke showed a reduction from 23% to 13.5% in the percentage of infracted tissue resulting from MCAO. Contrary to this result, doses of 10 and 30 mg/kg produced a significant increase to 31.7% and 29.4%, respectively, of the infarct size demonstrating a neurodamaging effect under these stroke conditions.

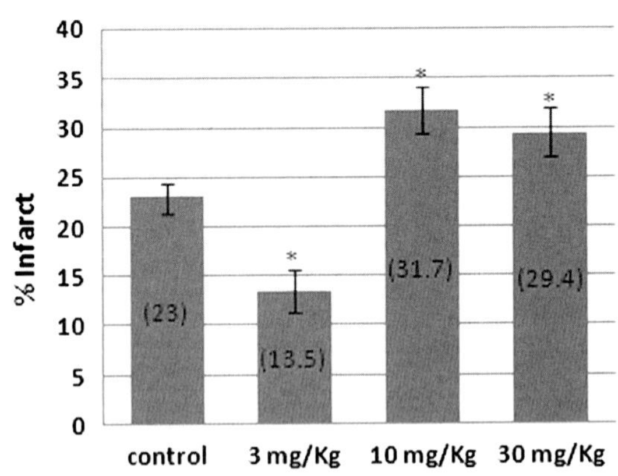

Figure 3. Effect of pentane extract from *Lepidium meyenii* (Maca) on % infarct in rats subjected to focal ischemic stroke. Values in parentheses represent the mean of the % infarct. Bars represent mean ± SEM. *Significantly $P < 0.05$ different from control.

This is a preliminary study of the effect of a pentane-extract of *Lepidium meyenii* administered intravenously in rats subjected to focal ischemic stroke. Previous pharmacological studies of the plant were performed with aqueous, hydroalcoholic or hexane extracts administered orally at equivalent doses without showing toxic effects. The pentane extract of Maca obtained by the method described contains mostly the lipo-soluble constituent alkaloids, benzylated amides (macamides), polyunsaturated oxoacids (macaenes), and benzylisothiocyanates. These compounds administered intravenously can likely reach the brain at higher concentration than other routes of administration. The results suggest that there are two different kinds of activity at the brain level in stroke conditions in rats, and possibly they depend on the different interaction of constituents with different cellular targets. One activity, at low doses, decreases the infarct volume indicating an inhibitory, antioxidative, or antiapoptotic mechanism that prevents cell death or protects neurons from ischemic insult. Another activity increasing the infarct volume, indicating that some excitatory, apoptotic, or neurotoxic processes are possibly activated at high doses. For instance, glucosinolates and isothiocyanates have reported pro-apoptotic and antiproliferative effects.[65,66]

The significant differences between the *in vitro* experiments that have not shown toxicity in cells at high concentrations, and the *in vivo* results showing deleterious effects at high doses may suggest new directions regarding potential mechanisms of action and toxicity that should be considered in

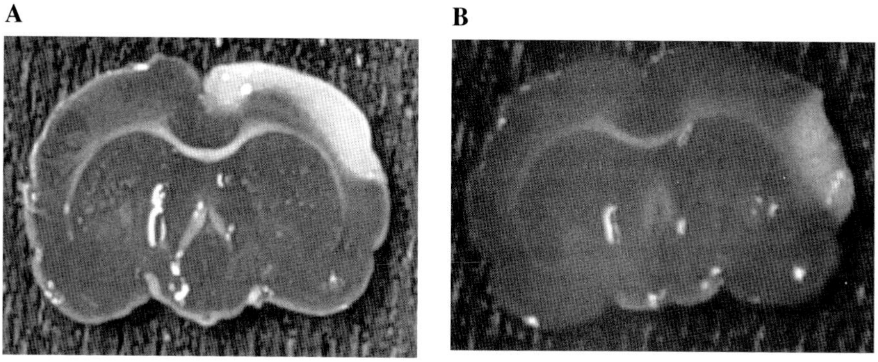

Figure 4. (**A**) Brain section of a rat subjected to focal ischemic stroke and treated with vehicle (control). (**B**) Brain section of a rat subjected to focal ischemic stroke and treated with pentane extract from *Lepidium meyenii* (Maca) at 3 mg/kg.

the future research on Maca. Other doses, different fractions of pentane extract, or isolated compounds need to be systematically evaluated for the neuroprotective mechanisms and toxicity to characterize the properties of *Lepidium meyenii*. The isolation and synthesis of derivatives may lead to the development of agents that can possibly be used to prevent or treat neurodegenerative diseases,[60] such as post-stroke, Alzheimer's disease,[67] and Parkinson's disease.[1]

Conflicts of interest

The authors declare no conflicts of interest.

References

1. Ravina, B.M., S.C. Fagan, R.G. Hart, *et al.* 2003. Neuroprotective agents for clinical trials in Parkinson's disease: a systematic assessment. *Neurology* **60:** 1234–1240.
2. Lo, E.H., M.A. Moskowitz & T.P. Jacobs. 2005. Exciting, radical, suicidal: how brain cells die after stroke. *Stroke* **36:** 189–192.
3. Garber, K. 2007. Stroke treatment–light at the end of the tunnel? *Nat. Biotechnol.* **25:** 838–840.
4. Lees, K.R. & J. Dawson. 2007. Advances in emerging therapies 2006. *Stroke* **38:** 219–221.
5. Love, S. 2003. Apoptosis and brain ischaemia. *Prog. Neuropsychopharmacol. Biol. Psychiatry* **27:** 267–282.
6. Unal-Cevik, I., M. Kilinc, A. Can, *et al.* 2004. Apoptotic and necrotic death mechanisms are concomitantly activated in the same cell after cerebral ischemia. *Stroke* **35:** 2189–2194.
7. del Zoppo, G.J. 2006. Stroke and neurovascular protection. *N. Engl. J. Med.* **354:** 553–555.
8. Hawkins, B.T. & T.P. Davis. 2005. The blood-brain barrier/neurovascular unit in health and disease. *Pharmacol. Rev.* **57:** 173–185.
9. Schabitz, W.R. & M. Fisher. 2006. Perspectives on neuroprotective stroke therapy. *Biochem. Soc. Trans.* **34:** 1271–1276.
10. Mehta, S.L., N. Manhas & R. Raghubir. 2007. Molecular targets in cerebral ischemia for developing novel therapeutics. *Brain Res. Rev.* **54:** 34–66.
11. Toledo, J. *et al.* 1998. Genetic variability of *Lepidium meyenii* and other Andean *Lepidium* species (Brassicaceae) assessed by molecular markers. *Ann. Bot.* **82:** 523–530.
12. Valentova, K. & J. Ulrichova. 2003. *Smallanthus sonchifolius* and *Lepidium meyenii* – prospective Andean crops for the prevention of chronic diseases. *Biomed. Pap. Med. Fac. Univ. Palacky Olomouc Czech. Repub.* **147:** 119–130.
13. Valerio, L.G., Jr. & G.F. Gonzales. 2005. Toxicological aspects of the South American herbs cat's claw (*Uncaria tomentosa*) and maca (*Lepidium meyenii*): a critical synopsis. *Toxicol. Rev.* **24:** 11–35.
14. Brinckmann, J. & E. Smith. 2004. Maca culture of the Junin Plateau. *J. Altern. Complement. Med.* **10:** 426–430.
15. Drewes, S.E., J. George & F. Khan. 2003. Recent findings on natural products with erectile-dysfunction activity. *Phytochemistry* **62:** 1019–1025.
16. Gonzales, G.F. & L.G. Valerio Jr. 2006. Medicinal plants from Peru: a review of plants as potential agents against cancer. *Anticancer Agents Med. Chem.* **6:** 429–444.
17. Cui, B., B.L. Zheng, K. He, *et al.* 2003. Imidazole alkaloids from *Lepidium meyenii*. *J. Nat. Prod.* **66:** 1101–1103.
18. Muhammad, I., J. Zhao, D.C. Dunbar, *et al.* 2002. Constituents of *Lepidium meyenii* 'maca'. *Phytochemistry* **59:** 105–110.

19. Piacente, S., V. Carbone, A. Plaza, *et al.* 2002. Investigation of the tuber constituents of maca (*Lepidium meyenii* Walp.). *J. Agric. Food Chem.* **50:** 5621–5625.
20. Ciska, E., B. Martyniak-Przybyszewska & H. Kozlowska. 2000. Content of glucosinolates in cruciferous vegetables grown at the same site for two years under different climatic conditions. *J. Agric. Food Chem.* **48:** 2862–2867.
21. Li, G., U. Ammermann & C.F. Quiros. 2001. Glucosinolate contents in maca (*Lepidium peruvianum* Chacon) seeds, sprouts and several derived commercial products. *Econ. Bot.* **55:** 255–262.
22. Dini, A. *et. al.* 1994. Chemical composition of *Lepidium meyenii. Food Chem.* **49:** 347–349.
23. Ganzera, M., J. Zhao, I. Muhammad, *et al.* 2002. Chemical profiling and standardization of *Lepidium meyenii* (maca) by reversed phase high performance liquid chromatography. *Chem. Pharm. Bull. (Tokyo)* **50:** 988–991.
24. McCollom, M.M., J.R. Villinski, K.L. McPhail, *et al.* 2005. Analysis of macamides in samples of maca (*Lepidium meyenii*) by HPLC-UV-MS/MS. *Phytochem. Anal.* **16:** 463–469.
25. Zhao, J., I. Muhammad, D.C. Dunbar, *et al.* 2005. New alkamides from maca (*Lepidium meyenii*). *J. Agric. Food Chem.* **53:** 690–693.
26. Tellez, M.R., I.A. Khan, M. Kobaisy, *et al.* 2002. Composition of the essential oil of *Lepidium meyenii* (Walp). *Phytochemistry* **61:** 149–155.
27. Bustos-Obregon, E., S. Yucra & G.F. Gonzales. 2005. *Lepidium meyenii* (maca) reduces spermatogenic damage induced by a single dose of malathion in mice. *Asian J. Androl.* **7:** 71–76.
28. Ruiz-Luna, A.C., S. Salazar, N.J. Aspajo, *et al.* 2005. *Lepidium meyenii* (maca) increases litter size in normal adult female mice. *Reprod. Biol. Endocrinol.* **3:** 16.
29. Chung, F., J. Rubio, C. Gonzales, *et al.* 2005. Dose-response effects of *Lepidium meyenii* (maca) aqueous extract on testicular function and weight of different organs in adult rats. *J. Ethnopharmacol.* **98:** 143–147.
30. Cicero, A.F., E. Bandieri & R. Arletti. 2001. *Lepidium meyenii* Walp. improves sexual behaviour in male rats independently from its action on spontaneous locomotor activity. *J. Ethnopharmacol.* **75:** 225–229.
31. Cicero, A.F., S. Piacente, A. Plaza, *et al.* 2002. Hexanic maca extract improves rat sexual performance more effectively than methanolic and chloroformic maca extracts. *Andrologia* **34:** 177–179.
32. Gonzales, G.F., M. Gasco, A. Cordova, *et al.* 2004. Effect of *Lepidium meyenii* (maca) on spermatogenesis in male rats acutely exposed to high altitude (4340 m). *J. Endocrinol.* **180:** 87–95.
33. Gonzales, G.F., J. Nieto, J. Rubio, *et al.* 2006. Effect of black maca (*Lepidium meyenii*) on one spermatogenic cycle in rats. *Andrologia* **38:** 166–172.
34. Gonzales, G.F., J. Rubio, A. Chung, *et al.* 2003. Effect of alcoholic extract of *Lepidium meyenii* (maca) on testicular function in male rats. *Asian J. Androl.* **5:** 349–352.
35. Gonzales, G.F., A. Ruiz, C. Gonzales, *et al.* 2001. Effect of *Lepidium meyenii* (maca) roots on spermatogenesis of male rats. *Asian J. Androl.* **3:** 231–233.
36. Rubio, J., M.I. Riqueros, M. Gasco, *et al.* 2006. *Lepidium meyenii* (maca) reversed the lead acetate induced—damage on reproductive function in male rats. *Food Chem. Toxicol.* **44:** 1114–1122.
37. Zheng, B.L., K. He, C.H. Kim, *et al.* 2000. Effect of a lipidic extract from *Lepidium meyenii* on sexual behavior in mice and rats. *Urology* **55:** 598–602.
38. Gonzales, G.F., A. Cordova, C. Gonzales, *et al.* 2001. *Lepidium meyenii* (maca) improved semen parameters in adult men. *Asian J. Androl.* **3:** 301–303.
39. Gonzales, G.F., A. Cordova, K. Vega, *et al.* 2003. Effect of *Lepidium meyenii* (maca), a root with aphrodisiac and fertility-enhancing properties, on serum reproductive hormone levels in adult healthy men. *J. Endocrinol.* **176:** 163–168.
40. Gonzales, G.F., A. Cordova, K. Vega, *et al.* 2002. Effect of *Lepidium meyenii* (maca) on sexual desire and its absent relationship with serum testosterone levels in adult healthy men. *Andrologia* **34:** 367–372.
41. Gonzales-Castaneda, C. & G.F. Gonzales. 2008. Hypocotyls of *Lepidium meyenii* (maca), a plant of the Peruvian highlands, prevent ultraviolet A-, B-, and C-induced skin damage in rats. *Photodermatol. Photoimmunol. Photomed.* **24:** 24–31.
42. Lopez-Fando, A., M.P. Gomez-Serranillos, I. Iglesias, *et al.* 2004. *Lepidium peruvianum* chacon restores homeostasis impaired by restraint stress. *Phytother. Res.* **18:** 471–474.
43. Zhang, Y., L. Yu, M. Ao, *et al.* 2006. Effect of ethanol extract of *Lepidium meyenii* Walp. on osteoporosis in ovariectomized rat. *J. Ethnopharmacol.* **105:** 274–279.
44. Gonzales, G.F., S. Miranda, J. Nieto, *et al.* 2005. Red maca (*Lepidium meyenii*) reduced prostate size in rats. *Reprod. Biol. Endocrinol.* **3:** 5.
45. Gonzales, G.F., V. Vasquez, D. Rodriguez, *et al.* 2007. Effect of two different extracts of red maca in male rats with testosterone-induced prostatic hyperplasia. *Asian J. Androl.* **9:** 245–251.
46. Rubio, J., M. Caldas, S. Davila, *et al.* 2006. Effect of three different cultivars of *Lepidium meyenii* (maca) on

learning and depression in ovariectomized mice. *BMC Complement. Altern. Med.* **6:** 23.

47. Rubio, J., H. Dang, M. Gong, *et al.* 2007. Aqueous and hydroalcoholic extracts of black maca (*Lepidium meyenii*) improve scopolamine-induced memory impairment in mice. *Food Chem. Toxicol.* **45:** 1882–1890.
48. Rubio, J., W. Qiong, X. Liu, *et al.* 2008. Aqueous extract of black maca (*Lepidium meyenii*) on memory impairment induced by ovariectomy in mice. *Evid Based. Complement. Alternat Med.* [Epub ahead of print].
49. Dording, C.M., L. Fisher, G. Papakostas, *et al.* 2008. A double-blind, randomized, pilot dose-finding study of maca root (*L. meyenii*) for the management of SSRI-induced sexual dysfunction. *CNS Neurosci. Ther.* **14:** 182–191.
50. Brooks, N.A., G. Wilcox, K.Z. Walker, *et al.* 2008. Beneficial effects of *Lepidium meyenii* (maca) on psychological symptoms and measures of sexual dysfunction in postmenopausal women are not related to estrogen or androgen content. *Menopause* **15:** 1157–1162.
51. Sandoval, M., N.N. Okuhama, Angeles F.M., *et al.* 2002. Antioxidant activity of the cruciferous vegetable maca (*Lepidium meyenii*). *Food Chem.* **79:** 207–213.
52. Valentova, K., D. Buckiova, V. Kren, *et al.* 2006. The *in vitro* biological activity of *Lepidium meyenii* extracts. *Cell Biol. Toxicol.* **22:** 91–99.
53. Bogani, P., F. Simonini, M. Iriti, *et al.* 2006. *Lepidium meyenii* (maca) does not exert direct androgenic activities. *J. Ethnopharmacol.* **104:** 415–417.
54. Valentova, K., D. Stejskal, J. Bartek, *et al.* 2008. Maca (*Lepidium meyenii*) and yacon (*Smallanthus sonchifolius*) in combination with silymarin as food supplements: *in vivo* safety assessment. *Food Chem. Toxicol.* **46:** 1006–1013.
55. Buckholtz, N.S. 1980. Neurobiology of tetrahydro-beta-carbolines. *Life Sci.* **27:** 893–903.
56. Gonzales, G.F. & C. Gonzales-Castaneda. 2008. The Methyltetrahydro-{beta}-carbolines in maca (*Lepidium meyenii*). *Evid. Based. Complement. Alternat Med.* **6:** 315–316.
57. Herraiz, T. 2000. Tetrahydro-beta-carbolines, potential neuroactive alkaloids, in chocolate and cocoa. *J. Agric. Food Chem.* **48:** 4900–4904.
58. Sacco, R.L., J.Y. Chong, S. Prabhakaran, *et al.* 2007. Experimental treatments for acute ischaemic stroke. *Lancet* **369:** 331–341.
59. Burov, Y.V., A.B. Uzdenskii & T.N. Robakidze. 2000. Comparative analysis of neuroprotective activity of new chemical agent Vp and piracetam. *Bull. Exp. Biol. Med.* **129:** 362–364.
60. Sarang, S.S., T. Yoshida, R. Cadet, *et al.* 2002. Discovery of molecular mechanisms of neuroprotection using cell-based bioassays and oligonucleotide arrays. *Physiol. Genomics* **11:** 45–52.
61. Chen, S.T., C.Y. Hsu, E.L. Hogan, *et al.* 1986. A model of focal ischemic stroke in the rat: reproducible extensive cortical infarction. *Stroke* **17:** 738–743.
62. Papadakis, M. & A.M. Buchan. 2006. Translational vehicles for neuroprotection. *Biochem. Soc. Trans.* **34:** 1318–1322.
63. Lau, K., W.G. McLean, D.P. Williams, *et al.* 2006. Synergistic interactions between commonly used food additives in a developmental neurotoxicity test. *Toxicol. Sci.* **90:** 178–187.
64. Hossmann, K.A. 2007. Cerebral ischemia: models, methods and outcomes. *Neuropharmacology.* **55:** 257–270.
65. Johnson, I.T. 2002. Anticarcinogenic effects of diet-related apoptosis in the colorectal mucosa. *Food Chem. Toxicol.* **40:** 1171–1178.
66. Leoni, O., R. Iori, S. Palmieri, *et al.* 1997. Myrosinase-generated isothiocyanate from glucosinolates: isolation, characterization and *in vitro* antiproliferative studies. *Bioorg. Med. Chem.* **5:** 1799–1806.
67. Shaughnessy, L., B. Chamblin, L. McMahon, *et al.* 2004. Novel approaches to models of Alzheimer's disease pathology for drug screening and development. *J. Mol. Neurosci.* **24:** 23–32.

Ann. N.Y. Acad. Sci. ISSN 0077-8923

ANNALS OF THE NEW YORK ACADEMY OF SCIENCES
Issue: *Neuroprotective Agents*

Physiological low dose of estrogen-protected neurons in experimental spinal cord injury

Supriti Samantaray,[1] Denise D. Matzelle,[1] Swapan K. Ray,[2] and Naren L. Banik[1]

[1]Division of Neurology, Department of Neurosciences, Medical University of South Carolina, Charleston, South Carolina. [2]Department of Pathology, Microbiology and Immunology, University of South Carolina School of Medicine, Columbia, South Carolina

Address for correspondence: Naren L. Banik, PhD, Department of Neurosciences (Neurology), Medical University of South Carolina, 96 Jonathan Lucas Street, MSC606, Suite 309CSB, Charleston, SC 29425. baniknl@musc.edu

A protective role for estrogen against neurodegeneration and neurotrauma has received enormous attention in recent years, unraveling multiple facets and thus establishing this steroid as a multiactive neuroprotectant. The present study briefly reports our findings on the neuroprotective efficacy of physiologically relevant low doses of estrogen in experimental spinal cord injury (SCI) in rats. The current finding further corroborates our earlier results on efficacy of pharmacological/supraphysiological levels of estrogen in SCI and adds to the significance of conducting preclinical studies on estrogen efficacy in SCI.

Keywords: estrogen; neuroprotection; spinal cord injury

Introduction

Spinal cord injury (SCI) is a complex assault with varying degrees of neurological deficit and loss of function depending upon the severity of the injury. Although methylprednisolone is administered in acute SCI, it remains controversial and the actual benefits of the steroid have lately been questioned.[1,2] Consequently, there is an urgent need for development of efficient drug for treatment of SCI. Our laboratory has long explored the diverse mechanisms of tissue destruction following SCI in rats and is currently involved in testing the efficacy of different neuroprotective drugs for treatment of SCI. A major and well-acknowledged issue in such research is formulation of a combination therapy or a multiactive drug as a choice for promoting therapeutic benefits in the complex multifaceted process of tissue destruction during SCI. Estrogen is such a candidate drug that has been reported by us in a series of *in vitro* and *in vivo* studies using supraphysiological doses of estrogen.[3–8] However, considering the various hormonal properties of estrogen that may be limited in its beneficial effects in the predominantly male SCI population, we are currently focused on testing the lower physiological doses of estrogen for its efficacy in SCI. The readers are advised to look at the large array of neuroprotective efficacy of estrogen especially in SCI in a review article published in this volume, where we have succinctly presented the efficacy of estrogen in the field. Here, we briefly report that physiological low doses of estrogen can protect neurons in the spinal cord after moderately severe injury in rats.

Materials and methods

Induction of spinal cord injury in rats and treatment with estrogen

SCI was induced in adult male Sprague-Dawley rats using the modified weight-drop method.[9] Animal care, surgery, and induction of SCI were conducted in accordance with the Guide for the Care and Use of Laboratory Animals of the US Department of Health and Human Services (National Institutes of Health, Bethesda, MD) and were approved by the Institutional Animal Care and Use Committee (IACUC) at the Medical University of South Carolina (Charleston, SC). Laminectomy was

doi: 10.1111/j.1749-6632.2009.05360.x

performed at T10; the spine was immobilized, and an impounder was gently placed onto the dura. Dropping a 5 g weight from a height of 8 cm induced a moderately severe 40 g cm force injury. Sham operated animals underwent laminectomy alone. Low dose estrogen (10 μg/kg/day and 200 μg/kg/day) was delivered by osmotic pumps implanted subcutaneously either via treatment bolus at 15 min plus osmotic pump continuously delivering estrogen until sacrifice at 48 h. At 48 h postinjury, rats were anesthetized and sacrificed by decapitation. Following decapitation, the original laminectomy was extended and three 1-cm segments of spinal cord (SC) were removed, representing the lesion segment, the rostral penumbra, and the caudal penumbra.

Collection of SC samples and immunofluorescent stainings

Harvested SC samples were immediately frozen in tissue embedding media (HistoPrep, Fisher Scientific, Suwanee, GA) at −70° C and processed for immunofluorescent stainings. TUNEL assay for cell death was done according to our previously reported method[10] followed by double immunofluoresecent stainings with the neuronal marker anti-NeuN antibody (Chemicon, Temecula, CA; 1:100). TUNEL-positive neurons were tracked with rhodamine-conjugated anti-digoxigenin IgG primary antibody raised in sheep (Roche Molecular Biochemicals, Indianapolis, IN) and fluorescein conjugated anti-mouse IgG secondary antibody raised in horse (Vector, Burlingame, CA) as reported earlier.[11] Sections were finally mounted with the anti-fade mounting medium Vectashield (Vector) and images were captured with a fluorescence non-confocal microscope using ImagePro Plus software (Media Cybernetics).

Results

Assessment of neuronal integrity was carried out in different treatment groups following acute SCI (Fig. 1). Representative photomicrographs from both the dorsal horn and ventral horn containing sensory neurons and motoneurons, respectively, showed a significant number of them to be TUNEL-positive in vehicle SCI as compared to the uninjured sham SC. Estrogen (200 μg) treatment alone did not show any discernable effects compared to sham, however, estrogen treatment (10 and 200 μg) in acute SCI rats significantly attenuated the number of TUNEL-positive neurons in the caudal penumbra, as demonstrated by reduced co-localization of TUNEL with NeuN staining (Fig. 1).

Discussion

The present study supports our earlier reports[5,7] on the beneficial effects of estrogen after SCI. In this study, our primary goal was to define a physiological low dose of the steroid that could still render neuroprotective effects. The present study showed that both 10 and 200 μg doses were neuroprotective after acute SCI. Estrogen administration was beneficial to neurons in the caudal penumbra where the neurons die largely by apoptotic mechanisms.[12] Both the sensory neurons in dorsal horn as well as the motoneurons in the ventral horn were protected, thus suggesting that some common protective mechanisms are activated by estrogen regardless of the neuronal subtype specificity. SCI is due to mechanical injury in the vast majority of cases and revival of functional loss implies recovery of the total neuronal population in the dorsal and ventral horn. The present study is highly clinically relevant because estrogen effects on both the sensory and motoneuron were assessed and found to be protected. Furthermore, our study showed neuroprotective effects with both the doses, a lower 10 μg and a higher 200 μg, thus suggesting that receptor-mediated mechanisms are operative. It also narrows down the required dose to a physiological low profile thus, limiting the undesired side reactions of the steroid. It would be worthwhile to emphasize that present study used 17β-estradiol, the endogenous format of the steroid, and that it was applied postinjury; thus, making it more reasonable to expect translational benefits of the study to human SCI. The neuroprotective efficacy of estrogen in the present study may certainly be explained as result of multiple mechanisms that are triggered by the low dose of estrogen that renders modification of the microenvironment in caudal penumbra by multiple other aspects. Ongoing research in our laboratory is addressing the molecular mechanisms of such protection and exploring different administration paradigm in both acute and chronic SCI regimen to validate estrogen in preclinical testing following SCI.

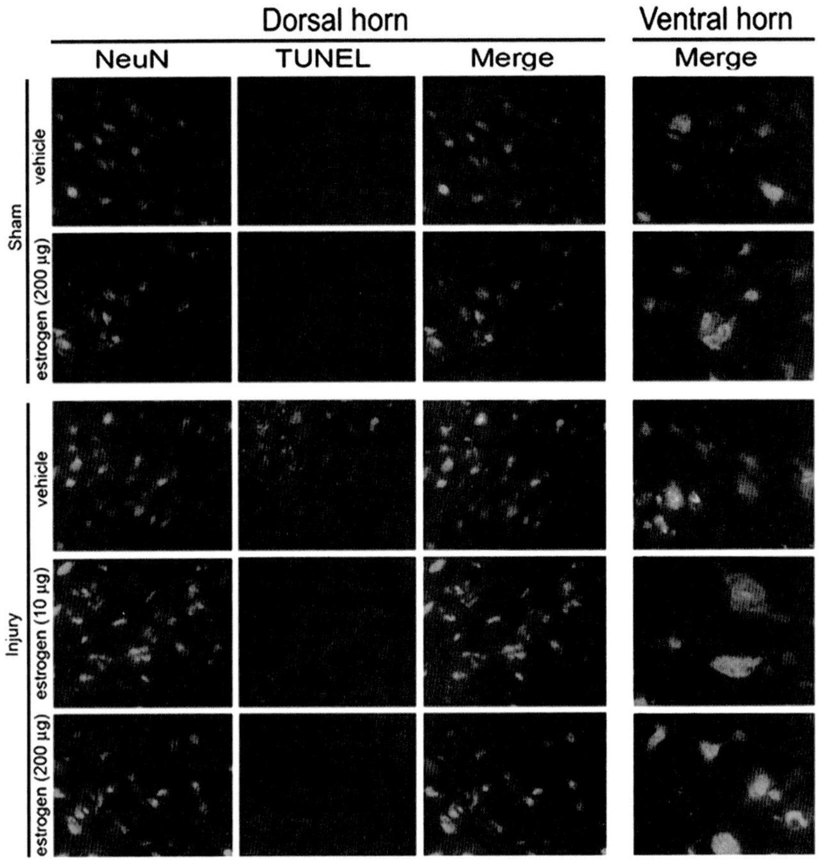

Figure 1. Double immunofluorescent stainings showed that low dose estrogen rendered neuroprotection in acute spinal cord injury (SCI) in rats. Coronal slices (5–7 μm) of spinal cord (SC) from caudal penumbra were double stained with neuronal marker NeuN (*green*) and TUNEL (*red*) to assess the neuronal death. Spinal cords from sham-vehicle animals showed healthy neurons—smaller sensory neurons in dorsal horn and larger motoneurons in ventral horn. SC slices from sham animals receiving estrogen (200 μg) were similar to sham vehicle and none of the groups showed any TUNEL-positive neurons. However, TUNEL staining in SC of injury-vehicle animals depicted significant neuronal death (*yellow* merge), which was protected upon estrogen treatment (10–200 μg). Panels of individual stains are shown in dorsal horn, whereas the merged panel alone is represented for ventral horn.

Conflicts of interest

The authors declare no conflicts of interest.

References

1. Miller, S.M. 2008. Methylprednisolone in acute spinal cord injury: a tarnished standard. *J. Neurosurg. Anesthesiol.* **20:** 140–142.
2. Rozet, I. 2008. Methylprednisolone in acute spinal cord injury: is there any other ethical choice? *J. Neurosurg. Anesthesiol.* **20:** 137–139.
3. Sur, P. *et al.* 2003. Estrogen attenuates oxidative stress-induced apoptosis in C6 glial cells. *Brain Res.* **971:** 178–188.
4. Sribnick, E.A. *et al.* 2007. Estrogen improves locomotor function following spinal cord injury. *Int. Soc. Neurochem.* **102**(S1): 203.
5. Sribnick, E.A. *et al.* 2006. Estrogen treatment of spinal cord injury attenuates calpain activation and apoptosis. *J. Neurosci. Res.* **84:** 1064–1075.
6. Sribnick, E.A. *et al.* 2004. 17β-estradiol attenuates glutamate-induced apoptosis and preserves electrophysiologic function in primary cortical neurons. *J. Neurosci. Res.* **76:** 688–696.

7. Sribnick, E.A. *et al.* 2005. Estrogen attenuated markers of inflammation and decreased lesion volume in acute spinal cord injury in rats. *J. Neurosci. Res.* **82:** 283–293.
8. Sribnick, E.A., S.K. Ray & N.L. Banik. 2006. Estrogen prevents glutamate-induced apoptosis in C6 glioma cells by a receptor-mediated mechanism. *Neuroscience* **137:** 197–209.
9. Perot, P.L., Jr. *et al.* 1987. Therapeutic model for experimental spinal cord injury in the rat: I. Mortality and motor deficit. *Cent. Nerv. Syst. Trauma* **4:** 149–159.
10. Ray, S.K. *et al.* 2000. Combined TUNEL and double immunofluorescent labeling for detection of apoptotic mononuclear phagocytes in autoimmune demyelinating disease. *Brain Res. Protoc.* **5:** 305–311.
11. Samantaray, S. *et al.* 2008. Melatonin attenuates calpain upregulation, axonal damage and neuronal death in spinal cord injury in rats. *J. Pineal Res.* **44:** 348–357.
12. Sribnick, E.A. *et al.* 2009. Estrogen as a promising multiactive agent for the treatment of spinal cord injury. In *Handbook of Neurochemistry and Molecular Neurobiology: Brain and Spinal Cord Trauma*, 3rd edn. A Lajtha, Ed., N.L. Banik & S.K. Ray, Vol. Eds.: 581–597. Springer. New York.

ANNALS OF THE NEW YORK ACADEMY OF SCIENCES
Issue: *Neuroprotective Agents*

Neuroprotective efficacy of estrogen in experimental spinal cord injury in rats

Supriti Samantaray,[1] Eric A. Sribnick,[1] Arabinda Das,[1] Nakul P. Thakore,[1] Denise Matzelle,[1] Shan P. Yu,[2] Swapan K. Ray,[3] Ling Wei,[2] and Naren L. Banik[1]

[1]Division of Neurology, Department of Neurosciences, Medical University of South Carolina, Charleston, South Carolina. [2]Department of Anesthesiology, Emory University, Atlanta, Georgia. [3]Department of Pathology, Microbiology and Immunology, University of South Carolina School of Medicine, Columbia, South Carolina

Address for correspondence: Naren L. Banik, PhD, Department of Neurosciences (Neurology), Medical University of South Carolina, 96 Jonathan Lucas Street, MSC606, Suite 309CSB, Charleston, SC 29425. baniknl@musc.edu

Spinal cord injury (SCI) leads to neurological deficits and motor dysfunction. Methylprednisolone, the only drug used for treating SCI, renders limited neuroprotection and remains controversial. Estrogen is one of the most potent multiactive neuroprotective agents and it is currently under investigation in our laboratory for its efficacy in SCI. The present review briefly summarizes our earlier findings on the therapeutic potential of pharmacological/supraphysiological levels of estrogen in SCI and outlines our ongoing research, highlighting the efficacy of physiological levels of estrogen against neuronal injury, axonal degeneration, and gliosis and also the molecular mechanisms of such neuroprotection in experimental SCI. Furthermore, our ongoing studies designed to explore the different translational potential of estrogen therapy suggest that this multiactive steroid may act as an adjunct therapy to promote angiogenesis, thus enhancing the functional recovery following chronic SCI. Taken together, these studies confirm that estrogen is a potential therapeutic agent for treating SCI.

Keywords: axonal degeneration; calpain; estrogen; neuroprotection; spinal cord injury

Introduction

Spinal cord injury (SCI) is a serious neurotrauma that leads to lifelong disability for which no suitable therapeutic strategies exist so far.[1] In the US there are approximately 450,000 people living with SCI, and an additional 11,000 new SCI cases occur every year; the majority being males between the ages of 16–30, as reported by the Foundation for Spinal Cord Injury Prevention, Care, and Cure. Thus, SCI is sufficiently prevalent, highly debilitating, and a life-changing incident in otherwise healthy young individuals. Improvement of function in survivors of SCI is an enormous biomedical challenge not only to the clinicians, but also to the researchers.

An incomplete SCI is initially mild and causes minimal damage to the spinal cord (SC). However, this injury leads to complex pathologic processes, resulting in damaging secondary SCI. The physiology of secondary damage following SCI depicts deregulated intracellular and extracellular processes, initiating within minutes and propagating through hours and weeks after the primary assault. The final neurological deficit is determined by the extent of severity in which secondary injury deleteriously affects the healthy tissue and aggravates the primary damage. Hence, the main goal of any pharmacological treatment in acute SCI is to prevent and mitigate the detrimental secondary injury pathways, including the loss of cells due to apoptosis. Apoptosis or reversible death process in cells occurring in the periphery of lesion or penumbra is a tightly regulated physiological phenomenon and hence, treatable, as opposed to necrosis, which is an irreversible cell death process occurring within the lesion. Promotion of repair to the chronically injured SC and recovery of neurological function is the primary goal, but this is largely dependent on how early and effectively the primary care is rendered. Thus, the neuroprotective

doi: 10.1111/j.1749-6632.2009.05357.x

drugs hold enormous promises in the treatment of SCI.

Significant advances in experimental research have led to tremendous progress in unraveling the nature of SCI in the last few decades. A major focus over the years has been to use the corticosteroid methylprednisolone as a therapeutic agent for the treatment of SCI in humans. Unfortunately, data available from different clinical trials are controversial and qualitative.[2,3] Methylprednisolone treatment in SCI failed to get approval by the Food and Drug Administration that recommended it only as an "optional" treatment by "Guidelines for the Management of Acute Cervical Spine and Spinal Cord Injuries."[4] Besides, none of the treatments, such as thyroid releasing hormone, opioid antagonists, and the free radical scavengers in preclinical and clinical studies have been proven to be a major advantage in treatment of SCI.[5] The major barrier in development of effective SCI therapy lies in the complexity of multiple interlinked and interdependent damaging pathways involved in propagating the secondary injury process following SCI. Researchers have repeatedly emphasized the desperate need for the development of effective SCI therapeutic measures with either a combination of multiple neuroprotectants or with a single multiactive agent. Growing scientific evidence supports the hypothesis that estrogen is such a multiactive agent and may reduce inflammatory responses and increase viability and functionality of damaged neurons in the brain.[6–8] Recent results from our laboratory have further opened the possibility that estrogen therapy can be an efficient means to treat SCI in rats.[9,10]

Estrogen as a multiactive neuroprotectant

Multimodal neuroprotective efficacy of estrogen stems from diverse, yet interlinked mechanisms by which estrogenic steroids produce biological effects.[11] Classically, estrogen signals through a nuclear receptor, which targets transcription of mRNA and cognate protein expression.[12] Estrogen can also act via activation of its receptors ER-α and ER-β and downstream intracellular signaling through kinases.[6] It can act as an anti-inflammatory agent[13] and promote growth of micro vessels.[14] Estrogen can act directly at neurotransmitter receptor complexes or at ion channels resulting in altered neuronal current conductance or transcellular ion flux.[15] Thus, the hormone initiates generalized signaling pathways to the nuclear or membrane-localized effectors. Crosstalk between nuclear activation and membrane-associated events is likely. Estrogen also has important non-cell type-specific actions, such as antioxidation and conservation of endogenous free radical scavenging agents.[16] In a nutshell, diverse mechanisms of estrogen mediated neuroprotection may include genomic, receptor-dependent transcriptional regulation, and non-genomic rapid effects that may or may not be receptor mediated but involves regulation by kinases as well as other effects such as anti-inflammatory, antioxidative, and anti-apoptotic, making it a versatile neuroprotectant. Thus, estrogen may be a potential candidate and testing its efficacy against neurotrauma including SCI may be beneficial.

Furthermore, it is important to note that both ER-α and ER-β are distributed widely in the body in both genders. ER-α predominates in the uterus and mammary gland, whereas ER-β has significant roles in the central nervous, cardiovascular, and immune systems.[17] Such wide-scale distribution of the estrogen receptors infers greater access of low dose of estrogen to the receptors and underscores the possibility of beneficial effects of estrogen.

Estrogen protects different neural cells

Because an array of neural cells is damaged during the progression of SCI lesion, we tested the mechanisms of estrogen efficacy individually in monocultures and subsequently in neuron and glia co-cultures (our unpublished observations). Previous reports from our laboratory have shown that supraphysiological doses of estrogen could combat multiple aspects of oxidative stress through a receptor independent mechanism in a rat astroglial cell line (C6) that resembles primary astrocytes.[18] Furthermore, C6 cells were shown to express estrogen receptors and were protected from glutamate-induced excitotoxic assault by treatment with nanomolar (nM) concentration of estrogen via receptor-mediated mechanism.[19] Likewise, low dose estrogen treatment also ameliorated apoptotic shrinkage and rendered functional protection to primary neuronal cultures exposed to glutamate toxicity, as confirmed by electrophysiological recordings of capacitance.[20] When co-cultured with glia, neurons could tolerate greater glutamate toxicity and estrogen treatment enhanced the protection through receptor-mediated mechanism (our unpublished observations).

Estrogen efficacy in experimental spinal cord injury

Extending our cell culture findings to experimental SCI in rats, we observed protection of the injured cord in acute phase.[9,10] Supraphysiological levels of estrogen attenuated inflammation, reduced or restricted the lesion volume, prevented axonal degeneration, and preserved myelin in acute experimental SCI. Moreover, the profound proteolytic events of the Ca^{2+}-activated proteinase calpain were reduced, which prevented the apoptosis of neurons largely present in caudal penumbra by estrogen treatment when administered immediately after SCI in rats.[9,10] In addition, similar high dose estrogen could mitigate the damage and restore functionality in chronic SCI in rats.[21] Such neuroprotective studies paved the path for further investigation of the clinical relevance on the efficacy of lower physiological doses of estrogen, applied immediately and at different times in the acute SCI paradigm. Subsequently, results from these studies helped to explore low dose estrogen efficacy in chronic SCI in rats. Indeed, estrogen mediated neuroprotection in SCI in rats was attained at much lower doses in subsequent studies in our laboratory.

Other protective effects of estrogen administration following SCI thus far include prevention of astrogliosis and microgliosis, reduction of proteolytic and apoptotic markers, and preservation of the axon-myelin structural unit. The estrogen-mediated attenuation of all these parameters is essential and important for recovery of neurological function following SCI. Functional recovery may be enhanced further by promoting microvessel growth and restoring blood supply, needed for cell survival as cells may die due to ischemia caused by disruption of blood vessels following the primary injury to SC. Because estrogen is known to promote angiogenesis and microvessel growth, its administration may help protect cells from ischemic damage following SCI. One of our goals is also to explore the angiogenic mechanism in both acute and chronic SCI.

Apart from our findings, there are a few studies from other laboratories that have addressed the estrogen efficacy in SCI. An increase in expression of the estrogen receptors ER-α and ER-β mRNA in lumbar SC motoneurons has been reported after axomotomy following sciatic nerve crush injury in bilaterally ovariectomized mice where exogenously supplied estrogen capsules (24 μg) rendered a sustained supraphysiological level of serum estrogen for the first three weeks.[22] Estrogen treatment induced gene expression resulting in acceleration of the growth and maturation of the axons. Furthermore, estrogen receptors were transported from the perikaryon into regenerating neurites, where they promoted local regeneration through the non-genomic ERK-activated signaling pathway.[22] Such protective effects of estrogen on motoneurons reflected well in experimental SCI in which it improved functional recovery in the injured rat, in part, by reducing apoptotic cell death with estrogen pretreatment (3–300 μg).[23] Furthermore, in a posttreatment paradigm in the same study, male rats were given a single injection of estrogen (100 μg/kg) immediately postinjury, which also showed significant recovery in locomotor activity coupled with decreased morphologic outcome. Subsequently adopting a 1 h post-SCI treatment regimen, the same group of researchers confirmed the steroid's neuroprotective mechanism being partly mediated by induction of Bcl-2 through PI3K/Akt-dependent CREB activation.[24] Estrogen also reduced the severity of autonomic dysfunction in SCI in male mice with administration of physiological dosage of estrogen in mice, wherein involvement of non-central/non-spinal mechanisms has been suggested.[25]

Protection by estrogen was further confirmed in SCI induced by complete crush injury. Estrogen effects in such severe SCI were assessed by comparing non-ovariectomized, ovariectomized control, and ovariectomized with low physiological level estrogen supplementation (corresponding to 20 pg/mL in blood) in premenopausal and postmenopausal female rats. The study reported improved behavioral (Basso, Beattie, and Bresnahan) scores, white matter sparing, and lower motor neuron survival by 21-day postinjury.[26] Another group reported that pretreatment with estrogen reduced the development of inflammation, tissue injury, neutrophil infiltration, expression of inducible nitric oxide synthase (iNOS), cycloxygenase-2 (COX-2) activity and several apoptotic markers associated with SC trauma[27] whereas we observed similar effects in a more preclinical posttreatment approach.[9,10,21]

The estrogen receptor antagonist ICI 182,780 has been used to confirm the estrogen-receptor involvement in neuroprotective action of estrogen following SCI.[27] A separate study by another group, who adopted our previously reported estrogen dosing regimen (a higher 4 mg/kg and a lower 100 μg/kg), highlighted a transient neuroprotective window through which estrogen protected SC by stimulating early cytokines release and astroglial responses.[28] These investigators suggested that such stimulations might prevent the spread of lesion and retard inflammatory cells to migrate into the surrounding tissue during the critical first week following SCI. The study reported improved locomotor-recovery over 4 weeks after injury and inferred them as probably the consequence of the transient hike in astroglial reactivity due to estrogen.[28]

As opposed to all the affirmative reports on estrogen efficacy following SCI, a solitary report suggests that gender differences in SCI are not estrogen-dependent and hence estrogen may not provide a viable therapy following SCI.[29] On the contrary, estrogen-related gender differences on the survival of rats following traumatic brain injury has been reported.[30] However, multiple reports on estrogen efficacy in experimental SCI conducted in diverse animal models spanning from acute through chronic models with various dosage regimens and confirming different aspects of neuroprotection certainly are in favor of the multiactive estrogen as a therapeutic agent. The results further validate its use as a promising candidate for the treatment of SCI.

A major challenge is establishment of the minimal effective dose taking into account the gender bias of the SCI victims and discerning the postinjury temporal window in which it will provide beneficial effect. To this end, our studies on postinjury treatment with estrogen, progressively lowering the dose from supraphysiological to physiological and with postinjury time-point of application, add greatly to the clinical relevance of estrogen as a promising agent in the treatment of SCI.

Conclusion

Although our ultimate goal is to unravel the molecular mechanisms by which estrogen prevents, preserves, and restores the injured SC and to make a coherent platform for preclinical testing, our findings thus far strongly suggests that estrogen can be an appropriate candidate for therapy following SCI. One of the major advantages of estrogen over methylprednisolone is that it is multiactive, angiogenic, and not controversial, and it is a natural endogenous hormone – which makes estrogen an ideal agent for the treatment of SCI.

Conflicts of interest

The authors declare no conflicts of interest.

References

1. Spinal Cord Injury: causes. In *Spinal Cord Injury*, 2009. Mayo Foundation for Medical Education and Research (MFMER).
2. Miller, S.M. 2008. Methylprednisolone in acute spinal cord injury: a tarnished standard. *J. Neurosurg. Anesthesiol.* **20:** 140–142.
3. Rozet, I. 2008. Methylprednisolone in acute spinal cord injury: is there any other ethical choice? *J. Neurosurg. Anesthesiol.* **20:** 137–139.
4. Hadley, M.N. *et al.* 2002. Guidelines for the management of acute cervical spine and spinal cord injuries. *Clin. Neurosurg.* **49:** 407–498.
5. Faden, A.I. & B. Stoica. 2007. Neuroprotection: challenges and opportunities. *Arch. Neurol* **64:** 794–800.
6. Brann, D.W. *et al.* 2007. Neurotrophic and neuroprotective actions of estrogen: basic mechanisms and clinical implications. *Steroids* **72:** 381–405.
7. Pozzi, S. *et al.* 2006. Estrogen action in neuroprotection and brain inflammation. *Ann. N.Y. Acad. Sci.* **1089:** 302–323.
8. Simpkins, J.W. & J.A. Dykens. 2008. Mitochondrial mechanisms of estrogen neuroprotection. *Brain Res. Rev.* **57:** 421–430.
9. Sribnick, E.A., *et al.* 2006. Estrogen treatment of spinal cord injury attenuates calpain activation and apoptosis. *J. Neurosci. Res.* **84:** 1064–1075.
10. Sribnick, E.A. *et al.* 2005. Estrogen attenuated markers of inflammation and decreased lesion volume in acute spinal cord injury in rats. *J. Neurosci. Res.* **82:** 283–293.
11. Vasudevan, N. & D.W. Pfaff. 2008. Non-genomic actions of estrogens and their interaction with genomic actions in the brain. *Front. Neuroendocrinol.* **29:** 238–257.
12. Marino, M., P. Galluzzo & P. Ascenzi. 2006. Estrogen signaling multiple pathways to impact gene transcription. *Curr. Genomics* **7:** 497–508.

13. Straub, R.H. 2007. The complex role of estrogens in inflammation. *Endocr. Rev.* **28:** 521–574.
14. Miller, V.M. & S.P. Duckles. 2008. Vascular actions of estrogens: functional implications. *Pharmacol. Rev.* **60:** 210–241.
15. Kelly, M.J. & E.R. Levin. 2001. Rapid actions of plasma membrane estrogen receptors. *Trends Endocrinol. Metab.* **12:** 152–156.
16. Nilsen, J. 2008. Estradiol and neurodegenerative oxidative stress. *Front. Neuroendocrinol.* **29:** 463–475.
17. Gustafsson, J.A. 2000. Novel aspects of estrogen action. *J. Soc. Gynecol. Invest.* **7:** S8-S9.
18. Sur, P., *et al.* 2003. Estrogen attenuates oxidative stress-induced apoptosis in C6 glial cells. *Brain Res.* **971:** 178–188.
19. Sribnick, E.A., S.K. Ray & N.L. Banik. 2006. Estrogen prevents glutamate-induced apoptosis in C6 glioma cells by a receptor-mediated mechanism. *Neuroscience* **137:** 197–209.
20. Sribnick, E.A., *et al.* 2004. 17β-Estradiol attenuates glutamate-induced apoptosis and preserves electrophysiologic function in primary cortical neurons. *J. Neurosci. Res.* **76:** 688–696.
21. Sribnick, E.A., *et al.* 2007. Estrogen improves locomotor function following spinal cord injury. *J. Neurochem.* **102**(Suppl 1): 203.
22. Islamov, R.R. *et al.* 2003. Effect of 17β-estradiol on gene expression in lumbar spinal cord following sciatic nerve crush injury in ovariectomized mice. *Brain Res.* **966:** 65–75.
23. Yune, T.Y. *et al.* 2004. Systemic administration of 17β-estradiol reduces apoptotic cell death and improves functional recovery following traumatic spinal cord injury in rats. *J. Neurotrauma* **21:** 293–306.
24. Yune, T.Y. *et al.* 2008. Estrogen-induced Bcl-2 expression after spinal cord injury is mediated through phosphoinositide-3-kinase/Akt-dependent CREB activation. *J. Neurotrauma* **25:** 1121–1131.
25. Webb, A.A. *et al.* 2006. Estrogen reduces the severity of autonomic dysfunction in spinal cord-injured male mice. *Behav. Brain Res.* **171:** 338–349.
26. Chaovipoch, P. *et al.* 2006. 17β-Estradiol is protective in spinal cord injury in post- and pre-menopausal rats. *J. Neurotrauma* **23:** 830–852.
27. Cuzzocrea, S. *et al.* 2008. Effect of 17β-estradiol on signal transduction pathways and secondary damage in experimental spinal cord trauma. *Shock* **29:** 362–371.
28. Ritz, M.F. & O.N. Hausmann. 2008. Effect of 17β-estradiol on functional outcome, release of cytokines, astrocyte reactivity and inflammatory spreading after spinal cord injury in male rats. *Brain Res.* **1203:** 177–188.
29. Swartz, K.R. *et al.* 2007. Gender differences in spinal cord injury are not estrogen-dependent. *J. Neurotrauma* **24:** 473–480.
30. Roof, R.L. & E.D. Hall. 2000. Estrogen-related gender difference in survival rate and cortical blood flow after impact-acceleration head injury in rats. *J. Neurotrauma* **17:** 1155–1169.

Ann. N.Y. Acad. Sci. ISSN 0077-8923

ANNALS OF THE NEW YORK ACADEMY OF SCIENCES
Issue: *Neuroprotective Agents*

Acetyl-L-carnitine reduces the infarct size and striatal glutamate outflow following focal cerebral ischemia in rats

Fakhreya Yousuf Jalal, Mark Böhlke, and Timothy J. Maher

Department of Pharmaceutical Sciences, Massachusetts College of Pharmacy and Health Sciences, Boston, Massachusetts

Address for correspondence: Fakhreya Yousuf Jalal, Department of Pharmaceutical Sciences, Massachusetts College of Pharmacy and Health Sciences, 179 Longwood Avenue, Boston, MA 02115. fakhreya.jalal@my.mcphs.edu

Acetyl-L-carnitine (ALCAR), an endogenous water soluble molecule, is synthesized in the brain and is involved in many aspects of neuronal activity, including metabolism and neuronal membrane formation and integrity. To determine ALCAR's neuroprotective effects, focal cerebral ischemia was induced using four models of middle cerebral artery occlusion (MCAO) and treatment with 0–400 mg/kg ALCAR (*i.p.*) prior to MCAO. While acute doses were without effect, pretreatment with chronic ALCAR (400 mg/kg/day for five days) significantly reduced infarct size. Lower chronic ALCAR doses were not effective. Additionally, elevations in microdialysate glutamate post-MCAO were attenuated by ALCAR treatment.

Keywords: cerebral ischemia; stroke; infarct size; ALCAR; microdialysis; glutamate

Introduction

Multiple lines of evidence have demonstrated glutamate's role as a mediator of neuronal cell death during ischemic stroke. Shortly after ischemia, neuronal depolarization causes the release of glutamate into the extracellular compartment, which overactivates glutamate receptors and leads to the influx of sodium and calcium, and eventually to the induction of several cell-death pathways.[1] Elevation in glutamate and K^+ levels following energy depletion induces a spreading depression at the boundary between the core and penumbra, which propagates to the penumbra, and contributes to an increase in infarct volume.[2] In addition, astrocytes, the major contributors to extracellular glutamate clearance, exhibit reversal of glutamate transporter function, which further aggravates the excitotoxic conditions.[3] In addition to glutamate, other neurotransmitters such as GABA, aspartate, taurine, and dopamine also contribute to the maturation of the injury following cerebral ischemia.[4]

The current study investigates the potential of the promising neuroprotective agent acetyl-L-carnitine (ALCAR) in the treatment of stroke. The endogenous water-soluble molecule ALCAR, [(R)-3-acetoxy-4-(trimethylammonio) butyrate], is synthesized in the brain from the reversible acetylation of carnitine,[5] and is well distributed throughout the brain (Fig. 1). In addition to its important role in fatty acid oxidation and energy metabolism,[6] ALCAR exerts several actions in the CNS. For example, in one study ALCAR improved memory and attention deficits associated with Down syndrome.[7] In addition, by modulating the activity of nerve growth factor (NGF), ALCAR might prevent age-related loss of NGF-binding capacity.[8] Other studies have reported the neuromodulatory effects of ALCAR on hippocampal synaptic structural dynamics.[9,10] ALCAR possesses considerable therapeutic benefits in various neuropathological conditions, such as Alzheimer's disease,[11] ischemia,[12] and diabetic neuropathy.[13]

ALCAR confers indirect protection from oxidative stress by reducing tissue lactic acidosis, which contributes to the formation of reactive oxygen species (ROS) following cerebral ischemia.[14] Despite the promising neuroprotective effects of ALCAR in different models of global ischemia,[12,15] limited studies have addressed its effects in stroke models and the underlying mechanisms of its neuroprotection.

doi: 10.1111/j.1749-6632.2009.05351.x

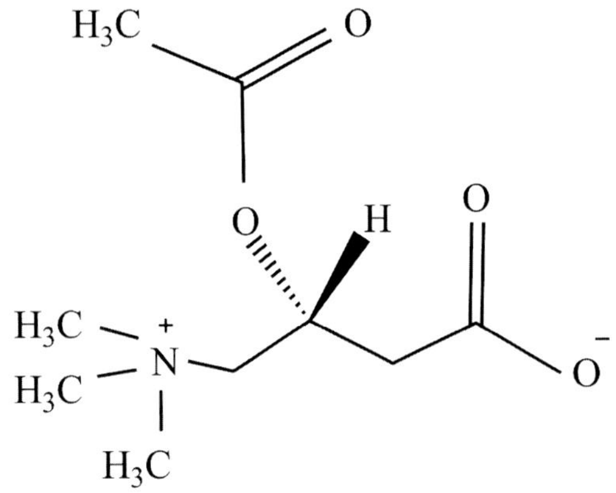

Figure 1. Chemical structure of acetyl-L-carnitine (ALCAR).

This study was therefore designed to determine the effect of ALCAR administration on brain infarct size, using four different middle cerebral artery occlusion (MCAO) procedures: (1) permanent distal occlusion of the middle cerebral artery (MCA) combined with a 60 min bilateral common carotid artery occlusion (CCAO)[16]; (2) permanent proximal occlusion of the MCA[17]; (3) intraluminal permanent MCAO; and (4) transient intraluminal suture with 90 min occlusion of the MCA followed by 48 h reperfusion.[18] In addition, a microdialysis technique was used to study the effect of ALCAR on striatal levels of glutamate when ALCAR was administered prior to stroke onset.

Materials and methods

All experimental procedures were conducted in accordance with the guidelines of the Institutional Animal Care and Use Committee (IACUC) of the Massachusetts College of Pharmacy and Health Sciences.

Animal preparation and experimental design in middle cerebral artery occlusion

Male Sprague-Dawley rats (Charles River Laboratories, Wilmington, MA) were used in all experiments and were housed in groups of two with *ad libitum* access to food (Rodent Diet 5001, LabDiet, Brentwood, MO) and tap water on a standard 12 h light/dark cycle. Rats were divided into two major groups, control (*i.p.* saline and MCAO) and ALCAR-treated (*i.p.* ALCAR and MCAO). Following anesthesia with chloral hydrate (400 mg/kg, *i.p.*), body temperature was monitored throughout the surgical procedures and maintained normothermic (37 ± 0.5° C) with a heating blanket. Acute (50, 200, or 400 mg/kg) and chronic (50, 200, or 400 mg/kg/day for five days) ALCAR (Sigma-Aldrich, St. Louis, MO) were first tested using permanent distal occlusion of the MCA combined with a 60 min bilateral CCAO. Following determination of the dose of ALCAR that produced a significant reduction in infarct size, this dose was also used in other models of focal cerebral ischemia: permanent MCAO (pMCAO)[17,18] and transient MCAO for 90 min followed by 48 h reperfusion.[18] ALCAR was given 30 min before the MCAO.

Permanent distal MCAO combined with 60 minute bilateral common carotid artery occlusion

Rats (325–350 g) were subjected to permanent occlusion of the distal MCA and temporary occlusion of both CCAs for 60 min as described by Chen *et al.*[16] Briefly, both CCAs were exposed by a midline cervical incision and were then isolated with 4-0 surgical silk ligatures. A vertical skin incision was made midway between the right eye and ear and the temporal muscles were retracted, followed by a temporal bone craniotomy. The right MCA was isolated and occluded with low-voltage electrical stimuli generated with bipolar forceps. Both CCAs were immediately occluded for 60 min. The CCAs were then reperfused for 24 h.

Permanent proximal MCAO

Rats (310–330 g) underwent occlusion of the proximal portion of the right MCA, according to the method of Tamura *et al.*[17] Briefly, the temporalis muscle was separated and the bone overlying the MCA was removed. The dura was opened and the MCA and its lenticulostriatal branch were electrocauterized just medial to the olfactory tract. The incision was closed and the rats were allowed to recover.

Permanent and transient MCAO by intraluminal suture

Focal cerebral ischemia was induced in rats (280–330 g) using the method of Longa *et al.*[18] A ventral midline incision was made to expose the CCA and external carotid artery (ECA). The arteries were ligated proximally and permanently with 6-0 silk and a 4-0 silicone rubber coated monofilament (diameter 0.19 mm, length 30 mm; Doccol Corporation, Redlands, CA) inserted into the ECA and advanced to the internal carotid artery (ICA) until resistance was felt and with some stretching of the ICA observed. The suture was kept in place for 24 h in the permanent model. In the transient model, the suture was slowly withdrawn to allow blood flow at 90 min following MCAO.

Ischemic infarct volume evaluation

Twenty-four or 48 h after reperfusion (permanent distal MCAO combined with 60 min bilateral CCAO model and transient intraluminal suture model, respectively) or 24 h after permanent MCAO (permanent proximal MCAO model and permanent intraluminal suture model), rats were deeply anesthetized, decapitated, and the brains were rapidly removed and placed in ice-cold phosphate buffer and then kept at -20° C for 15 min. Brains were sliced into 2 mm thick coronal sections and stained with 2% 2,3,5-triphenyltetrazolium chloride (TTC, Sigma-Aldrich, St. Louis, MO) for 20 min at 37° C. Following fixation in 10% formalin, the infarct areas (areas that lacked the red color stain of normal tissues) were quantified using Image J software. The volume of infarction in each animal was obtained by calculating the product of the average slice thickness (2 mm) and the infarcted area (the difference between the area of normal tissue in the ipsilateral brain hemisphere and the total area of the contralateral hemisphere) in all brain slices. The area of infarction was expressed as the percent area infarcted relative to the total area of the ipsilateral hemisphere.

Cerebral microdialysis

Microdialysis was used to measure the extracellular fluid (ECF) levels of striatal glutamate, which largely represents the ischemic core with minimal post-occlusion blood flow. Focal cerebral ischemia was induced using the permanent intraluminal suture model as previously described.[18] Rats were divided into three groups: (1) sham-operated group (saline-treated, no MCAO); (2) control group (saline-treated, MCAO); and (3) ALCAR-treated group (400 mg/kg/day, MCAO). All pretreatments were administered daily for five days.

Rats (270–290 g) were anesthetized with chloral hydrate (400 mg/kg) 24 h before MCAO, and a guide cannula for the CMA/12 microdialysis probe (CMA/Microdialysis, North Chelmsford, MA) was stereotaxically implanted into the right ventrolateral striatum (AP+0.7 mm, L-2.8 mm, V-6 mm relative to bregma), with the aid of an atlas, and secured to the skull with dental cement and screws.[19] Rats were then allowed to recover completely.

Twenty-four hours later, rats were anesthetized with chloral hydrate and kept under anesthesia during the entire 440 min experiment. Additional chloral hydrate was administered to rats as needed during the experiment, until the animals were sacrificed. The guide cannula was replaced with a CMA/12 probe with a membrane length of 3 mm (20,000 MW cutoff). Artificial cerebrospinal fluid (CSF) containing 145 mM NaCl, 2.7 mM KCl, 1.2 nM $CaCl_2{\cdot}2H_2O$, 1 mM $MgCl_2{\cdot}6H_2O$ and 2.0 mM Na_2HPO_4 was perfused at 2 μL/min with a microdialysis pump (Harvard Apparatus, Holliston, MA). Following 140 min of baseline collection, microdialysate samples were collected continuously at 20 min intervals for 60 min before MCAO, and until 240 min following MCAO. The last dose of saline (in the control group) and ALCAR (in the ALCAR-treated group) was injected 30 min before MCAO in the right brain hemisphere. Glutamate concentrations in the microdialysis samples were determined by HPLC analysis with calibration by external standards, as previously described.[20] Changes in glutamate levels after MCAO were calculated for each rat as the percent change from the average baseline value for that animal.

Statistical analysis

All values are expressed as mean ± SEM. One-way ANOVA followed by *post hoc* t-test with Bonferroni correction was used for comparison between groups in the Chen model animals. The nonparametric Mann-Whitney rank sum test was used to compare groups in the Tamura model. The Student's t-test was used to compare groups in intraluminal suture models. The mean transmitter outflow after the ischemic period between control and ALCAR-treated groups was examined using the nonparametric Mann-Whitney rank sum test. A P-value < 0.05 was considered statistically significant.

Results

Acute administration of ALCAR using the permanent distal occlusion of the MCA combined with a 60-min bilateral CCA occlusion (Chen model) caused all animals to experience infarctions in the ipsilateral cortical area, as revealed by loss of TTC staining (Fig. 2A). Cortical infarct volumes of animals administered acute ALCAR pre-injury treatments at doses of 50, 200, and 400 mg/kg (20.1 ± 2.1%, n = 8; 24.2 ± 2.5%, n = 9; 30.0 ± 1.9%, n = 8, respectively) 30 min prior to the onset of cerebral ischemia, were not significantly different from controls (25.2 ± 1.6%, n = 10, Figs. 2A and B). However, infarct volumes of animals receiving chronic 5 day pre-injury treatments with ALCAR at 400 mg/kg/day (9.0 ± 1.9%, n = 8, $P < 0.001$) were 64% less than those in the control group (25.1 ± 1.2%, n = 10, Figs. 3A and B). Chronic treatment with ALCAR at the lower doses of 50 mg/kg (26 ± 1.7%, n = 7) and 200 mg/kg (27.4 ± 1.9%, n = 7) had no significant effect on infarct size (Figs. 3A and B).

Occlusion of the right MCA using the proximal permanent occlusion model (Tamura model) resulted in infarction that was restricted to the right cortical and striatal regions. Chronic administration of ALCAR at 400 mg/kg/day for five days significantly attenuated the infarct volume to 14.6 ± 0.5% (n = 8, $P < 0.002$), compared to control (21.4 ± 1.2%, n = 9, Figs. 4A and B). Similarly, occlusion of the right MCA using the intraluminal

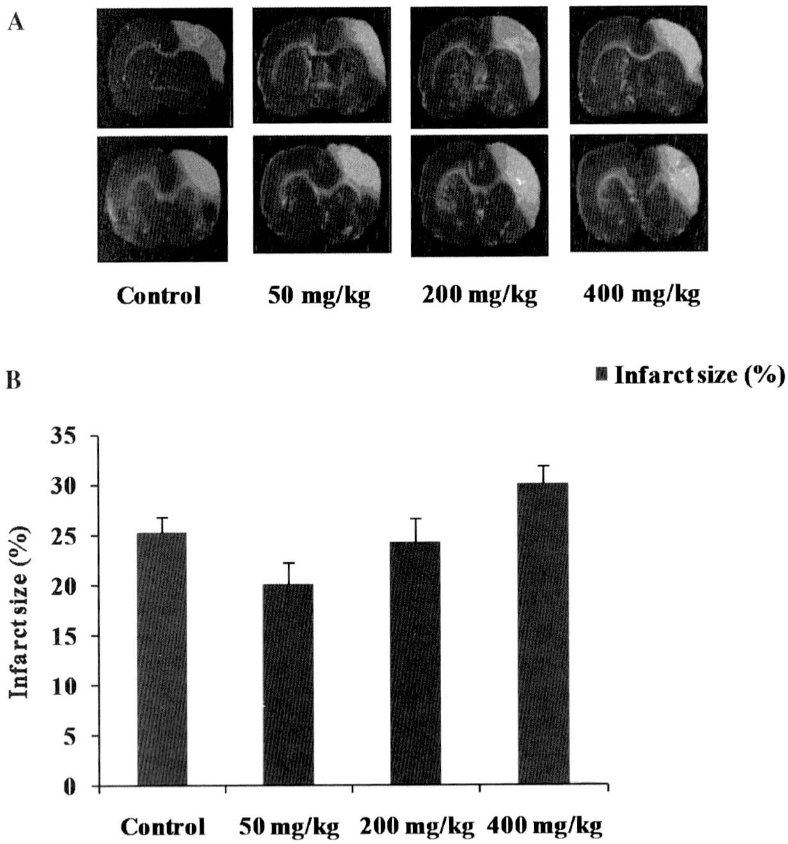

Figure 2. Effect of acute pre-injury administration of acetyl-L-carnitine (ALCAR) on infarct size. (A) 2,3,5-triphenyltetrazolium chloride (TTC) staining of cerebral infarct area in brain sections from saline and ALCAR (50, 200, 400 mg/kg) treated groups at 24 h post permanent distal occlusion of the middle cerebral artery (MCA) combined with 60 min bilateral common carotid artery occlusion. (B) Quantification of infarct size by TTC staining 24 h after the ischemic insult showed no significant difference between treated and control groups. Values are the means ± SEM.

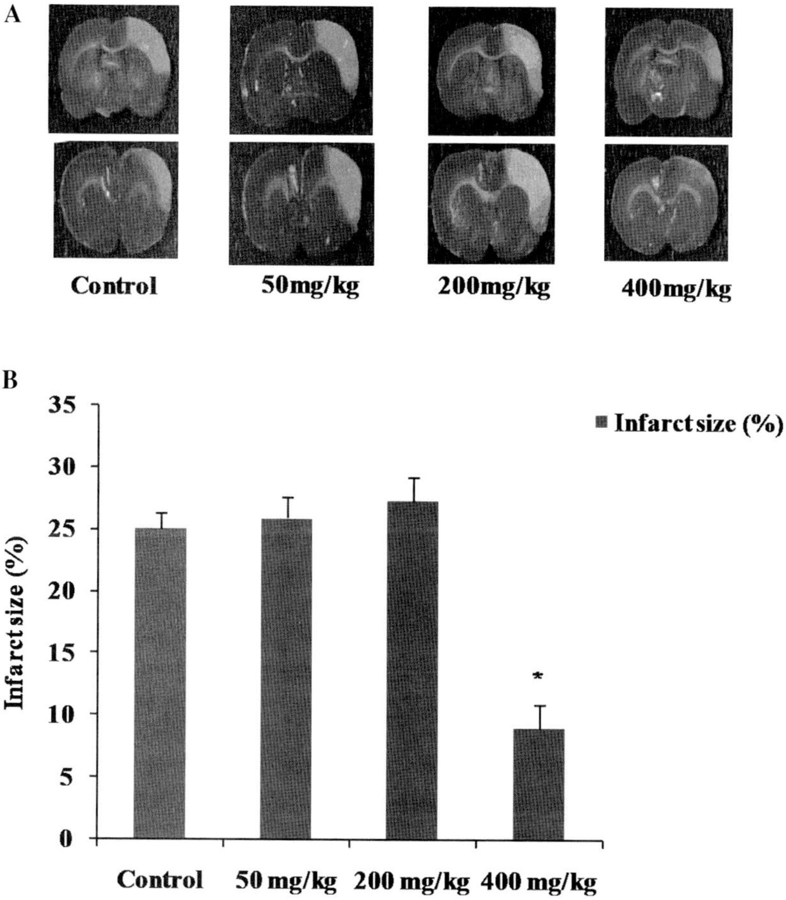

Figure 3. Effect of chronic pre-injury administration of acetyl-L-carnitine (ALCAR) on infarct size. (A) Histological evaluation by 2,3,5-triphenyltetrazolium chloride (TTC) stained brain sections demonstrating reduction in infarct size by pre-injury administration of ALCAR (400 mg/kg/day for five days); no effect was seen with ALCAR at 50 or 200 mg/kg/day for five days. (B) Percentage infarct size in saline-treated animals, and 50, 200, 400 mg/kg ALCAR for five days. Values are mean ± SEM. $^{*}P < 0.001$ compared to the control group.

suture models resulted in infarction in both cortical as well as in striatal regions. While a large volume of tissue injury was observed in the saline-treated control groups, chronic administration of ALCAR (400 mg/kg/day for five days) significantly attenuated the infarct volume in both permanent and transient MCA occlusion by 34% (27.1 ± 3.0%, $n = 7$, $P < 0.01$) and 40.5% (16.0 ± 2.4%, $n = 7$, $P < 0.005$), compared to respective saline-treated controls (41.0 ± 3.4%, $n = 7$; 26.9 ± 2.1%, $n = 7$, Figs. 5A and C, B and D).

Glutamate levels in the ECF microdialysates remained steady over the entire experimental period in the sham-operated group. A significant increase in glutamate levels appeared to demonstrate a biphasic response consisting of a steep increase within 30 min immediately after MCAO, followed by a noticeable reduction in the next 60 min, and a marked increase over the subsequent 120 min. Animals pretreated with ALCAR (400 mg/kg/day for five days, *i.p.*) exhibited significantly smaller elevations (87% reduction compared to controls, $P < 0.001$) in striatal ECF glutamate following MCAO (Fig. 6).

Discussion

The principal findings of this study can be summarized as follows: (1) chronic pre-injury administration of ALCAR decreased the infarct size in four

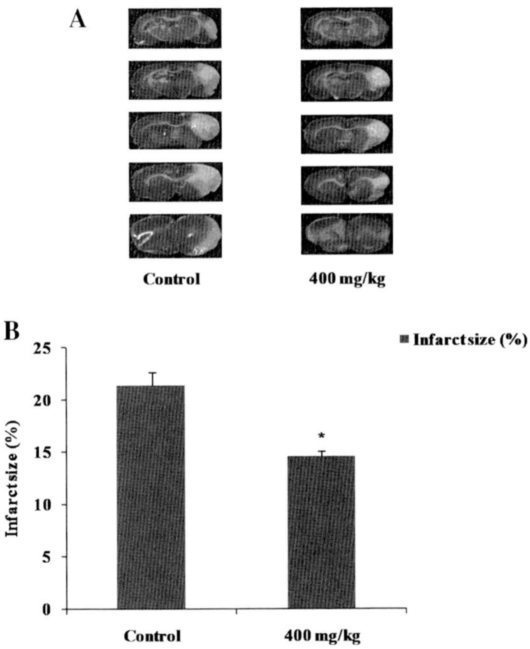

Figure 4. Effect of acetyl-L-carnitine (ALCAR) on the infarct size after proximal permanent focal cerebral ischemia. (A) 2,3,5-triphenyltetrazolium chloride (TTC) brain sections in ALCAR treated and control groups. (B) Percentage infarct size in saline and ALCAR (400 mg/kg/day for five days) groups. Values are mean ± SEM. $^*P < 0.002$ compared to the control group.

different models of focal cerebral ischemia; (2) permanent occlusion of the middle cerebral artery was associated with a significant accumulation of striatal glutamate; and (3) ALCAR reduced the striatal ECF levels of the excitatory amino acid glutamate.

It is well established that various models of stroke differ in their pathophysiological mechanisms as well as in location and size of lesion produced.[21] Due to the lack of an ideal model to mimic human stroke, ALCAR was tested in various models of focal cerebral ischemia in rats. This study is the first to determine the reduction in infarct size in all four models as a result of ALCAR administration to rats. Chronic, but not acute, administration of ALCAR significantly reduced infarct size in these different models (permanent and transient) of focal cerebral ischemia when given each day for five days before the ischemic insult, suggesting that ALCAR's efficacy is independent of the type of ischemia or of reperfusion. These observations also agree closely with findings presented by Shuaib and colleagues, that pretreatment with ALCAR resulted in significant protection of the cerebral cortex, hippocampus, and striatum in the gerbil model of transient forebrain ischemia.[15] However, another study reported that acute post-injury treatment with ALCAR did not decrease infarct size, but did improve neurological outcomes following focal cerebral ischemia.[22]

In general, in most stroke models neuroprotective agents preferentially protect cortical areas more than striatal areas.[23,24] However, our study demonstrated that ALCAR protection is not restricted to cortical infarction, but is also effective on neuronal tissue in the striatum.

It is well established that glutamate has a pivotal role in striatal cerebral damage resulting from ischemic cell death in different stroke models (permanent and transient).[25] We hypothesized that ALCAR would decrease infarct size by reducing ECF levels of the excitatory neurotransmitter glutamate. In agreement with this hypothesis, it was previously reported that talampanel, an AMPA (α-amino-3-hydroxyl-5-methyl-4-isoxazole-propionate) antagonist, demonstrated the beneficial effect of attenuating infarct size in various models of stroke.[26]

Among the different stroke models, the intraluminal suture model was selected for measurements of glutamate as it represents a model of ischemic damage with reproducible infarctions in both the frontoparietal cortex and lateral caudoputamen.[27] The advantage of this model over other models of stroke is that craniotomy, which is associated with operative trauma, is avoided.[28] In addition, this procedure consistently produces striatal damage due to occlusion of the MCA at its origin.[29] Our data revealed a biphasic response of ECF glutamate in which levels reached a peak at 30 min after MCAO, declined toward baseline values, followed by a sustained elevation for 120 min. This finding is consistent with that of Saleh *et al.*, who reported a similar biphasic release of glutamate after permanent MCAO.[30]

Three possible pathways might be involved in the elevation of ECF glutamate during ischemia: (1) an early stimulation of calcium-dependent synaptic exocytosis,[31] followed by (2) activation of voltage-dependent calcium channels,[32] and finally by (3) reverse activation of excitatory amino acid (EAA) transporters.[33] These events occur at different stages of the ischemic episode. Because all these

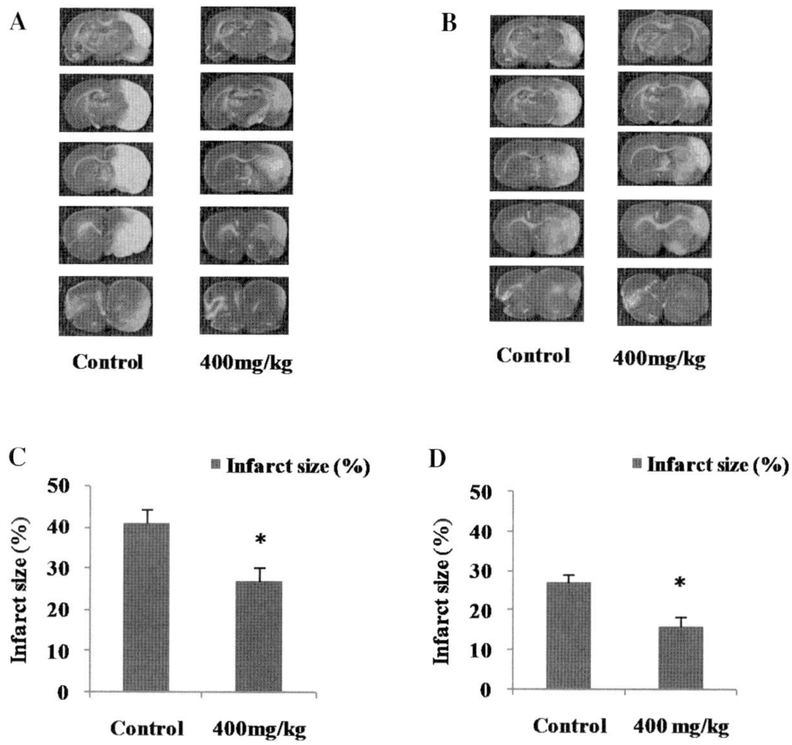

Figure 5. Protective effect of chronic administration of acetyl-L-carnitine ALCAR on infarct size, using permanent and transient intraluminal suture model. (A) 2,3,5-triphenyltetrazolium chloride (TTC)-stained brain coronal sections of ALCAR and saline-treated groups at 24 h post permanent middle cerebral artery occlusion (MCAO). (B) TTC-stained brain coronal sections of ALCAR and saline-treated groups at 48 h post infarct reperfusion in transient MCAO. (C) Infarct size (%) at 24 h after permanent MCAO of ALCAR-treated rats compared to saline-treated rats. (D) Percentage infarct size at 48 h in transient MCAO of ALCAR and control groups. Values are mean ± SEM. $^*P < 0.01$ (permanent), $^*P < 0.005$ (transient) compared to the control group.

processes are energy-dependent, glutamate release from synaptic terminals appears to be occurring immediately after the ischemic attack, prior to energy depletion. A drop in the levels of ATP during ischemia is responsible for the inhibition of calcium entry into the synaptic terminals,[34] which further inhibits glutamate release. At a later stage, the reduction in ATP levels affects the functions of both Na^+/Ca^+ exchangers and the Na^+/K^+ ATPase, facilitating disturbances in ionic gradients. Thus, excessive glutamate could be a result of the reversed action of glutamate transporters due to the collapse of Na^+ gradients.[35]

Proposed explanations for the biphasic release of glutamate were offered by Katayama *et al.*[31] when they reported that the transient increase in ECF glutamate levels is calcium-dependent and related to synaptic exocytotosis.[36] While the prolonged increase in glutamate levels that occurred in the second phase could be due to the breakdown of both neuronal and glial membranes, unlike neurons, astrocytes showed resistance to the glutamate-induced cell damage during ischemia.[37] One reason could be the presence of glycogen stores that maintain glucose levels.[38] Indeed, astrocytes have an important role in maintaining normal levels of glutamate via glutamate uptake in the brain,[39] and astrocytes have been shown to be neuroprotective in moderate ischemia or a slight increase in ECF levels of glutamate. On the contrary, in severe ischemic conditions, astrocytes were demonstrated to release glutamate through reversed glutamate transporter function, contributing to ischemic cell death.[40] It is worth noting that the primary factor involved in glutamate transporter reversal is energy depletion, which causes disturbances in ionic homeostasis.[41] Thus, the drop in

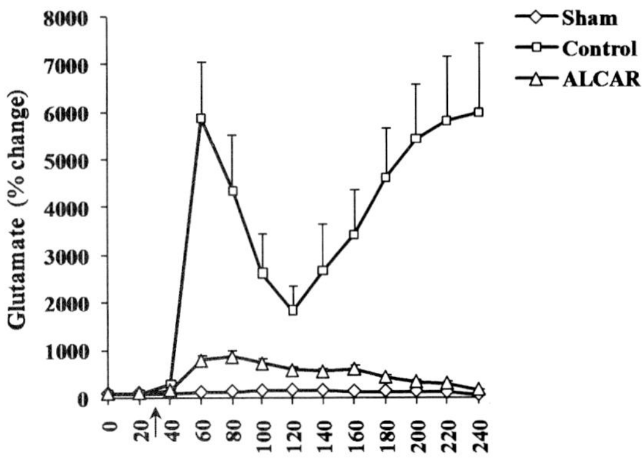

Figure 6. Effect of acetyl-L-carnitine (ALCAR) treatment (400 mg/kg/day for five days, *i.p.*) on the release of glutamate from rat striatum during permanent middle cerebral artery occlusion (MCAO). Each point is the mean ± SEM. Data are expressed as percent changes in glutamate outflow from the baseline value (mean of the first three samples). Permanent focal ischemia was achieved at the time denoted by the *arrow*. ◇ Sham-operated group ($n = 5$), □ Control group ($n = 7$), Δ ALCAR-treated group ($n = 7$).

ECF glutamate levels that was seen after a marked increase in the current study could be attributed to the role of transporters in astrocytes that normally keep ECF glutamate levels below a toxic level.

We have demonstrated that ALCAR administration counteracts ischemia-induced striatal outflow of glutamate for at least 220 min after the injury. One approach to overcome excitotoxic injury is to enhance glutamate uptake. Ceftriaxone, a beta-lactam antibiotic, was shown to upregulate excitatory amino acid transporter 2 (EAAT2)[42] and to decrease the injury volume in focal cerebral ischemia, when administered several days prior to the insult but not shortly after the ischemic event.[43]

The precise mechanisms responsible for the inhibition of glutamate by ALCAR are not understood at this time. As an energy facilitator, ALCAR might have an important role in normalizing glutamatergic neurotransmission by supplying glutamate transporters with ATP to effectively remove the excess ECF glutamate. Maintaining normal glutamate levels could also prevent the sustained activation of *N*-methyl-D-aspartate (NMDA) receptors and hence their downregulation.[44] ALCAR has been shown to exert protective effects against glutamate-induced excitotoxicity in hippocampal neuronal cell cultures.[45] This suggests that ALCAR protects against excitotoxicity-induced cell death via direct antagonism of glutamate receptors.

Cerebral ischemia is well known to be associated with the excessive release of free radicals.[46] One role of free radicals in brain injury appears to be to inhibit glutamate uptake primarily by oxidation of SH groups.[47] This explanation is supported by a study which demonstrated that the stimulation of glutamate receptors results in free radical production and in the inhibition of glutamate uptake in neuronal and glial co-cultures.[48] ALCAR has also been reported to exert an indirect antioxidant effect through the induction of antioxidant genes[14] and to increase the concentration of glutathione in the substantia nigra,[49] which might contribute to the protection of glutamate transporters during MCAO.

With its acetyl moiety, ALCAR promotes oxidative cerebral energy production and inhibits anerobic glycolysis and lactic acidosis, the latter two of which promote cell death.[50] Numerous studies have demonstrated post-injury neuroprotective effects of ALCAR in models of canine cardiac arrest and resuscitation.[12,51] The authors of these studies have theorized that the neuroprotective effects of ALCAR could result from the restoration of energy production and inhibition of anerobic glycolysis. In contrast, it has been observed that administration of ALCAR 30 min after reperfusion had no neuroprotective effect in a cardiac arrest resuscitation model, despite the reduction in lactate levels, which suggests a limited window for beneficial therapeutic effects of ALCAR administration.[52]

In conclusion, we report the correlation between the reduction in brain infarct size in the focal ischemia models, which represents an important feature related to chronic administration of ALCAR, and the *in vivo* neurochemical change which signifies its ability to protect the brain from ischemic insult, possibly by its ability to inhibit ECF glutamate accumulation during focal cerebral ischemia.

Conflicts of interest

The authors declare no conflicts of interest.

References

1. Frandsen, A. & A. Schousboe. 2003. AMPA receptor-mediated neurotoxicity: role of Ca2+ and desensitization. *Neurochem. Res.* **28:** 1495–1499.
2. Dirnagl, U., C. Iadecola & M.A. Moskowitz. 1999. Pathobiology of ischaemic stroke: an integrated view. *Trends Neurosci.* **22:** 391–397.
3. Kosugi, T. & K. Kawahara. 2006. Reversed actrocytic GLT-1 during ischemia is crucial to excitotoxic death of neurons, but contributes to the survival of astrocytes themselves. *Neurochem. Res.* **31:** 933–943.
4. Lin, B., M.Y. Globus, W.D. Dietrich, *et al.* 1992. Differing neurochemical and morphological sequelae of global ischemia: comparison of single- and multiple-insult paradigms. *J. Neurochem.* **59:** 2213–2223.
5. Ghelardini, C., N. Galeotti, M. Calvani, *et al.* 2002. Acetyl-L-carnitine induces muscarinic antinocieption in mice and rats. *Neuropharmacology* **43:** 1180–1187.
6. Lombardo, P., R. Scuri, E. Cataldo, *et al.* 2004. Acetyl-L-carnitine induces a sustained potentiation of the after-hyperpolarization. *Neuroscience* **128:** 293–303.
7. De Falco, F.A., E. D'Angelo, G. Grimaldi, *et al.* 1994. Effect of the chronic treatment with L-acetylcarnitine in Down's syndrome. *Clin. Ter.* **144:** 123–127.
8. Angelucci, L., M.T. Ramacci, G. Taglialatela, *et al.* 1988. Nerve growth factor binding in aged rat central nervous system: effect of acetyl-L-carnitine. *J. Neurosci. Res.* **20:** 491–496.
9. Bertoni-Freddari, C., P. Fattoretti, T. Casoli, *et al.* 1994. Dynamic morphology of the synaptic junctional areas during aging: the effect of chronic acetyl-L-carnitine administration. *Brain Res.* **656:** 359–366.
10. Bertoni-Freddari, C., P. Fattoretti, U. Caselli, *et al.* 1996. Acetylcarnitine modulation of the morphology of rat hippocampal synapses. *Anal. Quant. Cytol. Histol.* **18:** 275–278.
11. Spagnoli, A., U. Lucca, G. Menasce, *et al.* 1991. Long-term acetyl-L-carnitine treatment in Alzheimer's disease. *Neurology* **41:** 1726–1732.
12. Rosenthal, R.E., R. Williams, Y.E. Bogaert, *et al.* 1992. Prevention of postischemic canine neurological injury through potentiation of brain energy metabolism by acetyl-L-carnitine. *Stroke* **23:** 1312–1317; discussion 1317–1318.
13. Sima, A.A., H. Ristic, A. Merry, *et al.* 1996. Primary preventive and secondary interventionary effects of acetyl-L-carnitine on diabetic neuropathy in the bio-breeding Worcester rat. *J. Clin. Invest.* **97:** 1900–1907.
14. Zanelli, S.A., N.J. Solenski, R.E. Rosenthal, *et al.* 2005. Mechanisms of ischemic neuroprotection by acetyl-L-carnitine. *Ann. N.Y. Acad. Sci.* **1053:** 153–161.
15. Shuaib, A., T. Waqaar, T. Wishart, *et al.* 1995. Acetyl-L-carnitine attenuates neuronal damage in gerbils with transient forebrain ischemia only when given before the insult. *Neurochem. Res.* **20:** 1021–1025.
16. Chen, S.T., C.Y. Hsu, E.L. Hogan, *et al.* 1986. A model of focal ischemic stroke in the rat: reproducible extensive cortical infarction. *Stroke* **17:** 738–743.
17. Tamura, A., D.I. Graham, J. McCulloch, *et al.* 1981. Focal cerebral ischaemia in the rat: 1. Description of technique and early neuropathological consequences following middle cerebral artery occlusion. *J. Cereb. Blood Flow Metab.* **1:** 53–60.
18. Longa, E.Z., P.R. Weinstein, S. Carlson, *et al.* 1989. Reversible middle cerebral artery occlusion without craniectomy in rats. *Stroke* **20:** 84–91.
19. Paxinos, G. & C. Watson. 1982. *The Rat Brain in Stereotaxic Coordinates*. Academic Press. Sydney, Australia.
20. Karlsson, G.A., K.A. Chaitoff, S. Hossain, *et al.* 2007. Modulation of cardiovascular responses and neurotransmission during peripheral nociception following nNOS antagonism within the periaqueductal gray. *Brain Res.* **1143:** 150–160.
21. Durukan, A. & T. Tatlisumak. 2007. Acute ischemic stroke: overview of major experimental rodent models, pathophysiology, and therapy of focal cerebral ischemia. *Pharmacol. Biochem. Behav.* **87:** 179–197.
22. Lolic, M.M., G. Fiskum & R.E. Rosenthal. 1997. Neuroprotective effects of acetyl-L-carnitine after stroke in rats. *Ann. Emerg. Med.* **29:** 758–765.
23. Carmichael, S.T. 2005. Rodent models of focal stroke: size, mechanism, and purpose. *NeuroRx* **2:** 396–409.
24. Turski, L., H.H. Schneider, R. Neuhaus, *et al.* 2000. Phosphonate quinoxalinedione AMPA antagonists. *Restor. Neurol. Neurosci.* **17:** 45–59.
25. Takagi, K., M.D. Ginsberg, M.Y. Globus, *et al.* 1993. Changes in amino acid neurotransmitters and cerebral blood flow in the ischemic penumbral region following middle cerebral artery occlusion in the rat: correlation with histopathology. *J. Cereb. Blood Flow Metab.* **13:** 575–585.
26. Erdo, F., P. Berzsenyi & F. Andrasi. 2005. The AMPA-antagonist talampanel is neuroprotective in rodent models of focal cerebral ischemia. *Brain Res. Bull.* **66:** 43–49.
27. Garcia, J.H., K.F. Liu & K.L. Ho. 1995. Neuronal necrosis after middle cerebral artery occlusion in Wistar rats progresses at different time intervals in the caudoputamen and the cortex. *Stroke* **26:** 636–642; discussion 643.

28. Melani, A., L. Pantoni, C. Corsi, *et al.* 1999. Striatal outflow of adenosine, excitatory amino acids, gamma-aminobutyric acid, and taurine in awake freely moving rats after middle cerebral artery occlusion: correlations with neurological deficit and histopathological damage. *Stroke* **30:** 2448–2454; discussion 2455.
29. Garcia, J.H., S. Wagner, K.F. Liu, *et al.* 1995. Neurological deficit and extent of neuronal necrosis attributable to middle cerebral artery occlusion in rats. Statistical validation. *Stroke* **26:** 627–634; discussion 635.
30. Saleh, T.M., B.J. Connell, C. Legge, *et al.* 2004. Estrogen attenuates neuronal excitability in the insular cortex following middle cerebral artery occlusion. *Brain Res.* **1018:** 119–129.
31. Katayama, Y., T. Kawamata, T. Tamura, *et al.* 1991. Calcium-dependent glutamate release concomitant with massive potassium flux during cerebral ischemia *in vivo*. *Brain Res.* **558:** 136–140.
32. Seki, Y., P.J. Feustel, R.W. Keller, Jr., *et al.* 1999. Inhibition of ischemia-induced glutamate release in rat striatum by dihydrokinate and an anion channel blocker. *Stroke* **30:** 433–440.
33. Phillis, J.W., J. Ren & M.H. O'Regan. 2000. Transporter reversal as a mechanism of glutamate release from the ischemic rat cerebral cortex: studies with DL-threo-beta-benzyloxyaspartate. *Brain Res.* **868:** 105–112.
34. Camacho, A. & L. Massieu. 2006. Role of glutamate transporters in the clearance and release of glutamate during ischemia and its relation to neuronal death. *Arch. Med. Res.* **37:** 11–18.
35. Rossi, D.J., T. Oshima & D. Attwell. 2000. Glutamate release in severe brain ischaemia is mainly by reversed uptake. *Nature* **403:** 316–321.
36. Drejer, J., H. Benveniste, N.H. Diemer, *et al.* 1985. Cellular origin of ischemia-induced glutamate release from brain tissue *in vivo* and *in vitro*. *J. Neurochem.* **45:** 145–151.
37. Goldberg, W.J., R.M. Kadingo & J.N. Barrett. 1986. Effects of ischemia-like conditions on cultured neurons: protection by low Na+, low Ca2+ solutions. *J. Neurosci.* **6:** 3144–3151.
38. Swanson, R.A. 1992. Astrocyte glutamate uptake during chemical hypoxia *in vitro*. *Neurosci. Lett.* **147:** 143–146.
39. Rothstein, J.D., M. Dykes-Hoberg, C.A. Pardo, *et al.* 1996. Knockout of glutamate transporters reveals a major role for astroglial transport in excitotoxicity and clearance of glutamate. *Neuron* **16:** 675–686.
40. Dronne, M.A., E. Grenier, T. Dumont, *et al.* 2007. Role of astrocytes in grey matter during stroke: a modelling approach. *Brain Res.* **1138:** 231–242.
41. Longuemare, M.C. & R.A. Swanson. 1995. Excitatory amino acid release from astrocytes during energy failure by reversal of sodium-dependent uptake. *J. Neurosci. Res.* **40:** 379–386.
42. Rothstein, J.D., S. Patel, M.R. Regan, *et al.* 2005. Beta-lactam antibiotics offer neuroprotection by increasing glutamate transporter expression. *Nature* **433:** 73–77.
43. Chu, K., S.T. Lee, D.I. Sinn, *et al.* 2007. Pharmacological induction of ischemic tolerance by glutamate transporter-1 (EAAT2) upregulation. *Stroke* **38:** 177–182.
44. Rao, K.V. & I.A. Qureshi. 1999. Reduction in the MK-801 binding sites of the NMDA sub-type of glutamate receptor in a mouse model of congenital hyperammonemia: prevention by acetyl-L-carnitine. *Neuropharmacology* **38:** 383–394.
45. Forloni, G., N. Angeretti & S. Smiroldo. 1994. Neuroprotective activity of acetyl-L-carnitine: studies *in vitro*. *J. Neurosci. Res.* **37:** 92–96.
46. Peters, O., T. Back, U. Lindauer, *et al.* 1998. Increased formation of reactive oxygen species after permanent and reversible middle cerebral artery occlusion in the rat. *J. Cereb. Blood Flow Metab.* **18:** 196–205.
47. Trotti, D., N.C. Danbolt & A. Volterra. 1998. Glutamate transporters are oxidant-vulnerable: a molecular link between oxidative and excitotoxic neurodegeneration? *Trends Pharmacol. Sci.* **19:** 328–334.
48. Rao, S.D., H.Z. Yin & J.H. Weiss. 2003. Disruption of glial glutamate transport by reactive oxygen species produced in motor neurons. *J. Neurosci.* **23:** 2627–2633.
49. Fariello, R.G., T.N. Ferraro, G.T. Golden, *et al.* 1988. Systemic acetyl-L-carnitine elevates nigral levels of glutathione and GABA. *Life Sci.* **43:** 289–292.
50. Bogaert, Y.E., K.F. Sheu, P.R. Hof, *et al.* 2000. Neuronal subclass-selective loss of pyruvate dehydrogenase immunoreactivity following canine cardiac arrest and resuscitation. *Exp. Neurol.* **161:** 115–126.
51. Liu, Y., R.E. Rosenthal, P. Starke-Reed, *et al.* 1993. Inhibition of postcardiac arrest brain protein oxidation by acetyl-L-carnitine. *Free Radic. Biol. Med.* **15:** 667–670.
52. Rosenthal, R.E., Y.E. Bogaert & G. Fiskum. 2005. Delayed therapy of experimental global cerebral ischemia with acetyl-L-carnitine in dogs. *Neurosci. Lett.* **378:** 82–87.

Ann. N.Y. Acad. Sci. ISSN 0077-8923

ANNALS OF THE NEW YORK ACADEMY OF SCIENCES
Issue: *Neuroprotective Agents*

Posttreatment with uridine and melatonin following traumatic brain injury reduces edema in various brain regions in rats

Shruti V. Kabadi and Timothy J. Maher

Department of Pharmaceutical Sciences, Massachusetts College of Pharmacy and Health Sciences, Boston, Massachusetts

Address for correspondence: Dr. Timothy J. Maher, Department of Pharmaceutical Sciences, Massachusetts College of Pharmacy and Health Sciences, 179 Longwood Avenue, Boston, MA 02115. Timothy.Maher@mcphs.edu

Traumatic brain injury (TBI) is a major health problem and a significant cause of death, disability, and neurobehavioral deficits. We investigated the effect of posttreatment with uridine and melatonin, separate and in combination, on edema in various brain regions following TBI via lateral fluid percussion. Uridine (16 and 32 mg/kg, *i.p.*) and melatonin (200 mg/kg, *i.p.*), individually reduced edema in impacted striatum versus TBI. Combination treatment of uridine (32) and melatonin (200) decreased edema in impacted as well as non-impacted hippocampus (75.7 ± 0.5% and 75.4 ± 0.3%) and striatum (69.7 ± 1.2% and 72.6 ± 0.5%) respectively, as compared to the group that received vehicle following TBI. Combination of uridine (16) and melatonin (200) attenuated edema levels in impacted hippocampus (76.6 ± 0.4%) and striatum (71.7 ± 0.5% and 74 ± 0.3%, respectively). Combination of uridine and melatonin may be a possible treatment strategy for the damage caused by TBI and its neuroprotective potential needs to be evaluated further.

Keywords: uridine; melatonin; edema; traumatic brain injury (TBI)

Introduction

Traumatic brain injury (TBI), also known as brain trauma, is a significant cause of death, disability, and neurobehavioral deficits. Although TBI is a major medical problem, its underlying pathogenesis is incompletely understood. Primary damage occurs due to mechanical forces producing tissue deformation at the time of injury, leading to damage of blood vessels, axonopathy, neuronopathy, and causes initiation of complex cellular, inflammatory, neurochemical, and metabolic processes.[1] Secondary damage includes ischemic damage and cerebral swelling that leads to elevation of intracranial pressure, hydrocephalus, and infection.[1] The cellular and molecular changes include mitochondrial injury, DNA damage, astrocytosis, microglial activation, macrophage infiltration, increased expression of caspases and kinases, cell death and modulation of neurotransmission, causing excitotoxicity and their progression often leads to overt and subtle neurobehavioral deficits.[2–5]

Previous studies have demonstrated formation of cerebral edema within an acute period of 24 to 48 h following experimental brain injury.[6] Cerebral edema results from swelling of damaged cells and injury to blood vessels that forces fluid to enter the various regions of brain. Edema formation can be of three types: vasogenic (open barrier), cytotoxic (cellular, intact, or closed barrier), and interstitial (hydrocephalic).[7] Vasogenic brain edema is characterized by the structural and functional impairment of the blood-brain barrier[7] and involves accumulation of protein-rich exudates derived from plasma due to increased permeability of endothelial cells to albumin and other plasma proteins.[8] Cytotoxic brain edema, is characterized by sustained intracellular accumulation in both astrocytes and neurons without affecting the integrity of the blood-brain barrier.[7] This results from the

doi: 10.1111/j.1749-6632.2009.05352.x

increased permeability of sodium and potassium ions across the cell membrane, depletion of energy because of failure of the active ion pumps, such as the Na^+/K^+-ATPase pump, or uptake of osmotically active solutes.[7,8] Interstitial cerebral edema occurs due to hydrocephalus in which the edema fluid, derived from the cerebrospinal fluid, is forced into the paraventricular tissues due to increased hydrostatic pressure.[8,9] As a result of edema and congestion, there is brain swelling which causes a major increase in intracranial pressure and may lead to distortion, shift, and herniation of the brain.[1] The determination of edema levels is one of the useful parameters for assessing the extent of damage attributed to experimental TBI, and various studies using animal models of TBI have utilized elevations in edema formation in various brain regions as an appropriate and reliable outcome.[6–11] Other biochemical alterations resulting from TBI include degradation of phospholipids, such as phosphatidylcholine,[12] and cytoskeletal proteolysis.[13] Reactive oxygen species (ROS) cause damage in several parts of the brain after TBI by various mechanisms such as lipid peroxidation, protein oxidation, DNA damage, and damage to membrane structures and mitochondria.[14]

While a host of potential neuroprotective agents has been studied for the treatment of injury resulting from head trauma, only a few drugs have shown promising preliminary results and are under experimental study. Melatonin, an indoleamine hormone secreted by the pineal gland, plays an important role in directly scavenging free radicals released during oxidative stress.[15,16] In addition, melatonin enhances the activities of a variety of antioxidative enzymes,[17,18] stimulates the synthesis of glutathione,[19] reduces the electron leakage from mitochondrial electron transport chain,[20] and demonstrates synergism with other antioxidants.[21] Uridine, a natural pyrimidine, is biosynthesized by various mechanisms[20] and serves as a substrate for the salvage pathway of pyrimidine nucleotide synthesis, known as the Kennedy cycle. In this pathway, both uridine and cytidine act as precursors of cytidine triphosphate (CTP) and cytidine diphosphate-choline (CDP-choline, citicoline) that further result in the biosynthesis of neuronal membrane phospholipids, phosphatidylcholine (PC) and phosphatidylethanolamine (PE).[22,23]

In the present study, we hypothesized that post-treatment with a free radical scavenger, melatonin and a pyrimidine nucleoside, uridine, individually and in combination, attenuates edema levels in various brain regions after TBI induced via lateral fluid percussion.

Materials and methods

Materials

Male Sprague Dawley rats (300–350 g) were obtained from Charles River Laboratories (Wilmington, MA) and housed in 18 × 9.5 × 8.5 (inch) plastic cages in our animal facility with a 12 h light and 12 h dark schedule with *ad libitum* access to food and water. The chemicals: melatonin, uridine, and chloral hydrate were obtained from Sigma Aldrich, Inc. (St. Louis, MO). Uridine was dissolved in saline and administered at a volume of 1 mL/kg, whereas melatonin was dissolved in polyethylene glycol (PEG) 400: sterile water for injection (1:1 v/v) and injected at a volume of 2 ml/kg, to the rats via intraperitoneal route. The injury was performed using the fluid percussion device, FPD302 (Amscien Instruments, Richmond, VA). All the experimental procedures have been approved by the Institutional Animal Care and Use Committee of Massachusetts College of Pharmacy and Health Sciences, Boston.

Surgery

The rats were anesthetized with chloral hydrate (400 mg/kg, *i.p.*) and a midline incision was made exposing the skull. A craniotomy (diameter 4.8 mm) was performed at a position corresponding to to 4.7 mm posterior to the bregma and 3.5 mm lateral (referring to atlas of Watson and Paxinos) on the right side of skull. A plastic female luer lock fitting (Small Parts, Inc., Miramar, FL) was fixed on the exposed skull. TBI was performed via fluid percussion at a pressure corresponding to 2.5–2.8 atms. Body temperature was maintained throughout the surgery using a thermistor probe and a heating pad.

Groups and drug treatments

The treatments were administered via single dosing, 15 min postinjury. In the first part of the study, rats were divided into 4 groups: Sham+Vehicle ($n = 12$), Sham+Treatment ($n = 6$), TBI+Vehicle ($n = 12$), and TBI+Treatment ($n = 8$–10). The injured rats received either the vehicle (TBI+Vehicle) or one of the following *i.p.* treatments (mg/kg;

TBI+Treatment): uridine (16 or 32), or melatonin (100 or 200). The sham rats received either the vehicle (Sham+Vehicle) or treatment [uridine (32 mg/kg) or melatonin (200 mg/kg); Sham+Treatment]. The choice of doses for the combination treatment was made on the basis of the effect of these treatments on edema in various brain regions. In the second part of the study, rats were divided into groups: Sham+Vehicle ($n = 9$), Sham+Treatment ($n = 6$), TBI+Vehicle ($n = 9$), and TBI+Treatment ($n = 7$–8). The treatment group (TBI+Treatment) received a combination of uridine (16) with melatonin (200), or uridine (32) with melatonin (200) following injury. The Sham+Treatment group was administered a combination of uridine (32) and melatonin (200).

Determination of edema levels by wet weight/dry weight method

After 48 h, rats were sacrificed by carbon dioxide asphyxiation and brains were removed. The ipsilateral (right, impacted) and contralateral (left, non-impacted) cortex, hippocampus, and striatum were dissected and the mean percentage water content was determined using the wet weight/dry weight method (drying specifications: 105° C for 24 h).[11] The percentage water content (edema) was calculated by using the following relationship:

$$\% \text{ water content } (\% \text{ edema}) = \frac{(\text{wet weight} - \text{dry weight})}{\text{wet weight}} \times 100$$

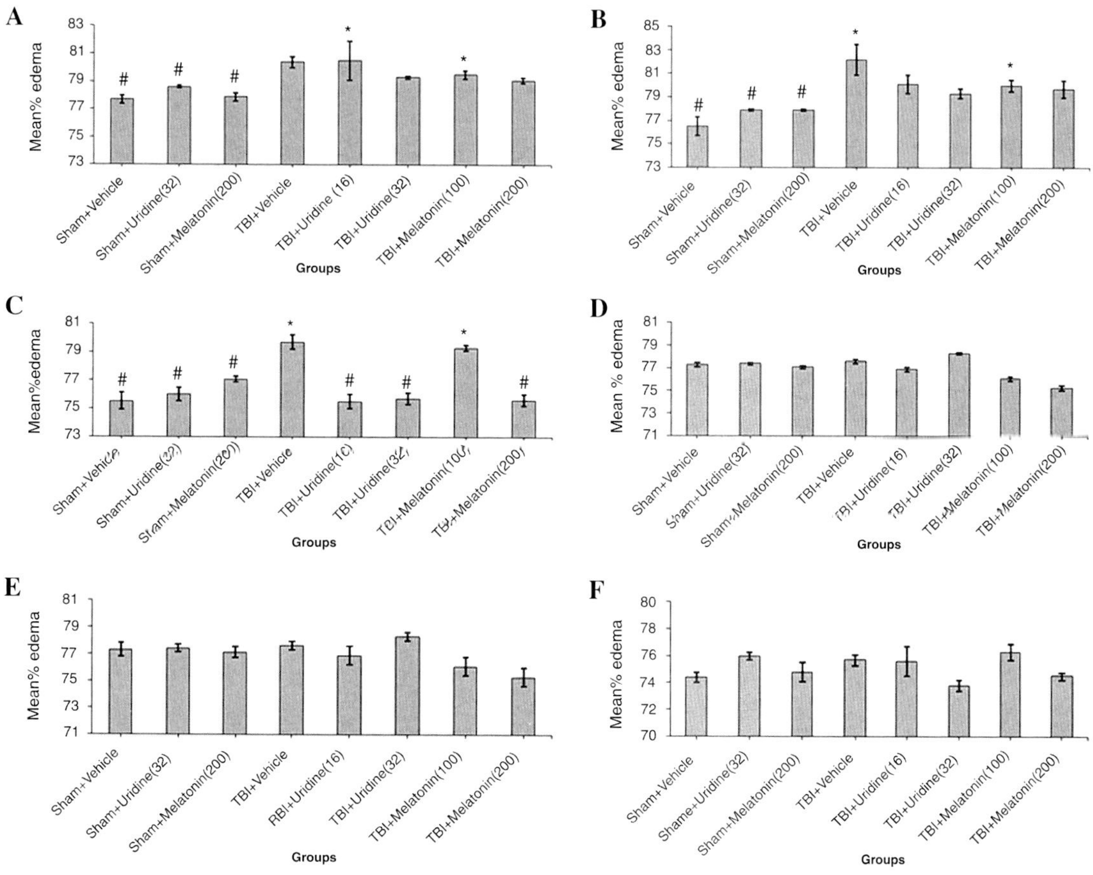

Figure 1. Effect of posttreatment of uridine and melatonin, individually on mean percentage edema in impacted (ipsilateral) cortex (**A**), hippocampus (**B**), striatum (**C**), non-impacted (contralateral) cortex (**D**), hippocampus (**E**), striatum (**F**), following TBI. ANOVA following Dunn's ($P < 0.05$; A–B,D–F) and Student–Newman–Keuls methods of multiple comparison testing ($P < 0.001$; C) versus Sham+Vehicle and TBI+Vehicle; *: significance versus Sham+Vehicle, #: significance versus TBI+Vehicle.

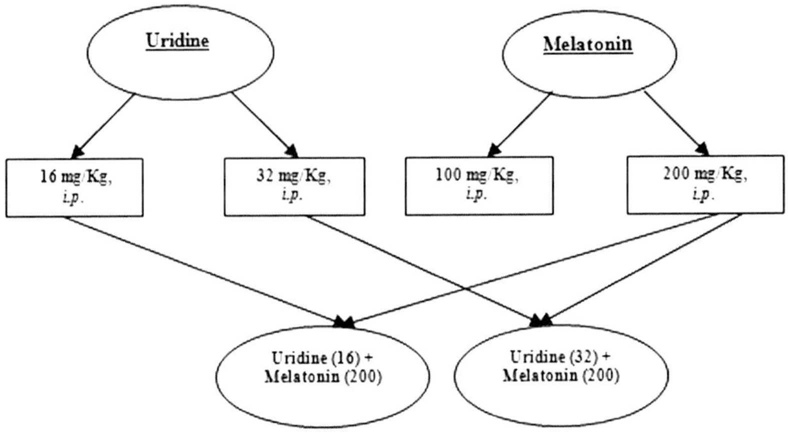

Figure 2. Proposed combinations of uridine (mg/kg) and melatonin (mg/kg): uridine (16) + melatonin (200), and uridine (32) + melatonin (200).

Data analysis

The data for percentage of edema was expressed as mean ± standard error of the means (SEM). All the groups were compared statistically by one-way analysis of variance (ANOVA) followed by suitable *post hoc* multiple comparison testing [Dunn's ($P < 0.05$) or Student–Newman–Keuls ($P < 0.001$)] using Sigma Stat (3.5) software.

Results

We observed that TBI via fluid percussion resulted in significant elevation ($P < 0.05$) in percentage edema values in cortex (79.4 ± 0.2–80.4 ± 0.4%), hippocampus (79.9 ± 0.2–82.2 ± 1.3%) and striatum (79.7 ± 0.5–81.1 ± 0.5%) on the impacted side in TBI+Vehicle rats, when compared to Sham+Vehicle group (77.7 ± 0.2%, 75.4 ± 0.5–76.5 ± 0.8%, 73.9 ± 0.7–75.5 ± 0.6%, respectively) in all the studies (Figs. 1A–C and 3A–C). As a result of administration of both doses (16 and 32 mg/kg) of uridine following TBI, we observed a significant reduction ($P < 0.05$) in edema only in impacted striatum (75.5 ± 0.5% and 75.7 ± 0.4%, respectively) when compared with TBI+Vehicle (79.7 ± 0.5%) (Fig. 1C). Similarly, posttrauma treatment with only the higher dose (200 mg/kg) of melatonin attenuated ($P < 0.05$) edema levels in impacted striatum (75.6 ± 0.4%) versus TBI+Vehicle group (Fig. 1C). In the non-impacted tissues, there was no significant difference between percentage water content of Sham+Vehicle (cortex: 78.1 ± 0.2%, hippocampus: 77.3 ± 0.5%, and striatum: 74.4 ± 0.4%) and TBI+Vehicle (cortex: 78.2 ± 0.2%, hippocampus: 77.6 ± 0.3%, and striatum: 75.7 ± 0.4%) rats and both uridine and melatonin, when administered individually, did not bring about any reduction in these levels (Figs. 1D–F).

On the basis of the above mentioned results, both doses of uridine and the higher dose of melatonin were selected and two combinations (mg/kg) were proposed for administration following TBI: Uridine (16) + Melatonin (200) {Combination 1}, and Uridine (32) + Melatonin (200) {Combination 2} (Fig. 2).

In the combination study, both combination 1 and 2 caused a significant attenuation ($P < 0.05$) of hippocampal (76.6 ± 0.4% and 75.7 ± 0.5%, respectively) and striatal (71.7 ± 0.5% and 69.7 ± 1.2%, respectively) edema on the impacted side versus TBI+Vehicle group (hippocampus: 79.9 ± 0.2%, striatum: 81.1 ± 0.5%, Figs. 3B,C). On the non-impacted side, both the combinations reduced ($P < 0.05$) striatal edema (74 ± 0.3% and 72.6 ± 0.5%, respectively) and only the group receiving combination 2 was observed to have significantly lower ($P < 0.05$) hippocampal edema levels (75.4 ± 0.3%), when compared with percentage edema values in TBI+Vehicle rats (striatum: 76.1 ± 0.3%, hippocampus: 78.3 ± 0.5%) (Figs. 3E,F). However, both the combination treatments failed to reduce cortical water content in impacted (79.5 ± 0.6% and 78.9 ± 0.1%, respectively) as well as non-impacted side (78.5 ± 0.1% and 77.9 ± 0.1%, respectively)

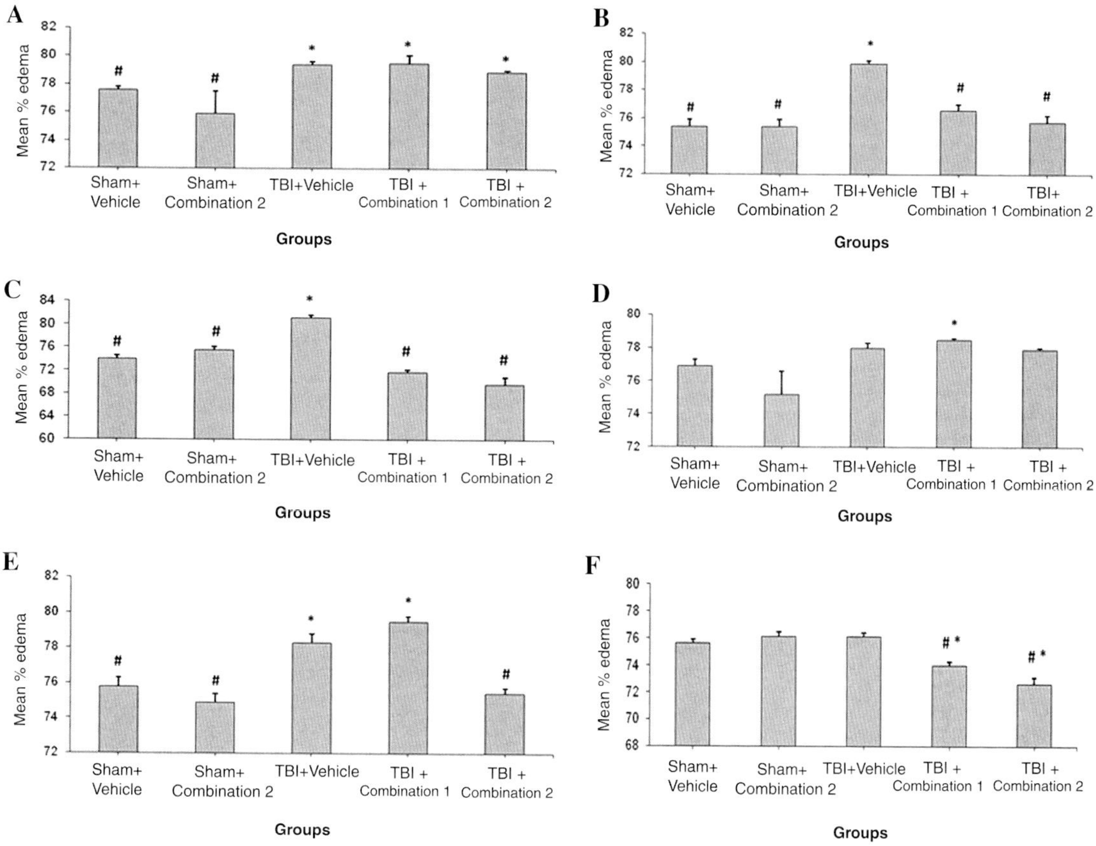

Figure 3. Effect of posttreatment of uridine (16 and 32 mg/kg) and melatonin (200 mg/kg), in combination on mean percentage edema in impacted (ipsilateral) cortex (**A**), hippocampus (**B**), striatum (**C**), non-impacted (contralateral) cortex (**D**), hippocampus (**E**), striatum (**F**) following TBI. ANOVA following Dunn's ($P < 0.05$; A,C–D) and Student–Newman–Keuls ($P < 0.001$; B,E and $P < 0.05$; F) methods of multiple comparison testing versus Sham+Vehicle and TBI+Vehicle; *: significance versus Sham+Vehicle, #: significance versus TBI+Vehicle.

versus TBI+Vehicle group (impacted: 79.4 ± 0.2%, non-impacted: 78 ± 0.3%) (Figs. 3A,D). A significant difference ($P < 0.05$) in non-impacted hippocampal edema values between Sham+Vehicle (75.8 ± 0.5%) and TBI+Vehicle (78.3 ± 0.5%) groups was observed (Fig. 3E). However, there was no difference in values of percentage water content in non-impacted cortex (Sham+Vehicle: 77.4 ± 0.2%, TBI+Vehicle: 78.0 ± 0.3%) and striatum (Sham+Vehicle: 75.6 ± 0.3%, TBI+Vehicle: 76.1 ± 0.3%) between these two groups (Figs. 3D,F). There was no significant difference between edema levels in Sham+Vehicle and Sham+Treatment in all the treatments for tissues on both impacted and non-impacted sides (Figs. 1 and 3).

Discussion

Our results indicate for the first time that posttreatment with uridine (16 and 32 mg/kg) and melatonin (200 mg/kg), both individually and in combination, can reduce posttraumatic edema in various brain regions. The injury resulted in a significant elevation in edema levels in ipsilateral cortex, hippocampus and striatum. Higher doses of both uridine and melatonin did not influence the brain edema in rats that did not receive injury, which indicates that these agents do not have any effect on brain water content under normal physiological conditions. The underlying mechanisms by which our treatments exhibit neuroprotection are unknown. However, these drugs have been tested in other models of oxidative stress and neurodegenerative diseases.

Numerous studies have demonstrated the antioxidant ability of melatonin in *in vivo* models of cerebral ischemia. Melatonin reduces the volume of cerebral infarction, malondialdehyde (MDA) and reduced glutathione levels, and improves motor performance after acute ischemic stroke in rats.[24–27] In addition, melatonin has been found to be beneficial in certain models of experimental head trauma. The administration of melatonin (200 mg/kg, *i.p.*) following severe TBI by weight-drop model in rats results in a significant reduction in MDA levels.[28] Posttreatment of melatonin (5 mg/kg, *i.p.*) in severe TBI decreases the levels of thiobarbituric acid reactive substances (TBARS) in immature rats.[29] Melatonin (100 mg/kg, *i.p.*) significantly decreases the contusion volume in rats with moderate TBI via cortical impact.[30] Posttreatment of melatonin (5 mg/kg, *i.p.*) after closed head injury in mice has been found to potentiate the activity of antioxidants in the brain.[31]

The neuroprotection observed following treatment with uridine is likely due to its conversion to CDP-choline. The administration of CDP-choline has shown beneficial results in experimental models of stroke and cerebral ischemia,[32] TBI,[33,34] intracerebral hemorrhage,[35] and cognitive impairment.[33,36,37] Posttreatment with CDP-choline significantly reduces the neuronal loss in the hippocampus, decreases cortical contusion volume and improves neurological recovery in rats subjected to TBI via cortical impact.[34] Microdialysis studies have shown that daily CDP-choline (100 mg/kg, *i.p.*) increases extracellular acetylcholine levels in dorsal hippocampus and neocortex, and significantly attenuates the motor and spatial memory deficits on daily administration to rats following TBI.[33] Administration of CDP-choline at a dose of 400 mg/kg, *i.p.* after TBI significantly reduces brain edema and inhibits breakdown of the blood-brain barrier in rats.[10] Because uridine is a precursor of phospholipid intermediates, it is indirectly a substrate for synthesis of neuronal membrane.[38,39] It has been demonstrated in humans that CDP-choline when administered orally at various doses leads to elevation in levels of plasma uridine.[40] In addition, administration of uridine causes hypothermia in mice.[41] Several studies indicate that hypothermia reduces the extent of histopathological damage resulting from TBI.[42–45] Thus, the observed neuroprotective effects in this study could be partly attributed to hypothermic conditions produced by uridine. Future studies are required to examine the neuroprotective mechanisms of action of uridine following TBI.

It is interesting to observe the edema-reducing ability of both the drugs, individually and in combination, particularly in the striatum. Uridine has been found to potentiate dopaminergic neurotransmission in the striatum.[46,47] Chronic administration of uridine (32 mg/kg, *i.p.*) reduces rotations induced by L-dopa and methamphetamine in 6-hydroxydopamine (OHDA)-striatal lesioned rats which indicates that high doses of uridine may alter drug-induced striatal dopaminergic activity.[47] In addition to being an antioxidant, melatonin binds to its respective receptors (MT1, MT2, and MT3) to exhibit its pharmacological activity. The neuroprotective effects of melatonin may also be due to the specific interactions of its indole moiety with its receptors.[48] Melatonin receptors are abundant in various regions of the brain and their activation has been linked to the promotion of viability, neuronal differentiation of neural stem cells and the regulation of production of neurotrophic factors, such as brain-derived neurotrophic factor.[49] A melatonin receptor agonist may exhibit a similar neuroprotective effect and thus, may be a good candidate for determination of the specific mechanism of action of melatonin.

The reduction of edema levels by melatonin and uridine in hippocampus is of great significance because TBI leads to impairment of cognitive ability.[50,51] Thus, our combination treatment may exhibit potential for the development of strategies against cognitive deficits resulting from brain trauma. However, reduction of brain edema by a particular neuroprotective agent may or may not correlate with improvement of neurobehavioral recovery. Studies have shown that administration of 100 mg/kg, *i.p.* of CDP-choline following TBI that attenuates edema only in ipsilateral cortex, and not in the hippocampus,[10] when administered daily postinjury causes a significant reduction in spatial memory performance deficits.[33]

Our results indicate that TBI via fluid percussion that causes elevation in edema levels in ipsilateral tissues may not necessarily result in the same in tissues on the contralateral side. It was only in the combination study that we observed a significant increase in hippocampal edema on the contralateral side following TBI, when compared with sham rats. Brain trauma results in laceration and diffuse vascular damage, particularly beneath the impact site which is referred to as coup contusion.[1] However, sometimes such pathophysiological damage is observed on the opposite side and is referred to as "countercoup" contusion.[1] From our results, it is not certain whether the damage goes on the contralateral side in all the tissues. The investigation of mechanisms involved in diffuse vascular disruption, axonal injury, and gliotic responses on the contralateral side can determine the extent of countercoup damage with certainty.

We determined the mean percentage edema levels by using wet weight/dry weight method. It is not clear whether our treatment reduces vasogenic or cytotoxic edema. Recent studies have suggested that cytotoxic edema, leading to astrocytic swelling predominantly occurs following TBI that mainly results from oxidative/nitrosative stress, mitochondrial permeability transition, and activation of mitogen-activated protein kinases (MAPK).[52–54] However, it has been reported that posttrauma glial swelling may be a result of cytotoxic mechanisms or/and breakdown of the blood-brain barrier.[10,55,56] The investigation of these processes may further shed some light on the mechanisms by which uridine and melatonin reduce regional brain edema.

In conclusion, our study is the first to demonstrate the neuroprotective effects of a combination of uridine amd melatonin on regional brain edema following TBI via fluid percussion in rats. Because the suggested mechanisms of action of both uridine and melatonin are different from each other, their combination may be effective in inhibiting the pathophysiological damage caused by TBI.

Conflicts of interest

The authors declare no conflicts of interest

References

1. Finnie, J.W. & P.C. Blumbergs. 2002. Animal models—traumatic brain injury. *Vet. Pathol.* **39:** 679–689.
2. Smith, D.H., X.H. Chen, J.E. Pierce, *et al.* 1997. Progressive atrophy and neuron death for one year following brain trauma in the rat. *J. Neurotrauma.* **14:** 715–727.
3. Williams, S., R. Raghupathi, M.A. MacKinnon, *et al.* 2001. *In situ* DNA fragmentation occurs in white matter up to 12 months after head injury in man. *Acta Neuropathol. (Berlin)* **102:** 581–590.
4. Cortez, S.C., T.K. McIntosh & L.J. Noble. 1989. Experimental fluid percussion brain injury: vascular disruption and neuronal and glial alterations. *Brain Res.* **482:** 271–282.
5. Raghavendra Rao, V.L., A. Dogan, K.K. Bowen, *et al.* 2000. Traumatic brain injury leads to increased expression of peripheral-type benzodiazepine receptors, neuronal death, and activation of astrocytes and microglia in rat thalamus. *Exp. Neurol.* **161:** 102–114.
6. Baskaya, M.K., A. Dogan, C. Temiz, *et al.* 2000. Application of 2,3,5-triphenyltetrazolium chloride staining to evaluate injury volume after controlled cortical impact brain injury: role of brain edema in evolution of injury volume. *J. Neurotrauma.* **17:** 93–99.
7. Unterberg, A.W., J. Stover, B. Kress, *et al.* 2004. Edema and brain trauma. *Neurosci.* **129:**1021–1029.
8. Betz, A.L., F. Iannotti & J.T. Hoff. 1989. Brain edema: a classification based on blood-brain barrier integrity. *Cerebrovasc. Brain Metab. Rev.* **1:** 133–154.
9. Katayama, Y. & T. Kawamata. 2003. Edema fluid accumulation within necrotic brain tissue as a cause of the mass effect of cerebral contusion in head trauma patients. *Acta Neurochir. Suppl.* **86:** 323–327.
10. Baskaya, M.K., A. Dogan, A.M. Rao, *et al.* 2000. Neuroprotective effects of citicoline on brain edema and blood-brain barrier breakdown after traumatic brain injury. *J. Neurosurg.* **92:** 448–452.
11. McIntosh, T.K., M. Thomas, D. Smith, *et al.* 1992. The novel 21-aminosteroid U74006F attenuates cerebral edema and improves survival after brain injury in the rat. *J. Neurotrauma.* **9:** 33–46.
12. Dhillon, H.S., D. Donaldson, R.J. Dempsey, *et al.* 1994. Regional levels of free fatty acids and Evans blue extravasation after experimental brain injury. *J. Neurotrauma.* **11:** 405–415.
13. Hicks, R.R., D.H. Smith & T.K. McIntosh. 1995. Temporal response and effects of excitatory amino acid antagonism on microtubule-associated protein 2 immunoreactivity following experimental brain injury in rats. *Brain Res.* **678:** 151–160.
14. Smith, S.L., P.K. Andrus, J.R. Zhang, *et al.* 1994. Direct measurement of hydroxyl radicals, lipid peroxidation, and blood-brain barrier disruption following unilateral cortical impact head injury in the rat. *J. Neurotrauma.* **11:** 393–404.

15. Tan, D.X., R.J. Reiter, L.C. Manchester, *et al.* 2002. Chemical and physical properties and potential mechanisms: melatonin as a broad spectrum antioxidant and free radical scavenger. *Curr. Top Med. Chem.* **2:** 181–197.
16. Hardeland, R. 2005. Antioxidative protection by melatonin: multiplicity of mechanisms from radical detoxification to radical avoidance. *Endocrine* **27:** 119–130.
17. Antolín, I., C. Rodríguez, R.M. Saínz, *et al.* 1996. Neurohormone melatonin prevents cell damage: effect on gene expression for antioxidant enzymes. *FASEB. J.* **10:** 882–890.
18. Rodriguez, C., J.C. Mayo, R.M. Sainz, *et al.* 2004. Regulation of antioxidant enzymes: a significant role for melatonin. *J. Pineal Res.* **36:** 1–9.
19. Winiarska, K., T. Fraczyk, D. Malinska, *et al.* 2006. Melatonin attenuates diabetes-induced oxidative stress in rabbits. *J. Pineal Res.* **40:** 168–176.
20. León, J., D. Acuña-Castroviejo, G. Escames, *et al.* 2005. Melatonin mitigates mitochondrial malfunction. *J. Pineal Res.* **38:** 1–9.
21. López-Burillo, S., D.X. Tan, *et al.* 2003. Melatonin, xanthurenic acid, resveratrol, EGCG, vitamin C and alpha-lipoic acid differentially reduce oxidative DNA damage induced by fenton reagents: a study of their individual and synergistic actions. *J. Pineal Res.* **34:** 269–277.
22. Connolly, G.P. & J.A. Duley. 1999. Uridine and its nucleotides: biological actions, therapeutic potentials. *Trends Pharmacol. Sci.* **20:** 218–225.
23. Cansev M. 2006. Uridine and cytidine in the brain: their transport and utilization. *Brain Res. Rev.* **52:** 389–397.
24. Pei, Z., S.F. Pang & R.T. Cheung. 2003. Administration of melatonin after onset of ischemia reduces the volume of cerebral infarction in a rat middle cerebral artery occlusion stroke model. *Stroke* **34:** 770–775.
25. Pei, Z., S.F. Pang & R.T. Cheung. 2002. Pretreatment with melatonin reduces volume of cerebral infarction in a rat middle cerebral artery occlusion stroke model. *J. Pineal Res.* **32:** 168–172.
26. Sinha, K., M.N. Degaonkar, N.R. Jagannathan, *et al.* 2001. Effect of melatonin on ischemia reperfusion injury induced by middle cerebral artery occlusion in rats. *Eur. J. Pharmacol.* **428:** 185–192.
27. Gupta, Y.K., G. Chaudhary & K. Sinha. 2002. Enhanced protection by melatonin and meloxicam combination in a middle cerebral artery occlusion model of acute ischemic stroke in rat. *Can. J. Physiol. Pharmacol.* **80:** 210–217.
28. Cirak, B., N. Rousan, A. Kocak, *et al.* 1999. Melatonin as a free radical scavenger in experimental head trauma. *Pediatr. Neurosurg.* **31:** 298–301.
29. Ozdemir, D., N. Uysal, S. Gonenc, *et al.* 2005. Effect of melatonin on brain oxidative damage induced by traumatic brain injury in immature rats. *Physiol. Res.* **54:** 631–637.
30. Sarrafzadeh, A.S., U.W. Thomale, S.N. Kroppenstedt, *et al.* 2000. Neuroprotective effect of melatonin on cortical impact injury in the rat. *Acta Neurochir. (Wien)* **142:** 1293–1299.
31. Beni, S.M., R. Kohen, R.J. Reiter, *et al.* 2004. Melatonin-induced neuroprotection after closed head injury is associated with increased brain antioxidants and attenuated late-phase activation of NF-kappaB and AP-1. *FASEB J.* **18:** 149–151.
32. Schäbitz, W.R., F. Li, K. Irie, *et al.* 1999. Synergistic effects of a combination of low-dose basic fibroblast growth factor and citicoline after temporary experimental focal ischemia. *Stroke* **30:** 427–431.
33. Dixon, C.E., X. Ma & D.W. Marion. 1997. Effects of CDP-choline treatment on neurobehavioral deficits after TBI and on hippocampal and neocortical acetylcholine release. *J. Neurotrauma.* **14:** 161–169.
34. Dempsey, R.J. & V.L. Raghavendra Rao. 2003. Cytidinediphosphocholine treatment to decrease traumatic brain injury-induced hippocampal neuronal death, cortical contusion volume, and neurological dysfunction in rats. *J. Neurosurg.* **98:** 867–873.
35. Clark, W., L. Gunion-Rinker, N. Lessov & K. Hazel. 1998. Citicoline treatment for experimental intracerebral hemorrhage in mice. *Stroke* **29:** 2136–2140.
36. Alvarez, X.A., M. Laredo, D. Corzo, *et al.* 1997. Citicoline improves memory performance in elderly subjects. *Meth. Find. Exp. Clin. Pharmacol.* **19:** 201–210.
37. Plataras, C., P. Angelogianni & S. Tsakiris. 2003. Effect of CDP-choline on hippocampal acetylcholinesterase and Na+,K(+)-ATPase in adult and aged rats. *Z. Naturforsch[C].* **58:** 277–281.
38. Cansev, M., C.J. Watkins, E.M. Van Der Beek, *et al.* 2005. Oral uridine-5′-monophosphate (UMP) increases brain CDP-choline levels in gerbils. *Brain Res.* **1058:** 101–108.
39. Richardson, U.I., C.J. Watkins, C. Pierre, *et al.* 2003. Stimulation of CDP-choline synthesis by uridine or cytidine in PC12 rat pheochromocytoma cells. *Brain Res.* **971:** 161–167.
40. Wurtman, R.J., M. Regan, I. Ulus, *et al.* 2000. Effect of oral CDP-choline on plasma choline and uridine levels in humans. *Biochem. Pharmacol.* **60:** 989–992.
41. Peters, G.J., C.J. van Groeningen, E.J. Laurensse, *et al.* 1987. Uridine-induced hypothermia in mice and rats

in relation to plasma and tissue levels of uridine and its metabolites. *Cancer Chemother. Pharmacol.* **20:** 101–108.

42. Dietrich, W.D. 1992. The importance of brain temperature in cerebral injury. *J. Neurotrauma.* **9:** S475–S485.
43. Dietrich, W.D., O.F. Alonso, R.B.M.Y. Globus, *et al.* 1994. Post-traumatic brain hypothermia reduces histopathological damage following concussive brain injury in the rat. *Acta Neuropathol.* **87:** 250–258.
44. Dietrich, W.D., R. Busto, M. Halley, *et al.* 1990. The importance of brain temperature in alterations of the blood-brain barrier following cerebral ischemia. *J. Neuropathol. Exp. Neurol.* **49:** 486–497.
45. Vitarbo, E.A., K. Chatzipanteli, K. Kinoshita, *et al.* 2004. Tumor necrosis factor alpha expression and protein levels after fluid percussion injury in rats: the effect of injury severity and brain temperature. *Neurosurg.* **55:** 416–425.
46. Farabegoli, C., E. Merlo Pich, M. Cimino, *et al.* 1988. Chronic uridine treatment reduces the level of [^{3}H]spiperone-labelled dopamine receptors and enhances their turnover rate in striatum of young rats: relationship to dopamine-dependent behaviours. *Acta Physiol. Scand.* **132:** 209–216.
47. Myers, C.S., H. Fisher & G.C. Wagner. 1995. Uridine reduces rotation induced by L-dopa and methamphetamine in 6-OHDA-treated rats. *Pharmacol. Biochem. Behav.* **52:** 749–753.
48. Mor, M., C. Silva, F. Vacondio, *et al.* 2004. Indole-based analogs of melatonin: *in vitro* antioxidant and cytoprotective activities. *J. Pineal Res.* **36:** 95–102.
49. Kong, X., X. Li, Z. Cai, *et al.* 2008. Melatonin regulates the viability and differentiation of rat midbrain neural stem cells. *Cell Mol. Neurobiol.* **28:** 569–579.
50. Baranova, A.I., M.D. Whiting & R.J. Hamm. 2006. Delayed, post-injury treatment with aniracetam improves cognitive performance after traumatic brain injury in rats. *J. Neurotrauma.* **23:** 1233–1240.
51. Browne, K.D., A. Iwata, M.E. Putt, *et al.* 2006. Chronic ibuprofen administration worsens cognitive outcome following traumatic brain injury in rats. *Exp. Neurol.* **201:** 301–307.
52. Norenberg, M.D., A.R. Jayakumar, K.V. Rama Rao, *et al.* 2007. New concepts in the mechanism of ammonia-induced astrocyte swelling. *Metab. Brain Dis.* **22:** 219–234.
53. Jayakumar, A.R., M. Liu, M. Moriyama, *et al.* 2008. Na-K-Cl cotransporter-1 in the mechanism of ammonia-induced astrocyte swelling. *J. Biol. Chem.* **283:** 33874–33882.
54. Jayakumar, A.R., K.V. Rama Rao, K.S. Panicker, *et al.* 2008. Trauma-induced cell swelling in cultured astrocytes. *J. Neuropathol. Exp. Neurol.* **67:** 417–427.
55. Bullock, R., W.L. Maxwell, D.I. Graham, *et al.* 1991. Glial swelling following human cerebral contusion: an ultrastructural study. *J. Neurol. Neurosurg. Psychiatry* **54:** 427–434.
56. Bramlett, H.M. & W.D. Dietrich. 2007. Progressive damage after brain and spinal cord injury: pathomechanisms and treatment strategies. *Prog. Brain Res.* **161:** 125–141.

Ann. N.Y. Acad. Sci. ISSN 0077-8923

ANNALS OF THE NEW YORK ACADEMY OF SCIENCES
Issue: *Neuroprotective Agents*

Ramelteon attenuates age-associated hypertension and weight gain in spontaneously hypertensive rats

Gregory F. Oxenkrug and Paul Summergrad

Department of Psychiatry, Tufts University School of Medicine and Tufts Medical Center, Boston, Massachusetts

Address for correspondence: Gregory F. Oxenkrug, Director, Psychiatry and Inflammation Program, Department of Psychiatry, Tufts University School of Medicine and Tufts Medical Center, Boston, MA 02111. goxenkrug@tuftsmedicalcenter.org

The neuroendocrine theory of aging suggests the common mechanisms of developmental (prereproductive) and aging (postreproductive) processes and identified a cluster of conditions (hypertension, obesity, dyslipidemia, type 2 diabetes, menopause, late onset depression, vascular cognitive impairment, impairment of immune defense, and some forms of cancer) as age-associated neuroendocrine disorders (AAND). Obesity, dyslipidemia, hypertension, and type 2 diabetes were later described as metabolic syndrome (MetS). Because melatonin attenuated development of MetS is age-dependent, that is, in young and old, but not in middle-aged rats, we studied the effect of the selective melatonin agonist, Ramelteon, on the two core symptoms of MetS/AAND: hypertension and body weight gain in spontaneously hypertensive (SHR) and normotensive Wistar-Kyoto male rats (WKY). SHR rats developed hypertension at the time of maximal weight gain that coincided with the onset of reproductive activity (8–10 weeks old). Chronic (but not acute) administration of Ramelteon (in drinking water, 8 mg/kg/day, from 4 to 12 weeks of age) attenuated age-associated increase of systolic blood pressure (tail-cuff method) by 45%, and age-associated body weight gain by 30%. Acute and chronic Ramelteon did not affect blood pressure and body weight in normotensive WKY rats. Ramelteon-induced attenuation of age-associated hypertension and weight gain suggests that Ramelteon might attenuate the other symptoms of MetS/AAND and might be useful in the treatment of MetS/AAND during puberty, menopause, and old age.

Keywords: Ramelteon; melatonin; hypertension; weight gain; aging; age; spontaneously hypertensive rats; metabolic syndrome; age-associated neuroendocrine disorders

Introduction

Melatonin is synthesized from serotonin mostly by the pineal gland. The rate limiting step of melatonin biosynthesis is serotonin-*N*-acetylation activated by noradrenaline via beta-1-adrenoreceptors. This step results in the formation of *N*-acetylserotonin (NAS), which is methylated into melatonin. Pineal melatonin synthesis follows a circadian rhythm: it is high during the night, and low during the day.

There is ample evidence that melatonin influences the cardiovascular system. Decreased blood melatonin levels were found in hypertensive patients.[1–3] Pineal melatonin levels decreased in spontaneously hypertensive rats (SHR)[4] while circadian rhythms of pineal melatonin production negatively correlated with the circadian blood pressure profile in hypertensive transgenic TGR (mREN2) rats carrying an additional mouse renin gene.[5]

Circadian rhythm of melatonin was advanced in patients with coronary heart disease in comparison with healthy subjects[2] and in SHR in comparison with normotensive Wistar-Kyoto rats (WKY).[6] The advance of melatonin circadian rhythm might contribute to the delayed normalization of melatonin biosynthesis in SHR subjected to the experimental jet lag syndrome.[7] The nighttime pineal levels of the immediate melatonin precursor, NAS, in 4-week-old (prehypertensive) SHR were higher than in the 12-week-old (hypertensive) SHR, while there were no age-associated changes of pineal NAS in WKY rats.[8] Isoproterenol, a beta-1-adrenoceptor agonist, induced higher pineal NAS levels in 4-week-old (prehypertensive) than in 12-week-old

doi: 10.1111/j.1749-6632.2009.05355.x

(hypertensive) SHR rats.[9] Pinealectomy resulted in transitional (up to 12 weeks) elevation of blood pressure in normotensive rats.[10,11]

Acute[12] and chronic administration of melatonin reduced blood pressure in normotensive men,[13–15] premenopausal women,[16] and postmenopausal women on estrogen replacement therapy.[17] Melatonin decreased blood pressure in male patients with hypertension,[18] and night blood pressure in patients with nocturnal hypertension.[19]

Melatonin and/or its immediate precursor, NAS, decreased blood pressure in SHR but not in normotensive WKY rats,[9,20,21] and in hypertensive Sprague-Dawley rats with metabolic syndrome.[22]

Melatonin administration to pregnant SHR rats decreased systolic blood pressure in their offspring[23] and inhibited hypertension and tachycardia in morphine withdrawal rats.[24] Melatonin attenuated pinealectomy-induced hypertension,[25] while pinealectomy attenuated the hypotensive effect of clorgyline, a selective monoamine oxidase type A inhibitor which stimulated melatonin biosynthesis.[26] Basal activity of the endogenous monoamine oxidase-A (MAO-A) inhibitor was three times higher in SHR than in WKY rats.[27] Cold-immobilization stress elevated the levels of the endogenous MAO-A inhibitor and induced higher pineal NAS levels in SHR than in WKY rats.[28]

Ramelteon is a potent and highly selective agonist of MT1/MT2 melatonin receptors with 3–16 times higher affinity for the melatonin MT1 and MT2 receptors than melatonin.[29]

We were interested in studying the acute and chronic effect of Ramelteon on blood pressure in SHR and WKY rats.

Methods

Animals

SHR and WKY rats (males) (Charles River Laboratories, Boston, MA) were housed two in one cage situated in an animal room at 22° C with a 14 h light (6:00–20:00)/10 h dark (20:00–6:00) cycle. All procedures using animals were in accordance with the Tufts University School of Medicine/Tufts Medical Center guidelines for animal studies and approved by the Institutional Animal Care Committee. All animals were fed with standard rat chow and had free access to drinking water.

Study protocol

Acute experiments. Ramelteon was dissolved in 1% dimethylsufoxide (DMSO)/water solution and administered by gavage (0.2 mL of solution/rat). Blood pressure was evaluated 30 min before and 1 and 2 h after administration of Ramelteon. Control rats were administered with 1% DMSO solution without Ramelteon. Acute experiments were conducted in female rats 8–10 weeks of age with three days interval between administration of each dose.

Chronic experiments. Ramelteon was dissolved in 1% DMSO/water solution and added to drinking water at a dose of 8 mg/kg/day/rat. Fresh solutions were prepared every day. Ramelteon was administered from 4 to 12 weeks of age. The control group of animals was treated with the DMSO/water solution without Ramelteon. Blood pressure was evaluated twice a week starting from 8 weeks of age. Body weight, food, and water intake were measured once a week.

Blood pressure measurements. Blood pressure was measured by tail plethysmography (tail-cuff method) in conscious rats using BP-2000 Blood Pressure Analysis System (Visitech Systems, Inc, Apex, NC). The measurements were performed during light time between 10:00 AM and 12:00 PM while the rats were kept in a temperature-regulated rat holder. Only systolic blood pressure measurements provided reproducible and reliable data. Therefore, values of diastolic blood pressure were not included in the analysis.

Statistical analysis

The results are expressed as the means ± standard deviation (SD). Statistical analysis was performed using unpaired Student's t-test for data from control and Ramelteon-treated rats. A difference was considered significant at $P < 0.05$.

Results

Acute experiments

Ramelteon (0.5, 3, and 5 mg/kg) did not affect blood pressure in both SHR and WKY rats (data not shown).

Chronic experiments

Addition of 1% DMSO/water solution with or without Ramelteon did not change water or food

Table 1. Effect of Ramelteon on systolic blood pressure in spontaneously hypertensive rats

	6 weeks	8 weeks	10 weeks	12 weeks
Control ($n = 9$)	154.7 ± 4.2#	175.6 ± 7.6	179.1 ± 12.8	182.8 ± 7.8
Ramelteon ($n = 9$)	152.7 ± 8.7#	175.8 ± 10.2	177.4 ± 9.8	168.8 ± 3.2*

Mean ± SD (mmHg). *: $P < 0.05$ versus 10 and 12 weeks Ramelteon and $P < 0.001$ versus 12 weeks control; #: $P < 0.01$ versus 8- 10- and 12-week-old rats.

consumption. Rats of both strains consumed 20 mL of drinking water and 30 g of rat chow/day/animal.

Blood pressure of 6-week-old SHR rats was within normal range in accordance with literature data. SHR rats developed hypertension by 8–12 weeks of age. Systolic blood pressure in 12-week-old control rats was higher than in 6-week-old animals by 18% (Table 1). The increase of systolic blood pressure in 12-week-old Ramelteon-treated rats was almost two times lower (10.5%).

Body weight of control SHR rats increased from 6 to 12 weeks by 70%, while in Ramelteon-treated rats body weight increased by 56% (Table 2).

Ramelteon had no effect on blood pressure and body weight in WKY (data not shown).

Discussion

There are two new findings resulting from our study: (1) chronic administration of Ramelteon slowed down age-associated increase of systolic blood pressure, and (2) chronic administration of Ramelteon slowed down age-associated increase of body weight in SHR rats.

The hypotensive effect of Ramelteon might be mediated via melatonin receptors because they were found in the brain centers involved in the regulation of the cardiovascular system, and in the peripheral vascular smooth muscles.[30] The two high-affinity membrane-associated human melatonin receptors, MT1 and MT2, have been cloned.[31] The involvement of melatonin receptors in regulation of blood pressure is further supported by the finding that the hypotensive effect of microinjection of melatonin into specific brain structures was almost completely prevented by luzindole, an antagonist of melatonin MT1/MT2 receptors.[32]

In the *ex vivo* experiments on isolated rat tail artery segments, melatonin in very low concentrations (10(−10) to 10(−7) M) potentiated phenylephrine-induced vasoconstriction while in higher concentrations (10(−7) to 10(−5) M) melatonin exerted vasodilation effect.[33] These results suggest that the vasoconstrictive effect of melatonin is mediated by MT1 receptors while the melatonin vasodilative effect is mediated by MT2 receptors. This suggestion was further supported by MT2 agonists-induced attenuation of the vasodilating effect of melatonin.[34]

Ramelteon showed very high affinity for MT1 and MT2 with Ki values of 14.0 and 112 respectively, making the affinities of Ramelteon for these receptors 3–16 times higher than those of melatonin.[29] Because Ramelteon has a higher affinity to MT1 than to MT2 receptors it is possible that *in vivo* its vasodilative effect (via MT2) is modulated by its vasoconstrictive effect (via MT1). This might explain the rather moderate (14 mmHg) decrease in blood pressure observed in our experiments. It is noteworthy that melatonin exerts a similar degree of hypotensive effect in humans.[19,34]

Some hypertensive patients lack a normal overnight decline ("dip") in blood pressure. These so-called nondippers are generally thought to be

Table 2. Effect of Ramelteon on body weight in spontaneously hypertensive rats

	6 weeks	8 weeks	10 weeks	12 weeks
Control ($n = 9$)	172.78 ± 9.39#	242.56 ± 9.42	274.89 ± 19.7	293.14 ± 9.38
Ramelteon ($n = 9$)	172.56 ± 9.57#	232.39 ± 9.58	253.79 ± 9.15*	269.78 ± 11.44**

Mean ± SD (g). #: $P < 0.01$ versus 12 weeks old; *: $P < 0.006$; and **: $P < 0.0001$ versus same age controls.

at higher risk for adverse cardiovascular events[35] and to benefit most from melatonin supplementation.[3,34] Ramelteon has a substantially longer half-life than melatonin,[36] and, in difference to melatonin and NAS, it has no significant effect on motor and cognitive performance measures in volunteers with a history of sedative abuse,[37] and on motor coordination in diazepam-primed mice.[38] Ramelteon may be better than melatonin in decreasing blood pressure, and, therefore, in reducing cardiovascular risk in hypertensive nondipper patients.

Our second finding is that Ramelteon attenuates age-associated body weight gain. This effect of Ramelteon might contribute to its hypotensive action. Literature data suggests that body growth and rising blood pressure are intimately linked, and hypertension results from an early disorder of growth.[39] Blood pressure and body weight in SHR rise with age (from birth to 8–12 weeks), and the time of maximal weight gain corresponded to the onset of a blood pressure spurt in SHR strain (approximately, at 50 days of age). In the same vein, caloric restriction lowered blood pressure[40] while methionine-deficient diet slowed down body weight gain and delayed the onset of hypertension (for 6 months) in SHR rats (Oxenkrug & Requintina, unpublished observation).

Ramelteon-induced attenuation of age-associated body weight gain in male SHR of prereproductive age might be of great importance independently of its hypotensive action.

The neuroendocrine theory of aging suggests the common mechanisms of developmental (prereproductive: from birth to onset of reproductive age) and aging (postreproductive: from the end of reproductive age to death) processes and identified certain conditions (hypertension, obesity, atherosclerosis, diabetes-II, metabolic immunosuppression) as AAND.[41–43] This theory predicts that Ramelteon (and/or melatonin) would decrease body weight gain during pre- and post-reproductive (menopausal females) periods but not during the reproductive period. Indeed, one year administration of Ramelteon did not affect body weight in monkeys of reproductive age,[44] while melatonin decreased weight in 10-month-old but not in 3-month-old rats.[45] It is noteworthy that melatonin partially prevented the increase of body weight and cholesterol in rat model of menopause (ovariectomized female rats),[46] and reduced hypertriglyceridemia (−39%), hyperinsulinemia (−33%) and hyperleptinemia (−43%), in type 2 diabetes (disease typical for postreproductive period) rats.[47]

Melatonin was effective in treatment of metabolic syndrome induced by high caloric diet or by antipsychotic drugs. Melatonin (supraphysiological doses of 10–30 mg/kg) decreased body weight gain and plasma glucose (13%), leptin (28%), and triglyceride (28%) levels in 10-month[48] and in 5–7-week-old[49] Sprague-Dawley rats fed a high-fat diet (a model closer to that observed in Western populations). Melatonin prevented an increase of plasma triglyceride levels (and systolic blood pressure) in Spraque-Dawley rats fed with high fructose (MetS model).[22]

Second-generation antipsychotics may be associated with weight gain, dyslipidemia, high blood pressure, and ultimately with cardiovascular disease, diabetes, and MetS.[50] Melatonin reversed olanzapine-induced reduction of melatonin and attenuated olanzapine-induced weight gain and increased visceral adiposity in female rats.[51]

Because we did not observe changes in food and water intake in Ramelteon-treated rats, it is most likely that its effect on body weight is related (similar to melatonin) to a decrease of intra-abdominal fat, and modulation of plasma levels of insulin, glucose, triglycerides, cholesterol, leptin,[45,48,49] and ghrelin, a rat stomach peptide antagonistic to leptin.[52]

MetS/AAND are associated with chronic inflammation and an abnormal pro-oxidant state.[53,54] The typical cytokine of chronic inflammation (Th 1 immune response) is interferon-gamma (IFNG) that increased in MetS/AAND. IFNG is the most powerful inducer of indole 2,3-dioxygenase (IDO), the rate-limiting enzyme of the kynurenine pathway of tryptophan metabolism. Activation of IDO shifted tryptophan metabolism from formation of melatonin to production of kynurenines,[55] and was observed in some conditions of MetS/AAND.[56,57] Therefore, MetS/AAND might be associated with melatonin deficiency, and be corrected by administration of melatonin[51] and/or its agonists. The involvement of melatonin receptors in melatonin-induced decrease of weight gain might be further confirmed by observation of the modulation of seasonal obesity in rodents by agonist/antagonist of MT1 and MT2 receptors.[58] In addition to melatonin receptors, melatonin might directly suppress kynurenine formation from tryptophan,[59] and inhibit production of pro-inflammatory cytokines.[60]

In conclusion, the results of our study suggested that Ramelteon attenuated age-associated development of hypertension and gain of body weight in male SHR rats. Their effects may be helpful in the treatment of the initial stages of hypertension (borderline hypertension) where weight reduction is recommended as an initial antihypertensive tool before introduction of pharmacological agents, and, especially, in nondipper hypertensive patients. Ramelteon might be also considered for an adjunct antihypertensive therapy.

Ramelteon might also be considered for prevention and treatment of MetS/AAND associated with development (prepubertal), aging (e.g., menopause), or induced by high caloric diets or psychotropic medications.

Acknowledgments

This study was supported by a grant from Takeda Pharmaceuticals, Inc. The authors are thankful for the excellent technical support provided by Ms. S. Borochin.

Conflicts of interest

The authors declare no conflicts of interest.

References

1. Jonas, M., D. Garfinkel, N. Zisapel, *et al.* 2003. Impaired nocturnal melatonin secretion in non-dipper hypertensive patients. *Blood Press.* **12:** 19–24.
2. Yaprak, M. *et al.* 2003. Decreased nocturnal synthesis of melatonin in patients with coronary artery disease. *Int. J. Cardiol.* **89:** 103–107.
3. Cagnacci, A. *et al.* 2005. Prolonged melatonin administration decreases nocturnal blood pressure in women. *Am. J. Hypertens.* **18**(12 Pt 1): 1614–1618.
4. Kawashima, K. et al. 1984. Melatonin in serum and the pineal of spontaneously hypertensive rats. *Clin. Exp. Hypertens. A* **6:** 1517–1528.
5. Enzminger, H. *et al.* 2001. Altered melatonin production in TGR(mREN2)27 rats: on the regulation by adrenergic agonists, antagonists and angiotensin II in cultured pinealocytes. *J. Pineal. Res.* **31:** 256–263.
6. Oxenkrug, G.F. & P.J. Requintina. 1992. Phase advanced circadian rhythm of the pineal melatonin biosynthesis in spontaneously hypertensive rats. *Biol. Psychiat.* **31:** 37S.
7. Oxenkrug, G.F. & P.J. Requintina. 2003. Melatonin and jet lag syndrome: experimental model and clinical implications. *CNS Spectrums.* **8:** 139–148.
8. Oxenkrug, G.F. 1998. N-acetylserotonin and the hypotensive effect of MAO-A inhibition (mini-review). *Vopr. Med. Khim.* **43:** 522–526.
9. Oxenkrug, G.F. 1999. Antidepressive and antihypertensive effects of MAO-A inhibition: role of N-acetylserotonin (a review). *Neurobiology* **792:** 213–224.
10. Zanoboni, A. & W. Zanoboni-Muciaccia. 1967. Experimental hypertension in pinealectomized rats. *Life Sci.* **6:** 2327–2331.
11. Cunnane, S.C. *et al.* 1980. Enhanced vascular reactivity to various vasoconstrictor agents following pinealectomy in the rat: role of melatonin. *Can. J. Physiol. Pharmacol.* **58:** 287–293.
12. Nishiyama, K. *et al.* 2001. Acute effects of melatonin administration on cardiovascular autonomic regulation in healthy men. *Am. Heart J.* **141:** E9.
13. Arangino, S. *et al.* 1999. Effects of melatonin on vascular reactivity, catecholamine levels, and blood pressure in healthy men. *Am. J. Cardiol.* **83:** 1417–1419.
14. Lusardi, P. *et al.* 1997. Effect of bedtime melatonin ingestion on blood pressure of normotensive subjects. *Blood Press Monit.* **2:** 99–103.
15. Kitajima, T. et al. 2001. The effects of oral melatonin on the autonomic function in healthy subjects. *Psychiatry Clin. Neurosci.* **55:** 299–300.
16. Cagnacci, A. *et al.* 1997. Potentially beneficial cardiovascular effects of melatonin administration in women. *J. Pineal. Res.* **22:** 16–19.
17. Cagnacci, A. 2001. Effect of exogenous melatonin on vascular reactivity and nitric oxide in postmenopausal women: role of hormone replacement therapy. *Clin. Endocrinol. (Oxf.)* **54:** 261–266.
18. Scheer, F.A. *et al.* 2004. Daily nighttime melatonin reduces blood pressure in male patients with essential hypertension. *Hypertension* **43:** 192–197.
19. Grossman, E. *et al.* 2006. Melatonin reduces night blood pressure in patients with nocturnal hypertension. *Am. J. Med.* **119:** 898–902.
20. Kawashima, K. *et al.* 1987. Antihypertensive action of melatonin in the spontaneously hypertensive rat. *Clin. Exp. Hypertens. A* **9:** 1121–1131.
21. K-Laflamme, A. *et al.* 1998. Impaired basal sympathetic tone and alpha1-adrenergic responsiveness in association with the hypotensive effect of melatonin in spontaneously hypertensive rats. *Am. J. Hypertens.* **11:** 219–229.

22. Leibowitz, A. *et al.* 2008. The role of melatonin in the pathogenesis of hypertension in rats with metabolic syndrome. *Am. J. Hypertens.* **2:** 348–351.
23. Kim, C.Y. *et al.* 2002. Effects of maternal-melatonin treatment on open-field behaviors and hypertensive phenotype in spontaneously hypertensive rats' (SHR) offspring. *Exp. Anim.* **51:** 69–74.
24. He, W. *et al.* 1998. Effect of melatonin on mean blood pressure and heart rate in morphine withdrawal rats. *Yao Xue Xue Bao* **33:** 727–730.
25. Karppanen, H. 1974. Studies of pinealectomy-induced hypertension in rats. Doctoral thesis, Helsinki.
26. Oxenkrug, G.F. *et al.* 1986. Possible melatonin involvement in the hypotensive effect of MAO inhibitors. *J. Neural Transm.* **66:** 271–280.
27. Oxenkrug, G.F. *et al.* 2000. The effect of cold immobilization stress on brain MAO A inhibitory activity and pineal N-acetyserotonin and melatonin in spontaneously hypertensive rats. *Stress Med.* **16:** 239–241.
28. Oxenkrug, G.F. & P.J. Requintina. 1998. The effect of MAO-A inhibition and cold-immobilization stress on N-acetylserotonin and melatonin in SHR and WKY rats. *J. Neural. Transm. [Suppl].* **52:** 333–336.
29. Kato, K. *et al.* 2005. Neurochemical properties of ramelteon (TAK-375), a selective MT1/MT2 receptor agonist. *Neuropharmacology* **48:** 301–310.
30. Viswanathan, M. *et al.* 1992. Differential expression of melatonin receptors in spontaneously hypertensive rats. *Neuroendocrinology* **56:** 864–870.
31. Dubocovich, M.L. *et al.* 2003. Molecular pharmacology, regulation and function of mammalian melatonin receptors. *Front Biosci.* **8:** 1093–1098.
32. Ding, C.N. *et al.* Effects of microinjection of melatonin and its receptor antagonists into anterior hypothalamic area on blood pressure and heart rate in rats. *Acta Pharmacol. Sin.* **22:** 997–1002.
33. Geary, G.G. *et al.* 1998. Effect of melatonin in the rat tail artery: role of K +channels and endothelial factors. *Br. J. Pharmacol.* **123:** 1533–1540.
34. Masana, M.I. *et al.* 2002. MT(2) melatonin receptors are present and functional in rat caudal artery. *J. Pharmacol. Exp. Ther.* **302:** 1295–1302.
35. Scheer, F.A. 2005. Potential use of melatonin as adjunct antihypertensive therapy. *Am. J. Hypertens.* **18**(12 Pt 1): 1619–1620.
36. Hardeland, R. *et al.* 2008. Melatonergic drugs in clinical practice. *Arzneimittelforschung* **58:** 1–10.
37. Johnson, M.W. *et al.* 2006. Ramelteon a novel hypnotic lacking abuse liability and sedative adverse effects. *Arch. Gen. Psychiatry* **63:** 1149–1157.
38. Miyamoto, M. 2006. Effect of ramelteon (TAK-375), a selective MT1/MT2 receptor agonist, on motor performance in mice. *Neurosci. Lett.* **402:** 201–204.
39. Schork, N.J. *et al.* 1994. Relationship of growth and blood pressure in inbred rats. *Am. J. Physiol.* **266**(3 Pt 2): R702–708.
40. Young, J.B. *et al.* 1978. Caloric restriction lowers blood pressure in the spontaneously hypertensive rat. *Metabolism* **27:** 1711–1714.
41. Dilman, V.M. 1971. Age-associated elevation of hypothalamic threshold to feedback control, and its role in development, ageing, and disease. *Lancet* **1:** 1211–1219.
42. Dilman, V.M. 1994. *Development, Aging and Disease: A New Rationale for an Intervention Strategy.* Harvard Acad. Publ. Zurich, Switzerland.
43. Dilman, V.M., I.P. Lapin & G.F. Oxenkrug. 1979. Serotonin and aging. In *Serotonin in Health and Disease,* Vol. 5. W. Essman, Ed.: 111–123. Spectrum Press, NY-London.
44. France, C.P. *et al.* 2006. Acute and chronic effects of ramelteon in rhesus monkeys (*Macaca mulatta*): dependence liability studies. *Behav Neurosci.* **120:** 535–541.
45. Rasmussen, D.D. *et al.* 2001. Aging-dependent changes in the effect of daily melatonin supplementation on rat metabolic and behavioral responses. *J. Pineal. Res.* **31:** 89–94.
46. Sanchez-Mateos, S. *et al.* 2007. Melatonin and estradiol effects on food intake, body weight, and leptin in ovariectomized rats. *Maturitas* **58:** 91–101.
47. Nishida, S. *et al.* Long-term melatonin administration reduces hyperinsulinemia and improves the altered fatty-acid compositions in type 2 diabetic rats via the restoration of Delta-5 desaturase activity. *J. Pineal. Res.* **32:** 26–33.
48. Puchalski, S.S. *et al.* 2003. Melatonin effect on rat body weight regulation in response to high-fat diet at middle age. *Endocrine* **21:** 163–167.
49. Prunet-Marcassus, B. *et al.* 2003. Melatonin reduces body weight gain in Sprague-Dawley rats with diet-induced obesity. *Endocrinology* **144:** 5347–5352.
50. Henderson, D.C. 2008. Managing weight gain and metabolic issues in patients treated with atypical antipsychotics. *J. Clin. Psychiatry* **69:** e04.
51. Raskind, M.A. *et al.* 2007. Olanzapine-induced weight gain and increased visceral adiposity is blocked by melatonin replacement therapy in rats. *Neuropsychopharmacology* **32:** 284–288.
52. Mustonen, A.M. *et al.* 2001. Preliminary evidence that pharmacologic melatonin treatment decreases rat ghrelin levels. *Endocrine* **16:** 43–46.

53. Festa, A. *et al.* 2000. Chronic subclinical inflammation as part of the insulin resistance syndrome: The Insulin Resistance Atherosclerosis Study (IRAS). *Circulation* **102:** 42–47.
54. Pacifico, L. *et al.* 2006. Increased T-helper interferon-gamma-secreting cells in obese children. *Eur. J. Endocrinol.* **154:** 691–697.
55. Oxenkrug, G.F. 2007. Genetic and hormonal regulation of the kynurenine pathway of tryptophan metabolism: new target for clinical intervention in vascular dementia, depression and aging. *Ann. N.Y. Acad. Sci.* **1122:** 35–49.
56. Brandacher, G. *et al.* 2007. Chronic immune activation underlies morbid obesity: is IDO a key player? *Curr. Drug Metab.* **8:** 289–295.
57. Brandacher, G. *et al.* 2006. Bariatric surgery cannot prevent tryptophan depletion due to chronic immune activation in morbidly obese patients. *Obes. Surg.* **16:** 54154–54158.
58. Le Gouic, S. *et al.* 1996. Effects of both a melatonin agonist and antagonist on seasonal changes in body mass and energy intake in the garden dormouse. *Int. J. Obes. Relat. Metab. Disord.* **20:** 661–667.
59. Walsh, H. A. & S. Daya. 1997. Inhibition of hepatic tryptophan-2,3-dioxygenase: superior potency of melatonin over serotonin. *J. Pineal. Res.* **23:** 20–23.
60. Perianayagam, M.C. *et al.* 2005. Immune modulating effects of melatonin, N-acetyl serotonin and N-acetyl dopamine. *Ann. N.Y. Acad. Sci.* **1053:** 386–393.

Ann. N.Y. Acad. Sci. ISSN 0077-8923

ANNALS OF THE NEW YORK ACADEMY OF SCIENCES
Issue: *Neuroprotective Agents*

Quinone reductase 2 and antidepressant effect of melatonin derivatives

Gregory F. Oxenkrug,[1] Sergey O. Bachurin,[2] Irina V. Prakhie,[1] and Nikolai S. Zefirov[2]

[1]Tufts University/Tufts Medical Center, Boston, Massachusetts. [2]Institute of Physiologically Active Compounds, Russian Academy of Sciences, Chernogolovka, Russia

Address for correspondence: Gregory F. Oxenkrug, Director, Psychiatry and Inflammation Program, Department of Psychiatry, Tufts University School of Medicine and Tufts Medical Center, Boston, MA 02111. goxenkrug@tuftsmedicalcenter.org

Melatonin and its immediate precursor, *N*-acetylserotonin (NAS), exert antidepressant effects in experimental models and clinical studies. We reported that melatonin and NAS decreased immobility time (an indicator of antidepressant activity) in the mouse tail suspension test. Melatonin type 3 receptor (MT3) was identified as the same protein as quinone reductase 2 (QR2) detoxifying and antioxidant enzyme. To further elucidate the role of QR2/MT3 in antidepressant action of NAS and melatonin, we studied the effect of QR2/MT3 agonist and antagonist in a tail suspension test. QR2/MT3 agonist 5-MCA-NAT decreased, while the QR2/MT3 antagonist prazosin increased the duration of immobility in the tail suspension test in a dose-dependent manner. Prazosin, in a dose that did not affect the duration of immobility, attenuated the antidepressant-like effect of NAS, melatonin, and typical tricyclic antidepressant, amitriptyline, in the tail suspension test. Our results suggest that the modulation of QR2/MT3 might contribute to mechanism(s) of antidepressant effect. New antidepressants might be searched among the agonists of QR2/MT3.

Keywords: melatonin; quinone reductase 2; *N*-acetylserotonin; tail suspension test; antidepressants; 5-MCA-NAT; prazosin

Introduction

We have previously suggested that stimulation of pineal melatonin biosynthesis might mediate the clinical antidepressant effect of the selective monoamine oxidase-A (MAO-A) inhibitors.[1] Animal and clinical studies confirmed the antidepressant effect of melatonin and its immediate precursor, *N*-acetylserotonin (NAS).[2–5]

Melatonin exerts its biological effects through two high affinity transmembrane G-protein-coupled receptors, MT1 and MT2.[6] Additionally, a low affinity cytosolic binding for the radiolabelled 2-[^{125}I]-iodomelatonin was identified and designated as MT3.[7] Pharmacological studies indicated that NAS has higher affinity to MT3 than melatonin.[8]

MT3 was identified as the same protein as human oxidoreductase 2 (QR2 protein).[9–11] 5-methoxycarbonylamino-*N*-acetyltryptamine (5MCA-NAT), MT3 agonist, and prazosin, and MT3 antagonist exert higher selectivity toward MT3 compared with MT1 and MT2[8] and specifically bind with the deep active-site cleft of QR2.[12,13]

QR2 (also known as *N*-ribosyldihydronicotinamide:quinone oxidoreductase 2) (EC 1.10.99.2) is a detoxifying and antioxidant enzyme.[14] Activation of QR2 may transform certain quinone substrates into more highly reactive compounds capable of causing cellular damage while QR2 knockdown K562 cells exhibit increased antioxidant and detoxification enzyme expression and reduced proliferation rates.[12,13] Therefore, inhibition (and not activation) of QR2 upregulates the expression of cellular antioxidant enzymes and cellular resistance to oxidative stress.

To further evaluate the possible mechanisms of antidepressant effect of melatonin and its derivatives we studied the effect of 5-MCA-NAT and prazosin on duration of immobility induced by melatonin and typical tricyclic antidepressant, amitriptyline, in mouse tail suspension test.

doi: 10.1111/j.1749-6632.2009.05354.x

Methods

The tail suspension test is a variant of the "behavioral despair" forced swimming test, in which immobility is induced by suspending an animal by the tail.[15] The test is based on the observation that a mouse suspended by the tail shows alternate periods of agitation and immobility. Unlike forced swimming, tail suspension-induced immobility is not accompanied by marked hypothermia or behavioral changes lasting longer than the test period itself, suggesting that the procedure is less stressful to the experimental animals. Tail suspension-induced immobility is genetically controlled and reflects a specific response to the test situation rather than a difference in basal motor activity.[16] The tail suspension test is useful as a rapid behavioral screening test for antidepressants.[15] Many clinically effective tricyclic, heterocyclic, and atypical antidepressants reduce the immobility that mice display after active and unsuccessful attempts to escape when suspended by the tail.[15,17] Among selective serotonin uptake inhibitors, clorimipramine, paroxetine, indalpine, fluvoxamine, and citaloprolam have shown clear activity in the tail suspension test.[15]

Male C57BL/6 mice (body wt 21 ± 25 g) were used in the study. They were housed, 10 per cage, in light-controlled chambers (12 h, light/12 h, dark cycle, lights on at 08:00, lights off at 20:00 h) with free access to food and water. C57BL/6 mice were selected for two reasons.

First, this strain was reported as one of the most suitable to be used in the tail suspension test due to its rather long baseline duration of immobility (100 s) contrary to the very short (6 s) observed in other strains.[16] Second, C57BL/6 mice combine the presence of melatonin receptors[18] with the virtual absence of enzymes of the pineal melatonin biosynthesis from serotonin.[19] Therefore, C57BL/6 mice were supposed to allow for the evaluation of the effects of the exogenous melatonin due to the presence of the melatonin receptors (or binding sites), without the interference of the endogenously produced melatonin. Each animal was tested in a chamber made out of white opaque plastic. The chamber was 17 cm wide × 25 cm high × 15 cm deep with a hook (4 cm) attached to the center of the ceiling. There was no front wall to allow for the observation of the mouse's behavior. The mouse was hung on the hook by an adhesive tape placed 15 mm from the extremity of its tail. The animal was positioned with its stomach towards the investigator to assure the observation of total immobility. The distance between the floor of the chamber and the nose of the animal was 10 cm. Immobility time was scored as a sum of the time periods during which the animal hung passively and motionless for at least 2 s. The total period of observation was 6 min. The experiments were conducted between 10:00 and 14:00 h in a quiet room. The source of light (50 W fluorescent bulb) was positioned 2 m above the experimental chamber. The animals were tested (without injections) several days before the experiment. Only those animals whose cumulative duration of immobility during a 6 min observation was no less than 100 s were selected for further experiments. Three animals were tested simultaneously. Each experimental group was composed of 9 animals. Drugs were dissolved in saline/twin (10%) solutions and administered (*i.p.*) at the doses indicated in Table 1. All control animals were injected with the vehicle and evaluated on the same day as the animals injected with the experimental drugs. Each experiment included one control and three experimental groups with combined number of 27 animals in control groups. Results were expressed as mean ± standard deviation (S.D.) (seconds) and statistically treated by ANOVA and Student t-test.

Results

The mean duration of immobility for all control groups combined was 202.52 ± 8.75 s (mean ± S.D.) ($n = 27$).

Melatonin (0.5 mg/kg) and NAS (15 mg/kg) decreased duration of immobility (153.24 ± 27.83, $P < 0.002$; and 130.67 ± 26.17, $P < 0.002$, respectively) as it was previously reported.[4]

5-MCA-NAT decreased the duration of immobility in a dose-dependent manner: low dose of 5-MCA-NAT (10 mg/kg) did not affect the duration of immobility while higher doses (25, and 50 mg/kg) decreased the duration of immobility (120.75 ± 12.56, $P < 0.002$; and 102.27 ± 17.56, $P < 0.002$) (Table 1).

Prazosin (0.5 mg/kg) increased duration of immobility 272.45 ± 16.72 ($P < 0.02$) but did not affect immobility in lower dose of 0.25 mg/kg (Table 1).

Prazosin in dose that did not affect duration of immobility (0.25 mg/kg) prevented decrease of

Table 1. The effect of quinone reductase ligands on duration of immobility in mouse tail suspension test

	Dose (mg/kg)	Duration of immobility % of control[a]	$P <$
Melatonin	0.5	75.7	0.02
Amitriptyline	10	58.2	0.002
Prazosin	0.5	135.3	0.002
Prazosin	0.25	92.4	ns
Melatonin +	0.5		
Prazosin	0.25	90.5	ns
NAS	15	64.5	0.002
NAS +	15 +		
Prazosin	0.25	93.6	ns
5-MCA-NAT	10	93.4	ns
5-MCA-NAT	25	59.6	0.002
5-MCA-NAT	50	50.5	0.002
5-MCA-NAT +	25 +		
Prazosin	0.25	94.5	ns
Amitriptyline +	10	60	<0.002
Prazosin	0.25		

[a]Drug effects expressed as percentages of control values: 202.52 ± 8.75 s; ns: not significant; all tested compounds were injected 30 min before the testing. Prazosin was injected 30 min before the other tested compounds.

immobility, induced by 5-MCA-NAT (25 mg/kg), NAS and melatonin, but not that of amitriptyline (Table 1).

Discussion

Literature and our data suggested that serotonin, noradrenaline, melatonin type 1 and type 2, and N-methyl-D-aspartate (NMDA) receptors contribute to mediation of antidepressant action (decrease duration of immobility) assessed by the tail suspension test.[20,21]

The major finding of the present study is that highly selective QR2/MT3 ligand, 5-MCA-NAT, exerts antidepressant-like activity (decreased duration of immobility in the tail suspension test). To the best of our knowledge, this is the first observation of the antidepressant-like activity of 5-MCA-NAT. Antidepressant-like activity of 5-MCA-NAT in the tail suspension test is, most likely, mediated via QR2/MT3 binding site since selective QR2/MT-3 antagonist, prazosin, prevented the effect of 5-MCA-NAT (Table 1).

The results of our study suggest that QR2/MT3 binding site might contribute to antidepressant effect of melatonin and NAS as well.[22] This suggestion is supported by data that prazosin attenuated melatonin- and NAS-induced decrease of duration of immobility in the tail suspension test (Table 1).

Other QR2/MT-3 agonists (i.e., QR2 inhibitors) might also exert antidepressant effects similar to 5-MCA-NAT. One of the most potent inhibitors of QR2 is resveratrol that (as 5MCA-NAT) specifically binds to the deep active-site cleft of QR2.[12] In addition to resveratrol's effect on the QR2/MT3 site, the antidepressant effect of resveratrol might depend on resveratrol-induced inhibition of indoleamine 2,3-dioxygenase, a rate-limiting enzyme of tryptophan metabolism along the kynurenine pathway.[23] Inhibition of kynurenine formation from tryptophan shifts tryptophan metabolism from the kynurenine pathway toward formation of serotonin,[24] the major substrate of antidepressant effect.[25] Resveratrol-induced inhibition of monoamine oxidase[26] might as well contribute to the shift of tryptophan metabolism from production of kynurenine toward serotonin formation because MAO inhibitors suppress the alternative enzyme of the kynurenine pathway, tryptophan 2,3-dioxygenase.[27] Besides activation of serotonin pathways,[20] antidepressant-like effect, that is, decreased duration of immobility in the tail suspension test, might be mediated by inhibition of NMDA receptors.[21] Considering that most (except one) products of kynurenine pathway are NMDA agonists, resveratrol (and maybe other QR2 inhibitors)-induced inhibition of indoleamine 2,3-dihydroxygenase might contribute to their antidepressant action. Among other QR2 agonists, NAS and melatonin, competitively inhibit tryptophan 2,3-dioxygenase.[27,28]

Modulation of QR2/MT3 sites is not involved in antidepressant mechanism of tricyclic antidepressants because prazosin did not affect amitriptyline-induced decrease of duration of immobility.

QR2/MT3 agonists, such as 5-MCA-NAT, might be effective as antidepressants in clinical settings. Their effect on 5-MCA-NAT (and other QR2/MT3 agonists) on tryptophan-kynurenine-serotonin metabolism might be worth future exploration.

Conflicts of interest

The authors declare no conflicts of interest.

References

1. Oxenkrug, G.F. 1991. The acute effect of monoamine oxidase inhibitors on serotonin conversion to melatonin. In *5-Hydroxytryptamine in Psychiatry: A Spectrum of Ideas.* M. Sandler, A. Coppen & S. Harnett, Eds.: 98–109. Oxford University Press, New York.
2. Skene, D. & B. Potgieter. 1981. Investigation of two models of depression. *S. Afr. J. Sci.* **77:** 180–182.
3. Requintina, P. *et al.* 1994. Synergistic sedative effect of selective MAO-A, but not MAO-B, inhibitors and melatonin in frogs. *J. Neural Transm. (Suppl.)* **41:** 141–144.
4. Prakhie, I.V. & G.F. Oxenkrug. 1998. The effect of nifedipine, Ca++ antagonist on activity of MAO inhibitors, N-acetylserotonin and melatonin in the mouse tail suspension test. *J. Neuropsychopharmac.* **1:** 35–40.
5. Dubocovich, M.L. *et al.* 1990. Antidepressant-like activity of the melatonin receptor antagonist, luzindole (N-0774), in the mouse behavioral despair test. *Eur. J. Pharmacol.* **182:** 313–325.
6. Dubocovich, M.L. 1995. Melatonin receptors: are there multiple subtypes. *Trends Pharmacol. Sci.* **16:** 50–56.
7. Molinari, E. *et al.* 1996. 2-[^{125}I]iodo-5-methoxycarbonylamino-*N*-acetyltryptamine: A selective radioligand for the characterization of melatonin ML2 binding sites. *Eur. J. Pharmacol.* **301:** 159–168.
8. Marco, M. *et al.* 1999. Melatonin receptors. *Curr. Med. Chem.* **6:** 501–518.
9. Mailliet, F. *et al.* 2005. Characterization of the melatoninergic MT_3 binding site on the NRH:quinone oxidoreductase 2 enzyme. *Biochem. Pharmacol.* **71:** 74–88.
10. Mailliet, F. *et al.* 2004. Organs from mice deleted for NRH:quinone oxydoreductase 2 are deprived of the melatonin binding site MT_3. *FEBS Lett.* **578:** 116–120.
11. Nosjean, O. *et al.* 2000. Identification of the melatonin-binding site MT_3 as the quinone reductase 2. *J. Biol. Chem.* **275:** 31311–31317.
12. Buryanovskyy, L. *et al.* 2004. Crystal structure of quinone reductase 2 in complex with resveratrol. *Biochemistry* **43:** 11417–11426.
13. Calamini, B. *et al.* 2008. Kinetic, thermodynamic and X-ray structural insights into the interaction of melatonin and analogues with quinone reductase 2. *Biochem. J.* **413:** 81–91.
14. Boutin, J.A. 2007. [Melatonin binding site MT3 is QR2: State of the art]. *J. Soc. Biol.* **201:** 97–103.
15. Steru, L. *et al.* 1987. The automated tail suspension test: a computerized device which differentiates psychotropic drugs. *Prog. NeuroPsychopharmacol. Biol. Psychiat.* **11:** 659–673.
16. Trulas, R. *et al.* 1989. Genetic differences in a tail suspension test for evaluating antidepressant activity. *Psychopharmacology* **99:** 287–288.
17. Kozlovski, V.L. & V. Prakhie. 1996. The effect of calcium channel blockers on the activity of antidepressants in the mouse tail suspension test. *J. Exp. Clin. Pharmacol.* **59:** 9–11.
18. Siuciak, J.A. *et al.* 1990. Autoradiographic localization of 2[I-125] iodomelatonin binding sites in the brains of C3H}HeN and C57Bl}6J strains of mice. *Eur. J. Pharmacol.* **180:** 387–390.
19. Ebihara, S. *et al.* 1986. Genetic control of melatonin synthesis in the pineal gland of mouse. *Science* **231:** 491–493.
20. O'Leary, O.F. *et al.* 2007. Depletion of serotonin and catecholamines block the acute behavioral response to different classes of antidepressant drugs in the mouse tail suspension test. *Psychopharmacology (Berl)* **192:** 357–371.
21. Mantovani, M. *et al.* 2003. Melatonin exerts an antidepressant-like effect in the tail suspension test in mice: evidence for involvement of N-methyl-D-aspartate receptors and the L-arginine-nitric oxide pathway. *Neurosci. Lett.* **343:** 1–4.
22. Oxenkrug, G.F. 2005. Antioxidant effects of N-acetylserotonin: possible mechanisms and clinical implications. *Ann. N.Y. Acad. Sci.* **1053:** 334–347.
23. Wirleitner, B. *et al.* 2005. Resveratrol suppresses interferon-γ-induced biochemical pathways in human peripheral blood mononuclear cells *in vitro. Immunol. Lett.* **100:** 159–163.
24. Oxenkrug, G.F. 2007. Genetic and hormonal regulation of the kynurenine pathway of tryptophan metabolism: new target for clinical intervention in vascular dementia, depression and aging. *Ann. N.Y. Acad. Sci.* **1122:** 35–49.
25. Lapin, I.P. & G.F. Oxenkrug. 1969. Intensification of the central serotoninergic processes as a possible determinant of the thymoleptic effect. *Lancet* **1:** 32–39.
26. Yáñez, M. *et al.* 2006. Inhibitory effects of cis- and trans-resveratrol on noradrenaline and 5-hydroxytryptamine uptake and on monoamine oxidase activity. *Biochem. Biophys. Res. Commun.* **344:** 688–695.
27. Samsonova, M.L. & G.F. Oxenkrug. 1972. Inhibition of substrate induction of TRY-pyrrolase in liver and increase in the content in 5-HT in brain under action of inhibitors of MAO. *Vopr. Med. Khim.* **17:** 198–201.
28. Walsh, H.A. & S. Daya. 1997. Inhibition of hepatic tryptophan-2,3-dioxygenase: superior potency of melatonin over serotonin. *J. Pineal. Res.* **23:** 20–23.

Ann. N.Y. Acad. Sci. ISSN 0077-8923

ANNALS OF THE NEW YORK ACADEMY OF SCIENCES
Issue: *Neuroprotective Agents*

Cerebrolysin reduces blood-cerebrospinal fluid barrier permeability change, brain pathology, and functional deficits following traumatic brain injury in the rat

Hari Shanker Sharma,[1] Sibilla Zimmermann-Meinzingen,[2] and Conrad E. Johanson[3]

[1]Laboratory of Cerebrovascular Research, Institute of Surgical Sciences, Department of Anaesthesiology & Intensive Care, University Hospital, Uppsala University, Uppsala, Sweden. [2]EVER Neuro Pharma, Unterach, Austria. [3]Department of Clinical Neuroscience, Brown Medical School, Rhode Island Hospital, Providence, Rhode Island

Address for correspondence: Hari Shanker Sharma, PhD (BHU), Dr. Med Sci (UU), Professor of Neurobiology (MRC), Docent in Neuroanatomy (UU), Frödingsgatan 12:28, SE-75421, Uppsala, Sweden. Sharma@surgsci.uu.se

Traumatic brain injuries (TBIs) induce profound breakdown of the blood-brain and blood-cerebrospinal fluid barriers (BCSFB), brain pathology/edema, and sensory-motor disturbances. Because neurotrophic factors, such as brain-derived neurotrophic factor (BDNF), insulin-like growth factor-1 (IGF-1), and glial cell-derived neurotrophic factor (GDNF), are neuroprotective in models of brain and spinal cord injuries, we hypothesized that a combination of neurotrophic factors would enhance neuroprotective efficacy. In the present investigation, we examined the effects of Cerebrolysin, a mixture of different neurotrophic factors (Ebewe Neuro Pharma, Austria) on the brain pathology and functional outcome in a rat model of TBI. TBI was produced under Equithesin (3 mL/kg, i.p.) anesthesia by making a longitudinal incision into the right parietal cerebral cortex. Untreated injured rats developed profound disruption of the blood-brain barrier (BBB) to proteins, edema/cell injury, and marked sensory-motor dysfunctions on rota-rod and grid-walking tests at 5 h TBI. Intracerebroventricular administration of Cerebrolysin (10 or 30 μL) either 5 min or 1 h after TBI significantly reduced leakage of Evans blue and radioiodine tracers across the BBB and BCSFB, and attenuated brain edema formation/neuronal damage in the cortex as well as underlying subcortical regions. Cerebrolysin-treated animals also had improved sensory-motor functions. However, administration of Cerebrolysin 2 h after TBI did not affect these parameters significantly. These observations in TBI demonstrate that early intervention with Cerebrolysin reduces BBB and BCSFB permeability changes, attenuates brain pathology and brain edema, and mitigates functional deficits. Taken together, our observations suggest that Cerebrolysin has potential therapeutic value in TBI.

Keywords: traumatic brain injury; brain edema; blood-brain barrier; blood-CSF barrier, choroid plexus; neuronal injury; cell death; Cerebrolysin; intracerebroventricular administration; sensory-motor function

Introduction

Traumatic brain injury (TBI) is one of the world's most devastating injuries, causing life-long disability in victims and impairing their quality of life permanently.[1,2] To date, there are no effective treatments or therapeutic procedures to significantly alleviate the sufferings of millions of brain-injury victims worldwide. Further research is needed to alleviate cognitive or functional deficits in these trauma patients to improve quality of life.

TBI can result from a deep penetrating wound into the skull that injures brain tissue.[3] However, other forms of TBI include severe blows to the skull from falls or gunshot.[4] Such wounds involve penetration or concussion. It is challenging in the laboratory to mimic the pathology encountered in clinical cases. Therefore, better experimental models are needed to enhance treatment opportunities.

Physical damage to brain causes swelling of the neurons, glia, and endothelial cells.[5] Such disrupted homeostasis leads to massive disturbances in sensory and cognitive functions.[6] Consequently,

doi: 10.1111/j.1749-6632.2009.05329.x

therapeutic strategies in TBI are needed to reduce brain swelling and neuronal damage for the purpose of enhancing functional outcome. Keeping these views in mind, our laboratory has developed a precise focal TBI model in rats in which the lesion is limited to cortical regions. This experimental procedure induces sensory and cognitive dysfunction similar to that seen in clinical cases.[7–9]

Using this model, we have shown that focal TBI results in massive breakdown of the blood-brain barrier (BBB) to protein tracers in both the injured and uninjured cortex.[7,8] Barrier disruption leads to pronounced edema formation and cell damage.[9] There are reasons to think that trauma-induced release of neurochemicals, for example, serotonin, prostaglandins, histamine, dynorphin, nitric oxide, and tumor necrosis factor-alpha, may adversely alter the BBB (see Refs. 10–13). Accordingly, efforts should be made to understand the role of these neurotransmitters and neuromodulators in modifying BBB function in TBI. Such information will likely have translational significance for the functional outcome of brain injuries in patients.

Recent observations indicate that growth hormones and neurotrophic factors, such as brain-derived neurotrophic factor (BDNF), glial cell-derived neurotrophic factor (GDNF), nerve growth factor (NGF), insulin-like growth factor (IGF) and neurotensin, given alone or in combination for spinal cord injury, attenuate cord pathology and improve functional outcome and motor paralysis (see Refs. 11, 14). Cerebrolysin is a mixture of various peptides and neurotrophic factors, and has a clinically proven neuroprotective role in stroke and Alzheimer's disease.[15,16] Thus, to extend these neuroprotective evaluations, we now analyze the possible protective role of Cerebrolysin in the TBI in our rat model. Our observations show that Cerebrolysin, when administered within early phases of TBI, confers remarkable neuroprotective effects on brain pathology and sensory-motor functions.

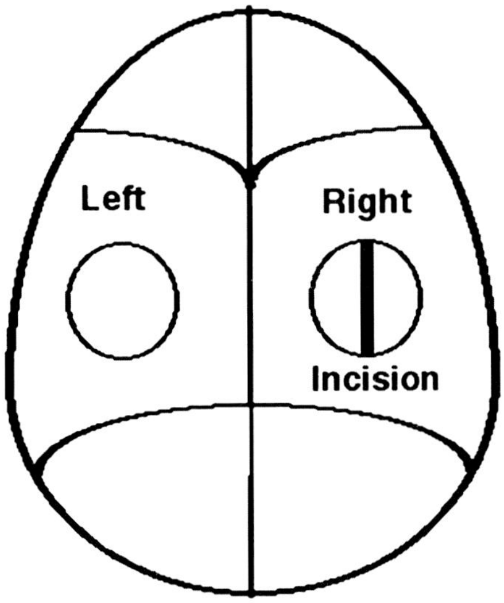

Figure 1. A model for traumatic brain injury (TBI) in rat. Under equithesin anesthesia, the parietal skull bone was exposed and a 4 mm^2 burr hole was made (O), and the underlying parietal cerebral cortex was exposed. A 3-mm deep and 5-mm long incision (I) was made on the right parietal cerebral cortex (for details see Refs. 7–9).

Materials and methods

Animals

Experiments were carried out on male Wistar rats (250–300 g) housed at controlled room temperature (21 ± 1° C) with a 12-h light and 12-h dark schedule. Food and tap water were supplied *ad libitum* before the experiment. All experiments were approved by the local Institutional Ethics Committee and conducted according to National Institute of Health (NIH) Guidelines for the care of experimental animals.

Traumatic brain injury

Under Equithesin anesthesia (3 mL/kg, i.p.) the animals were placed in a stereotaxic apparatus (Harvard Apparatus, Holliston, MA) and the parietal skull bones exposed. A burr hole was carefully made on both parietal bones (4 mm^2) without damaging the dura. Drilling was done at intermittent intervals and the skull often soaked with cold saline (4° C) to avoid warming of the skull bone and underlying brain tissue due to drilling-induced heat generation.[7,8] Also, the vibration due to drilling was minimized so that no concussive brain injury could occur due to technical reasons (see Refs. 7–9).

After opening the skull and exposing the parietal cerebral cortex, a 3-mm deep and 5-mm long stab injury was performed under stereotaxic guidance on the right parietal cortex (Fig. 1) as described earlier.[7,8] With a Gelco neurosurgical sponge (London, United Kingdom), bleeding from the cortical injury was soaked regularly until stopped, normally within a few minutes.[7,9] Both exposed (left side) and injured (right side) parietal cortices were covered with cotton soaked in saline at room temperature to avoid air-drying of cortical tissues.[7] Animals were allowed to survive 5 h after injury. Postoperative care was done according to NIH guidelines and those of the local Institutional Ethics Committee for animal care.

Control group

Animals with bilaterally-exposed parietal cerebral cortex without injury were used as sham controls, whereas intact animals were utilized as controls.[7–9]

Cerebrolysin treatment

Cerebrolysin (Ebewe Neuro Pharma, Austria) was administered in a dose of 10 or 30 μL into the left cerebral ventricle using an intracerebroventricular cannula either 1 h or 2 h after injury.[17] Sham rats identically received saline instead of Cerebrolysin.

Parameters measured

In Cerebrolysin- or saline-treated animals after injury the following parameters were measured in separate groups of rats ($n = 5$).

Blood-brain barrier permeability

The BBB permeability was quantified with Evans blue albumin (2% solution, 0.3 ml/100 g, i.v.) or radioiodine (^{131}I, 10 μCi/100 g, i.v.) as described earlier.[18] These tracers, administered under anesthesia into the right femoral vein at the end of the experiment, were allowed to circulate for 5–10 min. Then, after opening the right auricle, the intravascular tracers were flushed out with 0.9% sterile saline perfused through the heart at 100 mmHg pressure for 45 s.[18] Immediately before perfusion, about 1 mL of whole blood was withdrawn from the left ventricle of the heart for measuring radioactivity.

After perfusion, the cerebral cortex was excised and weighed. Cortical radioactivity was counted in a 3-inch Gamma counter (Packard, Meriden, CT). After radioactivity counting, some tissue samples were dissolved in a mixture of acetone and 0.5% sodium sulphate mixture to extract the Evans blue dye. The extracted Evans blue dye in each sample was measured colorimetrically as described earlier.[19,20] Before perfusion, a sample of cisternal cerebrospinal fluid (CSF) was also aspirated (50 to 100 μL) to determine radioiodine in the sample.[21,22]

Brain edema formation

In a separate group of rats, edema formation was assessed in the injured cerebral cortex. For this purpose, immediately after termination of the experiment, small pieces of cortical tissues were dissected out from both hemispheres. The major blood vessels and blood clots were removed quickly.[7–9] Tissue samples were immediately weighed and placed in an oven at 90° C for 72 h to obtain dry weight. Water content was calculated from the differences between wet and dry weight of the tissues as described earlier.[23]

Histopathology

In some rats ($n = 5$) neuronal damage was examined, using standard histological methods, in the cerebral cortex after TBI. For this purpose, following a brief saline rinse, animals were perfused with 4% paraformaldehyde through cardiac puncture.[23] Immediately after perfusion, the brains were dissected and placed in 4% paraformaldehyde at 4° C for one week. After one week of fixation, small tissue pieces were cut and embedded in paraffin. Approximately 3-μm thick sections were stained with Nissl or Hematoxylin and Eosin to detect nerve cell damage in control, injured, and Cerebrolysin-treated rats according to standard protocol.[23,24]

Sensory-motor functions

Trauma-induced alterations in sensory-motor function were examined using various tests in saline- or Cerebrolysin-treated rats (see below). These tests were performed in a blinded fashion, meaning that scores were taken by at least two independent observers not knowing the details of treatment or sham groups (see Refs. 25–27).

Rota-rod performance

The motor and cognitive function test was examined manually using Rota-rod performance (16 rpm). Rats were placed on a rota-rod (speed 16 rpm) and allowed to stay for 120 s. Rats falling from the rota-rod during a 120-s session after injury or treatment were recorded manually (see Ref. 25).

Inclined plane angle test

For this test, the rats were placed on an inclined plane maintained at 60° for 5 s. In order for rats to stay for 5 s on the inclined plane platform, the degree of the inclined plane was adjusted for injured-untreated or drug-treated rats (see Refs. 25–27). The degree at which rats could maintain their stay for 5 s was recorded manually.[25]

Grid-walking test

For this purpose, animals were placed on an inclined wire mesh (3 mm). The rats were allowed to climb for 60 s. The number of steps taken on this wire mesh was counted manually during this period and recorded for injured (untreated) and treated animals in a blind fashion by two independent observers as described earlier.[25–27]

Placement error

During climbing over the wire mesh, injured rats often placed their forelimbs into the mesh and could not hold them on the grids. This placement error was noted manually during a 60-s session and recorded for injured or treated rats in blinded fashion.[25]

Statistical analysis

ANOVA followed by Dunnet's test for multiple group comparison was used for statistical analysis of the data. Student's unpaired t-test was used to find out differences between control and experimental groups. Semiquantitative data (sensory-motor function) were examined using nonparametric Chi-square test. A P value < 0.05 was considered significant.

Results

Effect of Cerebrolysin on gross pathology

Cerebrolysin, when administered in high doses (30 μL) into the left cerebral ventricle after 5 min or 1 h injury, markedly reduced the visible edematous swelling of the injured cortex at 5 h compared to saline treatment. However, this effect was not seen when the drug was administered 2 h after brain injury. Administration of 10 μL Cerebrolysin was also effective in reducing brain edema when given 5 min or 1 h after injury but this effect was much less than for 30-μL infusion of Cerebrolysin (Table 1).

Cerebrolysin treatment also reduced the visual Evans blue staining after injury in animals that had a marked reduction in edema formation (Table 1). Thus, 10- and 30-μL Cerebrolysin doses reduced BBB leakage to Evans blue in cortical areas after injury if administered 5 min or 1 h, but not 2 h, after injury (see Table 1).

Effect of Cerebrolysin on BBB permeability

Injury to the cerebral cortex markedly increased the BBB permeability to Evans blue and radioiodine in the cortical areas at 5 h in both injured and uninjured cortical regions. This increase in the BBB permeability was most marked in the

Table 1. Effects of Cerebrolysin on gross cortical pathology after 5-h traumatic brain injury (TBI)

		Evans blue staining		Visual swelling	
Experiment type	n	Right injured	Left intact	Right injured	Left intact
Control	5	1	1	1	1
5-h brain injury	6	5	3	5	3
Saline + TBI	5	5	2	5	3
Cerebrolysin + TBI					
10 μL + 5 min	6	3	2	3	2
30 μL + 5 min	5	2	1	2	1
10 μL + 60 min	5	4	3	4	3
30 μL + 60 min	5	3	2	3	2
10 μL + 120 min	5	5	4	5	3
30 μL + 120 min	5	5	3	5	4

Values are from five to six rats (n) in each group. Visual grading: 1 = absent; 2 = mild; 3 = moderate; 4 = intense; 5 = severe. These grades were obtained by at least two independent observers in a blinded fashion (i.e., they did not know the details of treatment or there were no treatment groups).

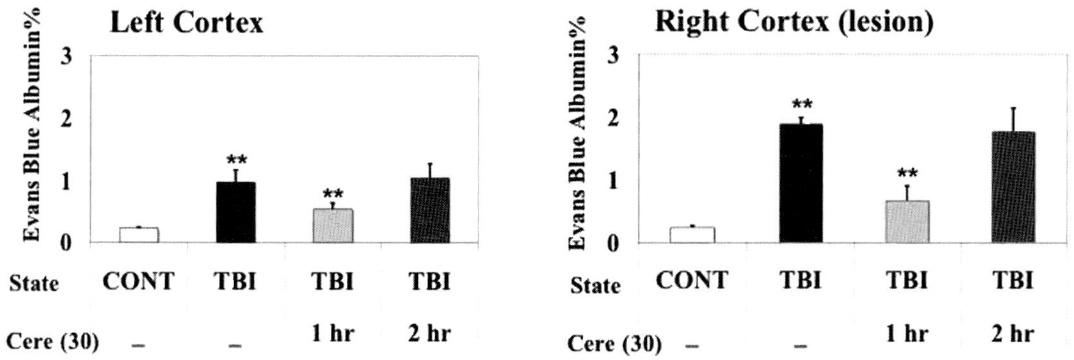

Figure 2. Effect of Cerebrolysin (Cere) treatment on traumatic brain injury (TBI) induced leakage of Evans blue albumin (EBA) in the right and left cortex. The dye entered into the brain was measured biochemically (see Ref. 35). Cerebrolysin treatment given intracerebroventricularly markedly attenuated EBA leakage in both the right and in left cortex after 5 h injury when administered 1 h after TBI. No significant effects can be seen when the Cerebrolysin was administered 2 h after TBI. ** $P < 0.01$, ANOVA followed by Dunnet's test from the control (CONT) group.

injured cortex. However, the contralateral cortex also showed a mild but significant increase in the extravasation of Evans blue and ^{131}I (Figs. 2 and 3).

Administration of Cerebrolysin (10 or 30 μL) either at 5 min or 1 h after TBI attenuated this increase in the BBB permeability to Evans blue and radioiodine seen in both hemispheres (Figs. 2 and 3). This effect was most pronounced in the contralateral cortical areas (Fig. 3). Cerebrolysin in high dose (30 μL) had greater effects in restoring cortical BBB dysfunction following TBI compared to the lower dose (10 μL; results not shown). Interestingly Cerebrolysin at 10 or 30 μL, when administered 2 h after TBI, did not significantly reduce BBB disruption to these tracers (Figs. 2 and 3).

Effect of Cerebrolysin on blood-cerebrospinal fluid barrier permeability

TBI also disrupted the blood-CSF barrier (BCSFB) at 5 h (Fig. 7). This is evident from the findings that cisternal CSF had a significant increase in radioiodine concentration compared to the non-traumatized control group (Fig. 7). Cerebrolysin treatment (30 μL) given either 5 min or 1 h after injury markedly reduced the CSF concentration of radioiodine (Fig. 7). However, administration of Cerebrolysin 2 h after trauma was ineffective in

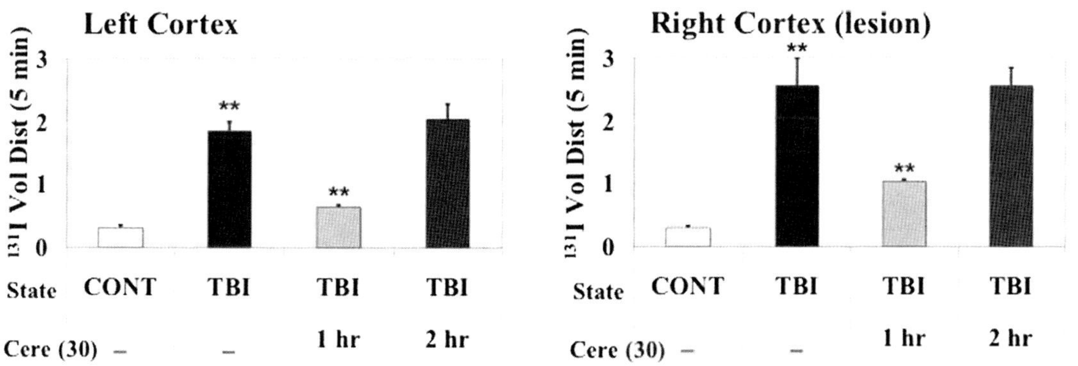

Figure 3. Effect of Cerebrolysin (Cere) treatment on traumatic brain injury (TBI) induced leakage of radioiodine (^{131}I) in the right and left cortex. Cerebrolysin treatment given intracerebroventricularly markedly attenuated radioiodine leakage in both right and in left cortex after 5 h injury when administered 1 h after TBI. No significant effects can be seen when the Cerebrolysin was administered 2 h after TBI. ** $P < 0.01$, ANOVA followed by Dunnet's test from the control (CONT) group.

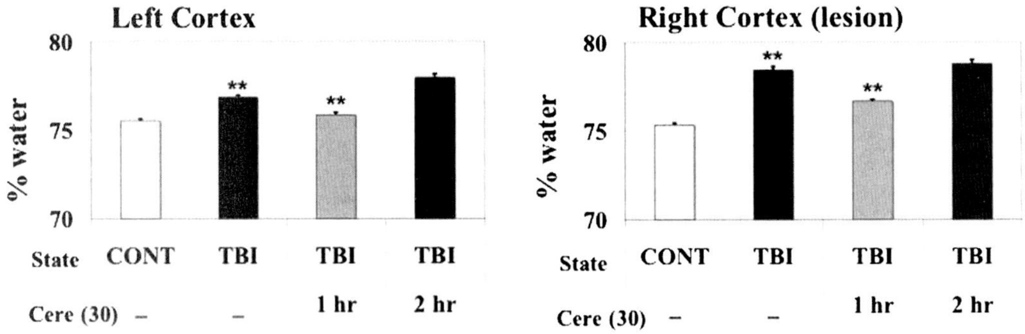

Figure 4. Effect of Cerebrolysin (Cere) treatment on traumatic brain injury (TBI) induced brain edema formation in the right and left cortex. Brain edema was measured using brain water content (see Refs. 7–9). Cerebrolysin treatment given intracerebroventricularly markedly attenuated brain water content in both right and in left cortex after 5 h injury when administered 1 h after TBI. No significant effects can be seen when the Cerebrolysin was administered 2 h after TBI. ** $P < 0.01$, ANOVA followed by Dunnet's test from the control (CONT) group.

reducing the CSF radioiodine content at 5 h post-TBI (Fig. 7).

Effects of Cerebrolysin on brain edema formation

TBI induced profound edema in both traumatized (injury side) and untraumatized (contralateral) cortical tissues over a 5-h period (Fig. 4). Thus, the cortical water content was increased significantly from the control values in the untreated injured groups. This increase in brain water content was significantly higher in the injured cortex compared to the uninjured side (Fig. 4). Intracerebroventricular administration of Cerebrolysin (10 or 30 μL), after 5 min or 1 h TBI, markedly reduced cortical water content dose-dependently in both the injured and uninjured hemispheres at 5 h (Fig. 4). However, Cerebrolysin treatment 2 h after trauma was ineffective in reducing brain water content in either directly injured or contralateral cortex (Fig. 4).

Effect of Cerebrolysin on brain pathology

Examination of cortical tissues showing edematous changes after trauma in both injured (incised) and uninjured hemispheres (non-incised) showed profound neuronal damages and distortions (Figs. 5 and 6). Thus, injured parietal cortical areas at 5 h

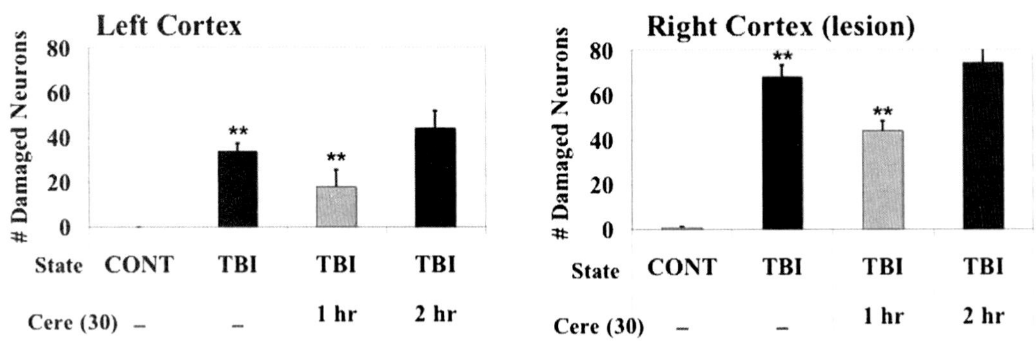

Figure 5. Effect of Cerebrolysin treatment on traumatic brain injury (TBI) induced neuronal damage in the right and left cortex. Neuronal damage was examined using histopathology employing Haematoxylin and Eosin or Nissl staining (see Refs. 7–9). Cerebrolysin treatment given intracerebroventricularly markedly attenuated neuronal damage in both right and in left cortex after 5 h injury when administered 1 h after TBI. No significant effects can be seen when the Cerebrolysin was administered 2 h after TBI. ** $P < 0.01$, ANOVA followed by Dunnet's test from the control (CONT) group.

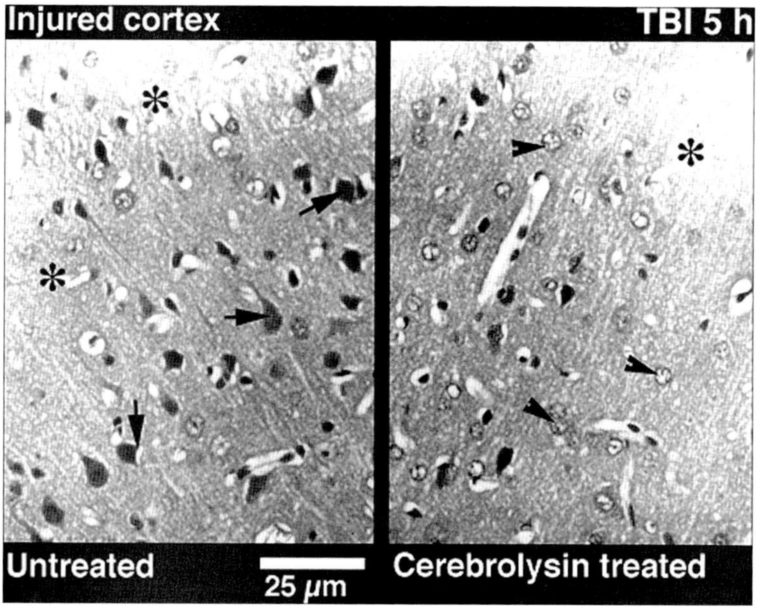

Figure 6. Neuronal damage (*arrows*) in the right injured cortex after 5 h traumatic brain injury (TBI) and its modification with Cerebrolysin treatment (1 h after TBI). Several neurons in untreated injured cortex showed marked damage (*arrows*) and sponginess and edema (*) are frequent in the neuropil (*left panel*). Treatment with Cerebrolysin markedly reduced the neuronal damage and edema formation in the injured cortex (*right panel*). Thus, several normal neurons (*arrow heads*) can be seen in the neuropil and incidences of edema or sponginess (*) were considerably reduced in Cerebrolysin-treated injured rat after 5 h TBI.

exhibited about 60 to 80 damaged neurons (per field analysis), whereas the uninjured cortex also showed 20 to 40 distorted nerve cells (Figs. 5 and 6). Cerebrolysin treatment (10 or 30 μL), given 5 min or 1 h after TBI, significantly reduced the numbers of damaged or distorted neurons in both the injured and uninjured parietal cortices (Figs. 5 and 6). This protective effect was most pronounced with the high dose of Cerebrolysin. The most marked effects of Cerebrolysin-induced neuroprotection were seen when the drug was administered 5 min after injury in high doses (results not shown). Uninjured cortex showed most pronounced neuroprotection by Cerebrolysin compared to the injured side (Figs. 5 and 6). On the other hand, no significant reduction in nerve cell damage was seen in injured animals when Cerebrolysin (10 or 30 μL) was administered 2 h after trauma (Figs. 5 and 6).

A representative example of cortical damage following TBI at 5 h, and its modification with Cerebrolysin treatment (30 μL, 1 h after injury), is shown in Figure 6. In Figure 6 it is evident that Cerebrolysin treatment markedly attenuated neuronal damage, edema formation, and sponginess in the neuropil. This effect is most pronounced in the contralateral parietal cortex compared to the ipsilateral (directly traumatized) cortex (Fig. 6).

Effect of Cerebrolysin on sensory-motor functions

TBI associated with edema formation and neuronal damage at 5 h post-trauma induction markedly altered motor and sensory functions (Figs. 8 and 9). Traumatized animals without Cerebrolysin manifested a marked deterioration of motor function on rota-rod performances and on grid-walking tests (Fig. 8). Thus, injured animals were able to stand on the rota-rod for about 30 s compared to 120 s in controls (Fig. 8). Furthermore, the injured animals also took markedly fewer steps (10 to 20) during 60 s of grid walking compared to 30 to 40 steps taken by normal rats (Fig. 8). The placement errors or falling of one or both forelimbs in the mesh were significantly higher in injured animals compared to none in normal rats (Fig. 9). The injured animals also showed less ability to stay for 5 s on an inclined

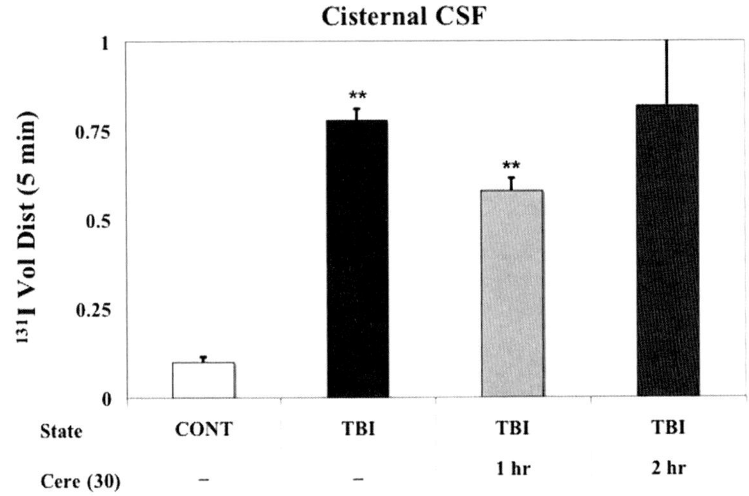

Figure 7. Early iodine leakage into CSF probably reflects increased permeability of choroid plexuses. Breakdown of the blood-cerebrospinal fluid barrier (BCSFB) in traumatic brain injury (TBI) and its modification with Cerebrolysin (Cere) treatment. TBI resulted in a marked increase in radioiodine (^{131}I) in the cisternal CSF as compared to control. Treatment with Cerebrolysin 1 h after TBI markedly reduced this radioiodine leakage in the cisternal CSF at 5 h TBI. ** = $P < 0.01$, ANOVA followed by Dunnet's test. CONT = control group.

plane, that is, at 25° to 30°, compared to normal rats which maintain position at an angle of 60° easily during the control test periods (Fig. 9).

Treatment with Cerebrolysin (30 μL) 1 h after injury markedly improved these motor and sensory functions in injured rats at 5 h (Figs. 8 and 9). Thus, Cerebrolysin-treated animals exhibited a higher score on rota-rod performances and grid-walking tests compared to untreated injured rats (Fig. 8). Furthermore, in Cerebrolysin-treated animals, the inclined plane angle was also significantly enhanced in these injured animals (average 50°) and the number of placement errors decreased remarkably (Fig. 9).

However, Cerebrolysin administration 2 h after injury did not alter these cognitive functions significantly compared to untreated injured animals (Fig. 9). Even so, some motor functions, for example, the grid-walking and rota-rod test performances, were still higher than the untreated injured animals in rats treated with Cerebrolysin at 2 h after injury (Fig. 8).

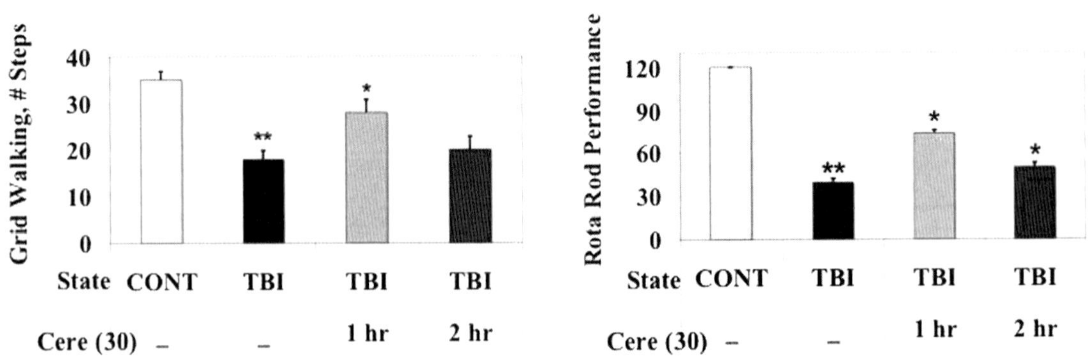

Figure 8. Improved motor and cognitive functions following traumatic brain injury (TBI) by Cerebrolysin (Cere) treatment. Cerebrolysin given 1 h after TBI markedly improved grid-walking test and rota-rod performances in rats with TBI seen at 5 h. This effect was also significant when the Cerebrolysin was given 2 h after TBI as seen on rota-rod performances. * = $P < 0.05$; ** = $P < 0.01$, ANOVA followed by Dunnet's test. CONT = control group.

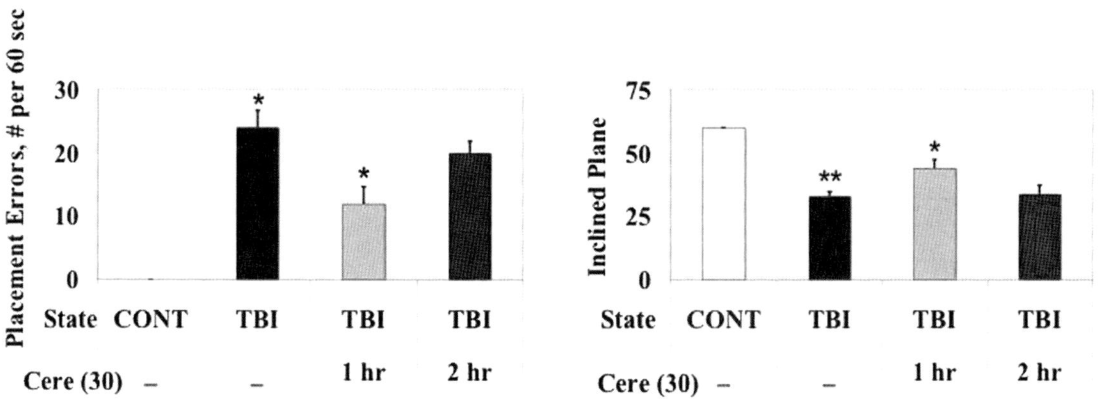

Figure 9. Improved motor and cognitive functions following traumatic brain injury (TBI) by Cerebrolysin treatment. Cerebrolysin given 1 h after TBI markedly reduced the placement errors and improved the inclined plane angle in rats with TBI at 5 h. This effect was not seen when the Cerebrolysin was given 2 h after TBI. * = $P < 0.05$; ** = $P < 0.01$, ANOVA followed by Dunnet's test. CONT = control group.

Discussion

The salient finding in this investigation is that Cerebrolysin administered in relatively high doses shortly after injury, within 5 to 60 min, is able to alleviate most of the brain pathology and cognitive and sensory dysfunctions tested in rats. However, a delay in Cerebrolysin administration from 1–2 h appears to be largely ineffective in reducing the consequences of brain pathology and functional outcome following TBI. Our observations further demonstrate that even lower doses could be effective if administered soon after brain injury (within 5 min). These new observations suggest that Cerebrolysin, depending on the dose and time of its administration, is capable of conferring neuroprotection against the detrimental effects of TBI.

Cerebrolysin is a mixture of neurotrophic factors and peptides that could act in the brain to attenuate oxidative or cellular stress.[15–17,28] A reduction in oxidative stress in TBI by Cerebrolysin appears to be one of the most important effects of the drug to induce neuroprotection.[28] Marked reduction in the consequences of TBI similar to that seen with a known antioxidant compound H-290/51 is in line with this idea.[24] Obviously, early inhibition or reduction of oxidative stress caused by trauma is needed for neuroprotection. This could be one of the reasons that a delayed administration of Cerebrolysin in TBI did not provide neuroprotection. To further support this concept, there is the need for further biochemical measurements of oxidative stress and related toxic agents in TBI following Cerebrolysin treatment. This is an experimental avenue currently being examined in our laboratory.

We used intracerebroventricular (icv) administration of Cerebrolysin on the contralateral side of the brain to induce neuroprotection in TBI. This route was chosen because CSF bulk flow is an active conduit in the brain. The ventricular supply pathway via the CSF circulation could be more effective than systemic administration of compounds (see Refs. 29–31), which has to cross the BBB. It is quite likely that drugs injected into the CSF pass rapidly into the brain parenchyma and reach a therapeutic concentration at the injury site. Obviously microhemorrhages, swelling of brain cells, and altered local tissue blood flow/metabolism will all restrict the availability of drugs to certain brain regions in sufficient concentrations when administered systemically.[12–14] Evidence is now presented that icv administration of Cerebrolysin is pharmacologically effective in TBI. This is supported by the dose-response data, that is, better neuroprotective effects are achieved in TBI when the drug was administered in high doses compared to low doses. A high concentration of drug distributed through CSF compartments can evidently reach brain tissue at a level to bestow substantial neuroprotective effects.

We observed time-related effects of Cerebrolysin on neuroprotection in TBI. Cerebrolysin injected into cerebral ventricles after 2 h TBI was ineffective in inducing neuroprotection. There are reasons to think that early phases of brain injury, for example, oxidative stress, lipid peroxidation, and other neurochemical changes, could be controlled well enough by early intervention with Cerebrolysin in high doses. Exogenous supplement of neurotrophic factors during early phases of CNS injuries are neuroprotective (see Ref. 32). Alternatively, more than 1 h after TBI the consequences of injury could lead to the emergence of other metabolic factors or toxins not adequately countered by neurotrophins. When considering this time frame post-injury, the lack of benefit of several neurotrophic factors in animal models of spinal cord injury support this idea.[33]

Our observations clearly show that TBI also induces breakdown of the BCSFB in the choroid plexus at the time of brain pathology. This indicates that a disrupted BCSFB also contributes to brain pathology (see Refs. 21, 22). Entry of serum proteins through opening of the BBB and BCSFB could easily spread to remote neuronal compartments leading to severe immune reactions and edema formation.[34,35] An increased uptake of serum proteins into the brain fluid compartments further accelerates edema formation and cell injury.[35,36] Thus, in TBI both the BBB and BCSFB play important roles in brain pathology progression. This idea is further supported by the present study using Cerebrolysin treatment. The administration of Cerebrolysin icv within an hour of TBI is not only able to attenuate BBB disruption, but also remarkably reduces BCSFB permeability to protein tracers. Therefore, following TBI, the drug-mediated prevention of these reductions (compromises) in cerebrovascular barrier integrity correlates well with the degree of neuroprotection. This indicates that to achieve neuroprotection, the maintenance of a normal functioning BBB and BCSFB is crucial in the face of injury. That the breakdown of the BBB and BCSFB in many neurological diseases associates with neurodegeneration is in line with our therapeutic transport/permeability model discussed above.

Reduction in brain edema by Cerebrolysin suggests that the drug is able to attenuate BBB and BCSFB permeability effectively leading to less edema formation after TBI. In this investigation a close correlation between less edema formation and the reduction in BBB and BCSFB leakage further supports this postulate.

Prevention of brain volume swelling, as well as the BBB or BCSFB dysfunctions, appears to be closely associated with minimizing cell injury and disturbances in sensory-motor function. Conversely, rats showing pronounced sensory-motor dysfunction after TBI exhibited marked BBB and BCSFB disturbances. A reduction in these sensory-motor deficits by Cerebrolysin occurred concurrently with less disruption of the barriers to protein and consequent brain cell damage. This fits to our hypothesis. Taken together, our observations show that trauma-induced BBB and BCSFB disruption greatly affects functional outcome and brain pathology. This point has not been emphasized, especially in a CSF context, in earlier investigations.

The mechanisms by which Cerebrolysin exerts its effects on the brain vasculature or neural tissues in attenuating cell damage are not yet clear. It appears that cellular stress caused by TBI may be attenuated by early intervention with Cerebrolysin treatment (see Refs. 37–39). A profound reduction in heat shock protein expression with Cerebrolysin treatment in hyperthermic brain injury points to the need for further investigations in this area.[39]

The probable mechanisms of barrier disruption and brain pathology following TBI in the uninjured (non-incised) hemisphere await elucidation. A pronounced increase in BBB permeability to protein tracers and brain edema formation in the left hemisphere after an injury to the right hemisphere suggest that a physical lesion alone is not sufficient to induce brain pathology.[7–9] The mechanism(s) of contralateral effects of TBI are likely to include diaschisis and transcallosal connections (see Ref. 41). The term "diaschisis" denotes specific changes in the CNS following a focal injury that are more widespread or lead to systemic alteration after trauma (see Ref. 41). Thus, injury-induced neurochemical or biological signals that could spread easily to the other hemisphere of the uninjured brain through CSF or through cerebral circulation could play significant roles.[10–12] A pronounced reduction in brain pathology in the left hemisphere with Cerebrolysin administration following TBI suggests that the icv cannula placement itself is not inducing any additional injury to the brain,[32] (see Ref. 40). It appears that icv administration of Cerebrolysin quickly spreads to the other side of the brain through CSF and or through the cerebral circulation to attenuate BBB dysfunction and brain edema in the injured side. This indicates that trauma-induced signals from the injured cortex are effectively neutralized with icv administration of Cerebrolysin.

Interestingly, Cerebrolysin also reduces the BCSFB permeability indicating that opening of the choroid plexus does not facilitate drug distribution to the brain tissues for effective therapeutic purposes. Thus, other mechanisms of CSF-drug transport across the brain tissues could be responsible for brain protection caused by Cerebrolysin in spite of a reduced BCSFB function. However, this is a subject that requires additional investigation.

Conclusion

In conclusion, our observations clearly show that Cerebrolysin has potential therapeutic effects in TBI. Cerebrolysin could quite effectively attenuate both brain pathology and functional disturbances following TBI if the drug could be administered in high concentrations into the cerebral circulation or brain ventricles during early phases of TBI.

Acknowledgments

The authors' research is supported by grants from Swedish Medical Research Council (2710, HSS); Astra-Zeneca, Mölndal (HSS), Sweden; National Institute of Health (NS27601, CEJ), USA; Alexander von Humboldt Foundation (HSS), Germany; Ebewe Neuro-Pharma, Austria Sweden (HSS); The University Grants Commission (HSS), New Delhi, India; and The Indian Council of Medical Research (HSS), New Delhi, India. The expert technical assistance of Kärstin Flink, Kerstin Rystedt, Franziska Drum, and Katherin Kern, the secretarial assistance of Aruna Sharma, and the graphical and editing contributions of Nancy and Julie Johanson are all greatly appreciated.

Conflicts of interest

The authors have no conflict of interest with any of the granting agencies mentioned above.

References

1. Colantonio, A., R. Croxford, S. Farooq, *et al.* 2009. Trends in hospitalization associated with traumatic brain injury in a publicly insured population, 1992–2002. *J. Trauma.* **66:** 179–183.
2. De Silva, M.J., I. Roberts, P. Perel, *et al.*, on behalf of the CRASH Trial Collaborators. 2008. Patient outcome after traumatic brain injury in high-, middle- and low-income countries: analysis of data on 8927 patients in 46 countries. *Int. J. Epidemiol.* **38:** 452–458.
3. Chan, W.W. & K.A. Choudhari. 2008. Penetrating head injury caused by a dart. *Ir. Med. J.* **101:** 255–256.
4. Abdolvahabi, R.M., S.A. Dutcher, J.M. Wellwood, *et al.* 2001. Craniocerebral missile injuries. *Neurol. Res.* **23:** 210–218. Review.
5. Batchelor, P.E., S. Tan, T.E. Wills, *et al.* 2008. Comparison of inflammation in the brain and spinal cord following mechanical injury. *J. Neurotrauma.* **25:** 1217–1225.
6. Whelan-Goodinson, R., J. Ponsford & M. Schönberger. 2008. Association between psychiatric state and outcome following traumatic brain injury. *J. Rehabil. Med.* **40:** 850–857.
7. Sharma, H.S., T. Winkler, E. Stålberg, *et al.* 2000. p-Chlorophenylalanine, an inhibitor of serotonin synthesis reduces blood-brain barrier permeability, cerebral blood flow, edema formation and cell injury following trauma to the rat brain. *Acta. Neurochir. Suppl.* **76:** 91–95.
8. Dey, P.K. & H.S. Sharma. 1983. Ambient temperature and development of traumatic brain oedema in anaesthetized animals. *Indian J. Med. Res.* **77:** 554–563.
9. Sharma, H.S. 2004. Histamine influences the blood-spinal cord and brain barriers following injuries to the central nervous system. In *Blood-Spinal Cord and Brain Barriers in Health and Disease.* H.S. Sharma & J. Westman, Eds.: 159–189, Elsevier. North Holland.
10. Sharma, H.S. 2008. New perspectives for the treatment options in spinal cord injury. *Expert Opin. Pharmacother.* **9:** 2773–2800. Review.
11. Sharma, H.S. 2007. A select combination of neurotrophins enhances neuroprotection and functional recovery following spinal cord injury. *Ann. N.Y. Acad. Sci.* **1122:** 95–111.
12. Sharma, H.S. 2005. Pathophysiology of blood-spinal cord barrier in traumatic injury and repair. *Curr. Pharm. Des.* **11:** 1353–1389. Review.
13. Sharma, H.S. 2004. Pathophysiology of the blood-spinal cord barrier in traumatic injury. In *Blood-Spinal Cord and Brain Barriers in Health and Disease.* H.S. Sharma & J. Westman, Eds.: 437–518. Elsevier. North Holland.
14. Sharma, H.S. 2007. Neurotrophic factors in combination: a possible new therapeutic strategy to influence pathophysiology of spinal cord injury and repair mechanisms. *Curr. Pharm. Des.* **13:** 1841–1874. Review.
15. Ren, J., D. Sietsma, S. Qiu, *et al.* 2007. Cerebrolysin enhances functional recovery following focal cerebral infarction in rats. *Restor. Neurol. Neurosci.* **25:** 25–31.

16. Ubhi, K., E. Rockenstein, E. Doppler, *et al.* 2009. Neurofibrillary and neurodegenerative pathology in APP-transgenic mice injected with AAV2-mutant TAU: neuroprotective effects of Cerebrolysin. *Acta. Neuropathol.* **117:** 699–712.
17. Windisch, M., A. Gschanes & B. Hutter-Paier. 1998. Neurotrophic activities and therapeutic experience with a brain derived peptide preparation. *J. Neural. Transm. Suppl.* **53:** 289–298.
18. Sharma, H.S. & P.K. Dey. 1986. Influence of long-term immobilization stress on regional blood-brain barrier permeability, cerebral blood flow and 5-HT level in conscious normotensive young rats. *J. Neurol. Sci.* **72:** 61–76.
19. Sharma, H.S. & P.K. Dey. 1987. Influence of long-term acute heat exposure on regional blood-brain barrier permeability, cerebral blood flow and 5-HT level in conscious normotensive young rats. *Brain Res.* **424:** 153–162.
20. Sharma, H.S. & P.K. Dey. 1986. Probable involvement of 5-hydroxytryptamine in increased permeability of blood-brain barrier under heat stress in young rats. *Neuropharmacology* **25:** 161–167.
21. Sharma, H.S. & C.E. Johanson. 2007. Intracerebroventricularly administered neurotrophins attenuate blood cerebrospinal fluid barrier breakdown and brain pathology following whole-body hyperthermia: an experimental study in the rat using biochemical and morphological approaches. *Ann. N.Y. Acad. Sci.* **1122:** 112–129.
22. Sharma, H.S. & C.E. Johanson. 2007. Blood-cerebrospinal fluid barrier in hyperthermia. *Prog. Brain Res.* **162:** 459–478. Review.
23. Sharma, H.S. & J. Cervós-Navarro. 1990. Brain oedema and cellular changes induced by acute heat stress in young rats. *Acta. Neurochir. Suppl. (Wien).* **51:** 383–386.
24. Sharma, H.S. & P.O. Sjöquist. 2002. A new antioxidant compound H-290/51 modulates glutamate and GABA immunoreactivity in the rat spinal cord following trauma. *Amino Acids* **23:** 261–272.
25. Sharma, H.S. 2006. Hyperthermia influences excitatory and inhibitory amino acid neurotransmitters in the central nervous system. An experimental study in the rat using behavioural, biochemical, pharmacological, and morphological approaches. *J. Neural. Transm.* **113:** 497–519.
26. Sharma, H.S. & A. Sharma. 2007. Nanoparticles aggravate heat stress induced cognitive deficits, blood-brain barrier disruption, edema formation and brain pathology. *Prog. Brain Res.* **162:** 245–273. Review.
27. Muresanu, D.F. & H.S. Sharma. 2007. Chronic hypertension aggravates heat stress induced cognitive dysfunction and brain pathology: an experimental study in the rat, using growth hormone therapy for possible neuroprotection. *Ann. N.Y. Acad. Sci.* **1122:** 1–22.
28. Calderón Guzmán, D., N. Osnaya Brizuela, R. García Álvarez, *et al.* 2008. Cerebrolysin and morphine decrease glutathione and 5-hydroxyindole acetic acid levels in fasted rat brain. *Biomed. Pharmacother.* **63:** 517–521.
29. Johanson, C.E., J.A. Duncan, 3rd, P.M. Klinge, *et al.* 2008. Multiplicity of cerebrospinal fluid functions: new challenges in health and disease. *Cerebrospinal. Fluid Res.* **5:** 10.
30. Johanson, C.E., J.A. Duncan, E.G. Stopa, *et al.* 2005. Enhanced prospects for drug delivery and brain targeting by the choroid plexus-CSF route. *Pharm. Res.* **22:** 1011–1037. Review.
31. Johanson, C.E., D.E. Palm, M.J. Primiano, *et al.* 2000. Choroid plexus recovery after transient forebrain ischemia: role of growth factors and other repair mechanisms. *Cell Mol. Neurobiol.* **20:** 197–216. Review.
32. Sharma, H.S., R. Patnaik, S. Patnaik, *et al.* 2007. Antibodies to serotonin attenuate closed head injury induced blood brain barrier disruption and brain pathology. *Ann. N.Y. Acad. Sci.* **1122:** 295–312.
33. Rossignol, S., M. Schwab, M. Schwartz, *et al.* 2007. Spinal cord injury: time to move? *J. Neurosci.* **27:** 11782–11792. Review.
34. Sharma, H.S., J. Westman & F. Nyberg. 1998. Pathophysiology of brain edema and cell changes following hyperthermic brain injury. *Prog. Brain Res.* **115:** 351–412. Review.
35. Sharma, H.S., J.A. Duncan & C.E. Johanson. 2006. Whole-body hyperthermia in the rat disrupts the blood-cerebrospinal fluid barrier and induces brain edema. *Acta. Neurochir. Suppl.* **96:** 426–431.
36. Sharma, H.S. & S.F. Ali. 2008. Acute administration of 3,4-methylenedioxymethamphetamine induces profound hyperthermia, blood-brain barrier disruption, brain edema formation, and cell injury. *Ann. N.Y. Acad. Sci.* **1139:** 242–258.
37. Sharma, H.S., T. Gordh, L. Wiklund, *et al.* 2006. Spinal cord injury induced heat shock protein expression is reduced by an antioxidant compound H-290/51. An experimental study using light and electron microscopy in the rat. *J. Neural. Transm.* **113:** 521–536.
38. Sharma, H.S., F. Nyberg, T. Gordh, *et al.* 2000. Neurotrophic factors influence upregulation of constitutive isoform of heme oxygenase and cellular stress response in the spinal cord following trauma. An experimental study using immunohistochemistry in the rat. *Amino Acids* **19:** 351–361.

39. Sharma, H.S., D.F. Muresanu, A. Sharma, *et al.* 2009. Cerebrolsyin attenuated's heat shock protein 72 kD response in heat stress. An experimental study in the brain. *Ann. N.Y. Acad. Sci.* (in press; This volume).
40. Wong, G.K., X.L. Zhu & W.S. Poon. 2005. Beneficial effect of Cerebrolysin on moderate and severe head injury patients: result of a cohort study. *Acta. Neurochir. Suppl.* **95:** 59–60.
41. Andrews, R.J. 1991. Transhemispheric diaschisis. A review and comment. *Stroke* **22:** 943–949.

Ann. N.Y. Acad. Sci. ISSN 0077-8923

ANNALS OF THE NEW YORK ACADEMY OF SCIENCES
Issue: *Neuroprotective Agents*

Cerebrolysin treatment attenuates heat shock protein overexpression in the brain following heat stress

An experimental study using immunohistochemistry at light and electron microscopy in the rat

Hari Shanker Sharma,[1] Dafin Muresanu,[2] Aruna Sharma,[1] and Sibilla Zimmermann-Meinzingen[3]

[1]Department of Surgical Sciences, Anaesthesiology & Intensive Care Medicine, University Hospital, Uppsala University, Sweden. [2]Department of Neurology, University of Medicine and Pharmacy "Iuliu Hatieganu", Cluj-Napoca, Romania. [3]EVER Neuro Pharma, Unterach, Austria

Address for correspondence: Hari Shanker Sharma, PhD (BHU), Dr. Med Sci (UU), Professor of Neurobiology (MRC), Docent in Neuroanatomy (UU); Frödingsgatan 12:28, SE-75421 Uppsala, Sweden. Sharma@surgsci.uu.se

The possibility that overexpression of heat shock proteins (HSPs) in the CNS represents a neurodestructive signal following hyperthermia was examined in a rat model using a potent neuroprotective drug, Cerebrolysin (Ebewe Pharma, Austria). Rats subjected to four hours of heat stress in a biological oxygen demand incubator at 38° C developed profound hyperthermia (41.23 ± 0.14° C) and overexpressed HSP 72 kD in several brain regions: cerebral cortex, hippocampus, cerebellum, thalamus, hypothalamus, brain stem, and spinal cord compared to controls. This HSP overexpression closely correlated with the leakage of blood-brain barrier permeability and vasogenic edema formation in these brain areas. HSP positive cells are largely confined in the edematous brain regions showing Evans blue leakage. Pretreatment with Cerebrolysin (5 mL/kg, i.v.) 30 minutes before heat stress markedly attenuated hyperthermia (39.48 ± 0.23° C, $P < 0.01$) and the induction of HSP to all the brain regions examined. Leakage of Evans blue albumin and increase in brain water content in these brain areas are also markedly reduced with Cerebrolysin pretreatment. These results are the first to show that Cerebrolysin, if administered before heat stress, attenuates hyperthermia induced stress reaction and HSP 72 kD induction. Taken together, these novel observations suggest that upregulation of HSP 72 kD in brain represents neurodestructive signals and a reduction in cellular stress mechanisms leading to decline in HSP expression is neuroprotective in nature.

Keywords: heat stress; Cerebrolysin; heat shock proteins (HSP 72 kD); blood-brain barrier; brain edema; brain pathology

Introduction

The role of heat shock proteins (HSPs) as a neuroprotective or neurodestructive signal following traumatic, ischemic, or metabolic insults to the central nervous system (CNS) is still not well characterized (see Refs. 1, 2). The term "heat shock proteins" is given due to the fact that sublethal heat shock (about 5° C above the normal body temperature) to *Drosophila melanogaster* resulted in the synthesis of this new class of proteins that are normally not present in normal tissues.[3] The name of heat shock protein was derived to this class of stress proteins on the basis of cell culture studies in which expression of HSP 72 kD was first seen when the medium was accidentally heated from 37° C to 45° C (see Refs. 4, 5). This abnormal expression of proteins following heat shock was termed "heat shock proteins" which is also sometimes referred to as "stress proteins" because upregulation of HSPs also occurs following ischemia, trauma, hypoxia, immobilization stress, chemical neurotoxicity, or even hypothermia.[6–9]

However, the functional significance of HSPs expression in the brain with regard to cell injury or cell survival is still not well known. A few

doi: 10.1111/j.1749-6632.2009.05330.x

studies showed that HSPs result in greater tolerance to normally lethal temperatures known as thermotolerance (see Refs. 1, 2, 6, 8) indicating that induction of HSPs is protective in nature. On the other hand, there are reasons to believe that induction of HSP occurs due to an increased threat to the cell survival.[6–9] Thus, depending on the magnitude and intensity of adverse stimuli, the cells start producing abnormal amount of HSPs.[10,11]

Interestingly, hyperthermia, stress, trauma, hypoxia, ischemia, and other forms of noxious insults to the CNS induces breakdown of the blood-brain barrier (BBB) permeability resulting in vasogenic brain edema formation and cell injury (see Refs. 8, 12–14). Thus, it is likely that HSP expression may reflect the consequences of BBB disruption and represent cellular stress and cellular injury signals that are able to induce HSP overexpression.[1–7]

However, upregulation of HSP by stress or injury signals does not indicate whether overproduction of HSP are beneficial or harmful in nature. One way to clarify this issue is to study effects of neuroprotective drugs on expression of HSP in various models of CNS insults. Keeping these views in consideration, we have undertaken a series of investigations to determine whether the role of HSP expression represents neuroprotective or neurodestructive signals in a wide variety of CNS insults in experimental animal models. In this investigation we examined the effects of Cerebrolysin, a known neuroprotective agent and a mixture of various neurotrophic factors and active peptides on HSP expression in hyperthermia induced brain injury. In addition, effects of Cerebrolysin on BBB disruption and brain edema formation in relation to HSP 70 expression were also examined in our rat model.

Materials and methods

Animals

Experiments were carried out on inbred male Charles Foster Rats (100–150 g) housed at controlled ambient temperature (21 ± 1° C) with 12 h light and 12 h dark schedule. Food and tap water were supplied *ad libitum* before the experiments. All investigations on animals were conducted according to National Institute of Health (NIH) guidelines for handling and care of experimental animals and approved by local Institutional Ethics Committee for animal care.

Heat stress

Rats were subjected to heat stress at 38° C for 4 h in a biological oxygen demand incubator (Adair Dutt & Co., New Delhi, India) (relative humidity 45–47%; wind velocity 20–25 cm/s) as described earlier.[15] This situation is very close to summer situations in many parts of Europe, Asia, and the United States (see Refs. 8, 15).

Cerebrolysin treatment

In a separate group of animals, Cerebrolysin (Ebewe Pharma, Unterach, Austria) was administered intravenously through a polyethylene cannula implanted aseptically in to the right jugular vein in rats 5–6 days before experiment.[16] We selected three different dose regimens of Cerebrolysin (1, 2.5, and 5 mg/kg, i.v.) in separate groups of rats 30 min before onset of heat stress.

Heat shock protein immunostaining

Heat shock protein (HSP) immunostaining was used to detect expression of HSP in selected brain regions after heat stress using a morphological approach.[13,17] For this purpose, immediately after heat exposure, rats were anesthetized with Equithesin (about 1 to 2 mL/kg, i.p.) and the intravascular blood was washed out with 0.9% cold saline through heart at 90 Torr perfusion pressure for 2 to 4 min (60 to 120 mL saline) using a constant infusion pump (Harvard Apparatus, Holliston, MA). After saline perfusion, the rats were perfused with cold 4% buffered paraformaldehyde for 6 to 10 min (200 to 300 mL fixative). After perfusion the animals were wrapped in aluminum foil and kept at 4° C in a refrigerator overnight. On the next day, the brains and spinal cord of these animals were taken out and placed in the same fixative at 4° C for 1 week.

Small pieces of brain tissues were cut and some of the pieces were embedded in paraffin using standard procedures and identical tissue pieces were placed on a Vibratome (Oxford Instruments, Oxford, United Kingdom) and about 40 μm thick sections were cut and collected in phosphate buffer solution in an incubation well.[17] About 3 μm thick paraffin sections were cut and placed on glass slides for further processing of HSP immunostaining.

Both Vibratome sections (free floating) and paraffin sections were incubated with mouse monoclonal HSP 72 kD antiserum (DAKO, Hamburg, Germany) in a concentration of 1:1000 or 1:5000 at 4° C overnight under constant vibrations. On the next day, the sections were washed according to standard procedures and the immunostaining was localized using peroxidase and antiperoxidase method as described in detail earlier.[17] Some sections were processed without HSP antibodies (negative controls) and stained similarly with peroxidase-antiperoxidase techniques. Immunostaining was examined with bright field light microscopy and photographed on a Kodak 100 ASA professional negative color film and processed in Kodak Laboratories (Stockholm, Sweden) professionally to obtain digital images on a CD-ROM as described earlier.[18] All images from control, experimental, and drug-treated animals were processed using a Macintosh computer (OX 10.3.4 System) using Adobe Photoshop version 7.0 employing identical color filters (see Ref. 18 for details).

Blood-brain barrier permeability

BBB permeability was examined using two well-known protein tracers, that is, Evans blue and radioiodine (^{131}I) that bind to serum albumin when administered into the systemic circulation (see Ref. 8). These tracers were administered into the right jugular vein (Evans blue 0.3 mL/100g, ^{131}I 10 μCi/100 g) at the end of heat exposure and allowed to circulate for 5 min.[15] The intravascular tracer was washed out with cold saline perfusion through the heart and the brains were dissected out. Small pieces of brains were weighed and counted in a Gamma counter (Packard, Meriden, CT). A reference sample of whole blood from the left ventricle was withdrawn immediately before saline perfusion. Extravasation of radioiodine was expressed as percentage of blood radioactivity (see Ref. 15). After counting the radioactivity, the samples were homogenized in mixture of acetone and 0.5% sodium sulphate to extract Evans blue dye in the sample. The dye extracted from brain was measured colorometrically in a spectrophotometer at 620 nm.[15–17] Calculation of dye content was done according to the standard curve for Evans blue prepared in the range of 0.01 to 2.0 mg% as described earlier.[15]

Brain edema

Brain edema in selected brain regions identical to those measured for BBB permeability was examined by changes in water content as described earlier (see Refs. 8, 15, 16). For this purpose, immediately after heat stress, the animals were decapitated and brains were removed and large vessels discarded. Selected brain regions were quickly removed, weighed, and placed in an oven at 90° C for 72 h to obtain their dry weight. Brain water content was calculated from the difference in the brain wet and dry weight.[15]

Thermal stress symptoms

Changes in rectal temperature using thermistor probes (Yellow Springfield, Dayton, OH) connected to a telethermometer (Aplab Electronics, London, United Kingdom), as well as behavioral signs of salivation and prostration were examined as thermal stress symptoms.[15]

Statistical analysis

ANOVA followed by Dunnet's test for multiple group and Chi Square test for semiquantitative data were used to evaluate statistical significance between different experimental groups. A P-value less than <0.05 was considered significant between the groups.

Results

Effect of Cerebrolysin on gross brain pathology in heat stress

When subjected to heat stress, rats treated with Cerebrolysin in lower doses exhibited disruption of the BBB to Evans blue and visual swelling at 4 h (Table 1; Fig. 4). Pretreatment with Cerebrolysin in high doses (5 mg/kg, i.v.) markedly reduced this visual swelling and blue staining of the brains after heat stress. This effect was most pronounced in animals that received a high dose of Cerebrolysin (5 mL/kg, i.v.) as compared to lower doses (1 or .5 mg/kg). Thus, in subsequent experiments only a high dose of Cerebrolysin (5 mg/kg) was used.

Effects of Cerebrolysin on heat shock protein expression

Subjection of animals to 4 h heat resulted in profound upregulation of HSP 72 kD in various brain areas (Table 2; Figs. 1 and 2). The cerebellum showed maximum number of HSP-positive cells in heat stress followed by cerebral cortex, hippocampus, brain stem, thalamus, hypothalamus, and spinal cord (see Fig. 3). Upregulation of HSP immunostaining is seen in both neuronal cytoplasm and in cell nucleus in several brain areas (Figs. 1 and 2).

Table 1. Effect of Cerebrolysin on heat stress induced gross brain pathology and thermal stress symptoms in rats

Experiment type	*n*	BBB leakage visual blue staining	Brain edema visual brain swelling	Rectal T °C	Salivation grade	Prostration grade
Control	4	nil	nil	36.86 ± 0.23	nil	nil
4 h heat stress (HS)	6	++++	++++	$41.48 \pm 0.12^{**}$	++++	++++
Cerebrolysin						
1 mL/kg, i.v.	4	nil	nil	36.65 ± 0.23	nil	nil
2.5 mL/kg, i.v.	5	nil	nil	36.67 ± 0.12	nil	nil
5 mL/kg, i.v.	5	nil	nil	36.71 ± 0.23	nil	nil
Cerebrolyisn+HS						
1 mL /kg, i.v.	6	+++	+++	$41.08 \pm 0.12^{**}$	+++	++++
2.5 mL/kg, i.v.	5	++	++	$40.67 \pm 0.23^{**}$	+++	+++
5 mL/kg, i.v.	6	+/−?	+	$39.89 \pm 0.13^{**}$	++	++

nil = absent, ++++ = severe, +++ = moderate, ++ = mild, + = faint, +/−? = not clear
** = $P < 0.01$, ANOVA followed by Dunnet's test for multiple group comparison.

In cortex, immunostaining of axons and dendrites are also seen. Control rats did not show any marked HSP positive cells. Occasionally, a few cells can be seen in some areas of the brain that took relatively much weaker immunostaining than heat stressed animals (Fig. 1; Table 2).

Pretreatment with Cerebrolysin markedly attenuated the number of HSP positive cells in the brain (see Fig. 2; Table 2). Thus, in Cerebrolysin treated animals only some cells in the various brain regions showed HSP immunoreaction (Figs. 2 and 3; Table 2).

Distribution of HSP positive cells in heat stressed animals was commonly seen in areas showing sponginess and edema (Fig. 1). The neurons that exhibit HSP expression also showed some

Table 2. Effects of Cerebrolysin (5 mg/kg, i.v.) on regional blood-brain barrier permeability, brain edema, and HSP expression in rats

	Brain regions					
Experiment type	Cerebral cortex	Hippocampus	Cerebellum	Thalamus	Hypothalamus	Spinal cord
Control group						
Evans blue mg %	0.24 ± 0.08	0.28 ± 0.04	0.18 ± 0.02	0.35 ± 0.10	0.44 ± 0.1	0.14 ± 0.04
[131]Iodine %	0.30 ± 0.06	0.30 ± 0.06	0.09 ± 0.004	0.45 ± 0.18	0.54 ± 0.23	0.19 ± 0.08
Water content %	74.34 ± 0.13	76.43 ± 0.21	75.34 ± 0.18	77.34 ± 0.23	76.45 ± 0.23	70.34 ± 0.23
HSP+ cells nr	2 ± 1	3 ± 2	1 ± 2	4 ± 6	3 ± 4	1 ± 2
4 h heat stress group						
Evans blue mg %	$2.34 \pm 0.10^{**}$	$1.45 \pm 0.12^{**}$	$2.89 \pm 0.09^{**}$	$1.35 \pm 0.12^{**}$	$0.98 \pm 0.09^{**}$	$0.84 \pm 0.10^{**}$
[131]Iodine %	$2.89 \pm 0.13^{**}$	$1.69 \pm 0.23^{**}$	$3.08 \pm 0.33^{**}$	$1.49 \pm 0.12^{**}$	$1.06 \pm 0.08^{**}$	$0.98 \pm 0.06^{**}$
Water content %	$78.43 \pm 0.21^{**}$	$79.89 \pm 0.43^{**}$	$79.56 \pm 0.08^{**}$	$79.45 \pm 0.10^{**}$	$78.89 \pm 0.12^{**}$	$73.79 \pm 0.12^{**}$
HSP+ cells nr	$220 \pm 24^{**}$	$160 \pm 34^{**}$	$289 \pm 35^{**}$	$174 \pm 23^{**}$	$98 \pm 14^{**}$	$56 \pm 12^{**}$
Cerebrolysin+4 h heat stress						
Evans blue mg %	$0.89 \pm 0.44^{*}$	$0.67 \pm 0.34^{*}$	$0.89 \pm 0.43^{*}$	$0.78 \pm 0.33^{*}$	$0.54 \pm 0.13^{*}$	$0.56 \pm 0.12^{*}$
[131]Iodine %	$0.96 \pm 0.34^{**}$	$0.89 \pm 0.34^{*}$	$0.98 \pm 0.23^{**}$	$0.89 \pm 0.44^{*}$	$0.67 \pm 0.23^{*}$	$0.67 \pm 0.23^{*}$
Water content %	$76.34 \pm 0.21^{**}$	$77.34 \pm 0.12^{**}$	$76.69 \pm 0.54^{**}$	$78.45 \pm 0.23^{**}$	$77.12 \pm 0.32^{**}$	$71.34 \pm 0.22^{**}$
HSP+ cells nr	$24 \pm 8^{*}$	$30 \pm 12^{*}$	$45 \pm 12^{*}$	$38 \pm 8^{**}$	$45 \pm 9^{**}$	$43 \pm 12^{**}$

Values are mean ± SD, * $P < 0.05$, ** $P < 0.01$, ANOVA followed by Dunnet's test.

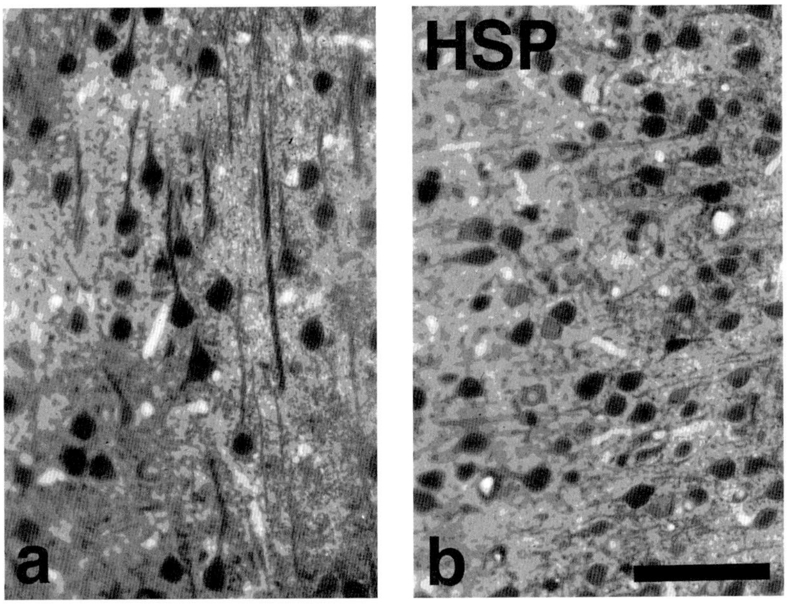

Figure 1. Heat shock protein (HSP) 72 kD expression in the cerebral cortex of rats subjected to 4 h heat stress. Marked upregulation of HSP positive neurons and dendrites can be seen in the parietal cortex (a) and in the temporal cortex (b). Bar = 30 μm.[1,2]

deterioration (Fig. 1). In Cerebrolysin treated animals, the HSP expression was weak and most of the neurons showed milder distortion than seen in untreated heat stressed rats exhibiting HSP positive immunostaining (Figs. 2 and 3).

Effects of Cerebrolysin on BBB permeability

Rats subjected to 4 h heat stress showed a profound increase in the BBB permeability to Evans blue and radioiodine in various brain regions as compared to control groups (see Table 2; Fig. 4). The cerebellum showed the greatest increase in the BBB permeability to proteins followed by cortex, hippocampus, thalamus, hypothalamus, and spinal cord (Table 2). In general, there was a greater leakage of radioiodine compared to Evans blue albumin in most of the brain regions in heat stress (Table 2).

Pretreatment with Cerebrolysin (5 mg/kg, i.v.) markedly reduced the BBB leakage in these heat stressed animals at 4 h (Table 2). Only a mild but significant increase in extravasation of Evans blue and radioiodine from control values could be seen in Cerebrolysin treated animals in heat stress (Table 2). In Cerebrolysin treated stressed animals the extravasation of radioiodine was also higher than Evans blue content in many brain regions (Table 2).

Effects of Cerebrolysin on brain edema formation

The brain areas associated with leakage of proteins following 4 h heat stress exhibited profound edema formation as seen by measurement of brain water content (Table 2; Fig. 4). The cerebellum showed the most marked increase in brain water followed by cortex, hippocampus, thalamus, hypothalamus, and spinal cord in heat stress (Table 2).

Pretreatment with Cerebrolysin significantly attenuated this increase in brain water content in heat stressed animals as compared to untreated stressed groups (Table 2).

Correlation between HSP expression, brain edema, and BBB permeability

Regression analysis showed a very tight correlation between HSP 72 kD expression in the cortex with Evans blue albumin leakage and brain edema formation irrespective of control, heat stress, or treatment with Cerebrolysin in heat stress (Fig. 5). Also, a close correlation was observed between leakage of Evans blue and brain edema formation in various groups of heat stress rats in untreated and Cerebrolysin treated animals (Fig. 4).

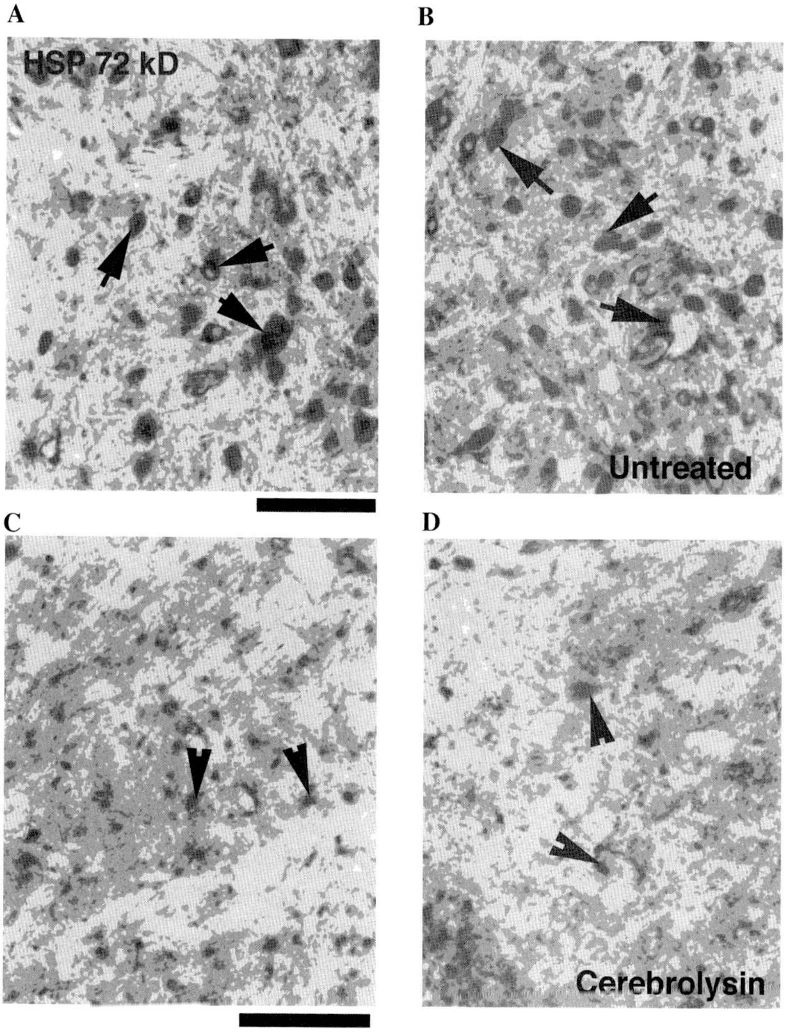

Figure 2. Vibratome sections from the cerebral cortex of rats subjected to 4 h heat stress at 38°C showing upregulation of heat shock protein (HSP) 72 kD in neurons (*arrows*) and in possibly a few glial cells (A,B). The immunoreactivity is present in neuronal cell cytoplasm and in many cases the nucleus was not stained. Pretreatment with Cerebrolysin markedly attenuated heat stress induced HSP upregulation (*arrow heads*) in identical areas of rat cerebral cortex (C,D). Bars: A,B = 25 μm, C,D = 20 μm.

Effects of Cerebrolysin on stress symptoms

Heat stress induced profound hyperthermia and behavioral symptoms, for example, salivation and prostration after 4 h exposure (Table 1, Fig. 4). Pretreatment with Cerebrolysin in high doses (5 mL/kg, i.v.) markedly attenuated these stress symptoms. Hyperthermia induced by heat stress and signs of behavioral salivation and prostration were significantly reduced by Cerebrolysin pretreatment (see Table 1). However, low doses of Cerebrolysin (1 mg or 2.5 mg) were ineffective in reducing heat stress induced hyperthermia or behavioral symptoms (Table 1).

Discussion

The present results for the first time show that Cerebrolysin, a mixture of potent neurotrophic factors and peptides, if given in high doses before heat stress is able to thwart HSP upregulation in the brain and spinal cord. Furthermore, our investigations show that this prevention of HSP overexpression with

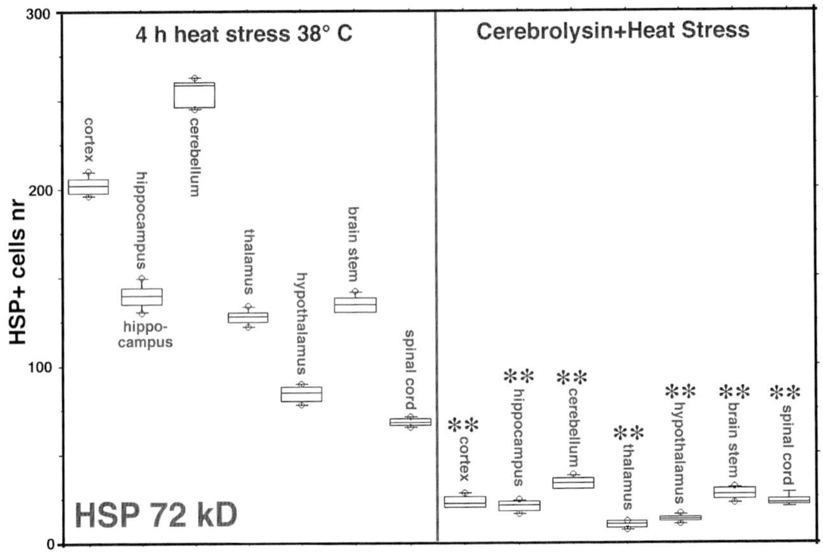

Figure 3. Semiquantitative analysis of heat shock protein (HSP) positive cells (neuronal and glial cells) in various regions of the rat brain after 4 h heat stress and its modification with Cerebrolysin pretreatment. ** $P < 0.01$, compared with untreated stressed rat, Chi Square test.

Cerebrolysin is associated with a reduction in the BBB disruption and brain edema. These observations suggest that overexpression of HSP represents severe stressful situations and could result from altered microvascular permeability disturbances and formation of brain edema.[8,9,12–17] This idea is further supported by the findings that Cerebrolysin in lower doses was not effective in reducing either the HSP responses in brain following heat stress or the BBB disruptions or brain edema formation. This indicates that BBB disruption and brain edema are important signals for HSP expression in heat stress. Furthermore, this study shows that high doses of Cerebrolysin could also attenuate brain pathology in heat stress, a finding not reported earlier.

The possible mechanism by which Cerebrolysin attenuates HSP response in heat stress and induces neuroprotection is unclear. However, available evidence shows that Cerebrolysin in high doses is able to reduce thermal stress symptoms. The magnitude of hyperthermia was considerably reduced with Cerebrolysin following heat stress as compared to the untreated group. A reduction in body temperature after heat stress is likely to reduce hyperthermia-induced alterations in cellular and molecular cascades in the CNS.[13–17] A reduction in the BBB breakdown seen in Cerebrolysin treatment in heat stress further supports this hypothesis.

Hyperthermia is known to release several neurochemicals in the brain including serotonin, prostaglandins, histamine, and opioid peptides.[1,2,8,9,12,15,16] These neurochemicals are known mediators of BBB permeability and brain edema.[12–18] Thus it is quite likely that a reduction in the magnitude of hyperthermia with Cerebrolysin pretreatment will also attenuate the release of these neurochemicals in the CNS. Attenuated release of these neurochemicals may reduce their effect on cerebral vessels, thus reducing the BBB disruption (see Refs. 15–18). Alternatively, Cerebrolysin treatment may alter the cellular and molecule response of microvessels to these neurochemicals leading to less disruption of the BBB in heat stress.[19,20]

Extravasation of proteins into the CNS microfluid environment leads to vasogenic edema formation.[21–23] The increase in brain water content in the areas showing disruption of the BBB to Evans blue and radioiodine found in the present investigation further supports this hypothesis. Because Cerebrolysin treatment in high doses also reduced the BBB breakdown to proteins in heat stress, a reduction in brain edema formation under such circumstances is quite likely.

That the formation of brain edema and disruption of the BBB permeability is associated with HSP expression, and that Cerebrolysin is quite effective in

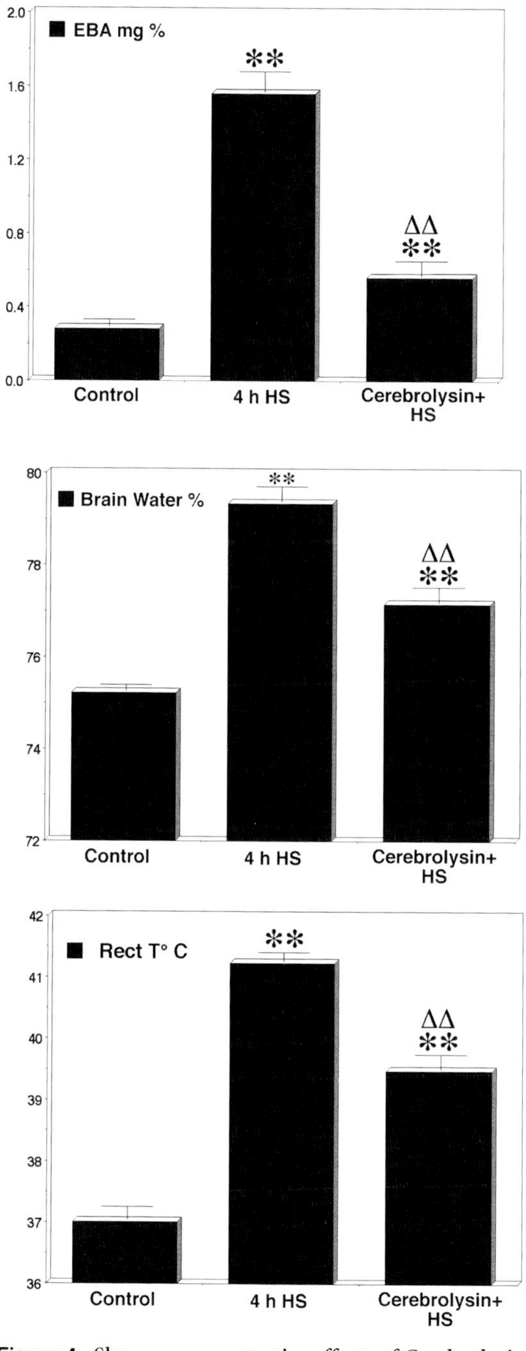

Figure 4. Shows neuroprotective effects of Cerebrolysin on Evans blue albumin leakage (*top panel*), brain edema formation (*middle panel*), and hyperthermia (*lower panel*) after 4 h heat stress (HS) in rats. ** = $P < 0.01$ from control group. DD = $P < 0.01$ compared with heat stressed rats, ANOVA followed by Dunnet's test.

attenuating these cascades, is further evident with our correlation study in heat stress. We observed a very tight correlation between HSP expression and brain edema formation and BBB breakdown in the cerebral cortex in heat stress with or without Cerebrolysin treatment (Fig. 4). This indicates that breakdown of the BBB to proteins will induce vasogenic edema and the spread of edema fluid into the brain could induce one of the strongest signals for HSP upregulation.[1,2,13,16,17] Thus, drugs that could block or reduce spread of edema fluid in the CNS will also be able to attenuate HSP expression (see Refs. 1, 2). The ability of Cerebrolysin to significantly reduce the HSP expression together with brain edema formation and BBB breakdown in heat stress clearly supports the above hypothesis.

The extracellular fluid microenvironment of the CNS is well controlled by the presence of an intact BBB (see Refs. 8, 9). The BBB maintains the homeostasis of the extracellular microenvironment in which neurons and glial cells are suspended strictly within a narrow limit.[1] Any alterations in the BBB function will alter the composition of the extracellular fluid microenvironment leading to dysfunction of the neuronal and non-neuronal cells. Leakage of serum proteins or other serum components into the extracellular fluid compartment due to BBB breakdown could thus markedly affect the physiological functions of the neurons and the glial cells.[21–23] It is quite likely that the sudden influx of serum components, including proteins, within the neuronal and glial cell microenvironment imposes severe stress on these cells.[21] As a result, these neuronal and/or glial cells react abnormally resulting in HSP overexpression. This abnormal stress reaction leading to HSP overproduction is clearly supported by our investigation in which intense HSP reaction is localized in damaged or distorted neurons.[1–5] When these basic cellular stress mechanisms are reduced by Cerebrolysin treatment, expression of HSP in the brain is considerably reduced.

Alternatively, a reduction in systemic stress will also attenuate stress signals to the brain leading to less expression of HSP in cells and tissues. This idea is supported by the fact that Cerebrolysin treatment reduced the magnitude of hyperthermia and thermal stress symptoms in animals and exhibited much less HSP expression than the untreated stressed rats. A reduction in thermal stress symptoms is thus able

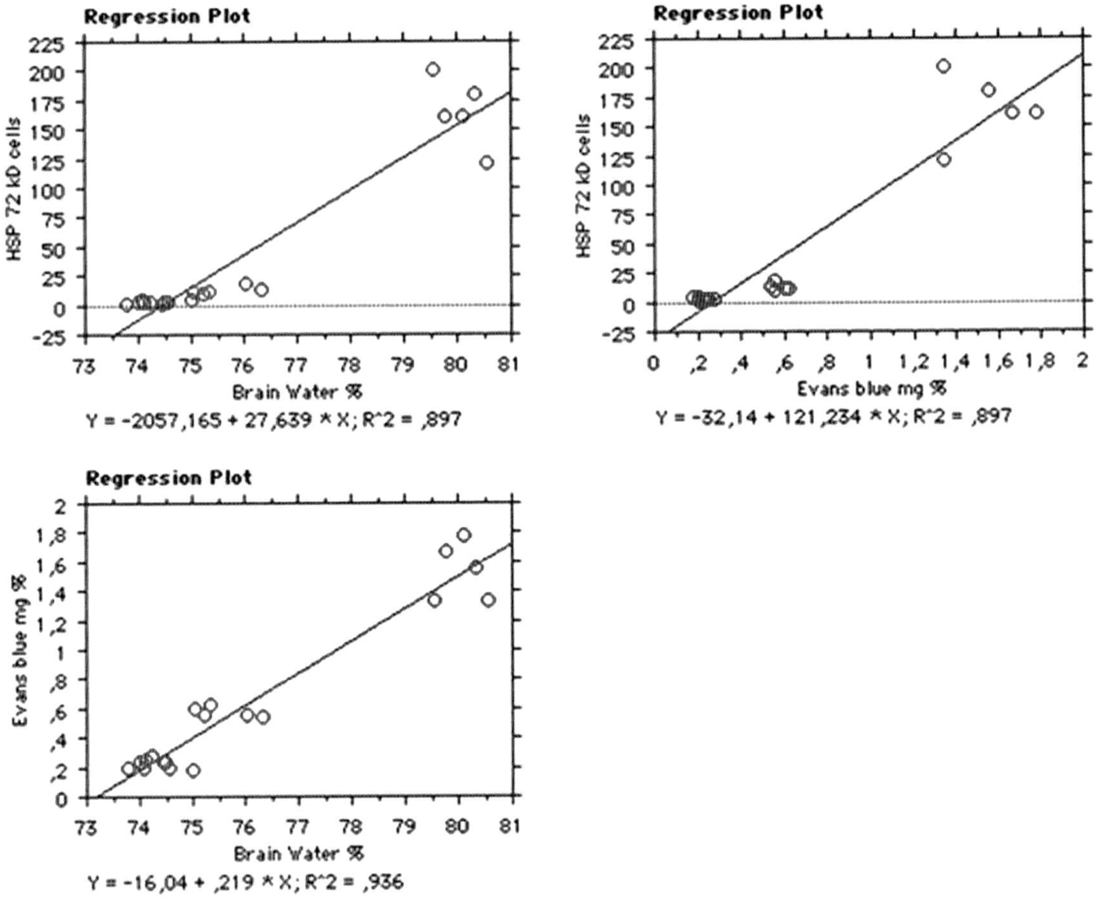

Figure 5. Shows tight correlation between heat shock protein (HSP) 72 positive cells with brain water content (*top left panel*), HSP positive cells with Evans blue leakage (*top right panel*), and Evans blue leakage and brain edema formation (*lower panel*) in control. 4 h heat stressed rats and their modification with Cerebrolysin treatment.

to alleviate some of the adverse reactions in the brain following heat stress.[1,2,8,15]

It is possible that Cerebrolysin could easily gain access into the brain of heat stressed rats and also induce neuroprotection at the cellular and molecular levels. Because Cerebrolysin is a mixture of various neurotrophic factors and active peptides,[19,20] it is likely that the drug could act on neuronal membranes and receptors to attenuate stress signals in the brain leading to less expression of HSP in Cerebrolysin treated heat stressed animals. A reduction in HSP expression following spinal cord injury by brain derived neurotrophic factors is in line with this idea.[24,25] Our observations thus indicate that in the absence of a sufficient cellular or molecular signal in drug-treated animals, the CNS components did not get sufficient cellular stress signals to induce HSP overexpression.

HSPs are not only induced by hyperthermia but also by a wide variety of insults including ischemia, hypoxia, heavy metals, and amino acid analogs, all of which cause HSP overproduction in cells and tissues in the CNS and in the periphery (see Refs. 1–5). The Hsp70 family is comprised of both constitutively expressed and stress-inducible HSP 70 (HSP 72 kD). In the present investigation we used only the inducible iso form of HSP 70 (HSP 72 kD) in hyperthermia experiments.[15–17] At the molecular level, HSPs work for protein quality control and during this process, it may be that due to various stress signals, these HSPs could be overexpressed in degenerating cells.[4,6,8] Increased expression of the inducible isoform of HSP in various neurodegenerating diseases is in line with this idea (see Refs. 1, 2). However, the HSPs as a cause or effect of these degenerating cells is still not well established and requires further investigation.[1,2,26] Keeping these views in consideration, our present study has opened a new avenue in HSP research and suggests that overexpression of HSP 72 kD may represent adverse signals in the cells. Furthermore, Cerebrolysin could be able to thwart stress-induced overexpression of HSP 72 kD in hyperthermia. Because Cerebrolysin is used currently in various neurological diseases to induce neuroprotection, based on our investigation, it appears that the drug could also be useful in treating hyperthermia related brain pathology in the future.

Conclusion

In conclusion, our study demonstrates that hyperthermia induced BBB dysfunction and brain edema could actively contribute to HSP overexpression. This indicates that HSP may represent neuronal excitation or neuronal stress in situations of brain pathology. Whether upregulation of HSP in cells by itself induces any neuroprotection in brain is unclear from our study. However, our investigation clearly shows that when various neurodestructive signals, for example, leakage of plasma proteins and other serum neurotoxins, were restricted by Cerebrolysin treatment, HSP expression by the brain cells was much less evident. Taken together, these observations suggest that neurodestructive signals are primarily responsible for HSP overexpression in CNS injuries.

Acknowledgments

This investigation is supported by Grants from Swedish Medical Research Council (nr. 2710, HSS); Göran Gustafsson Foundation, Stockholm, Sweden (HSS); Alexander von Humboldt Foundation, Bonn, Germany (HSS); Society for Study on Neuroplasticity and Neuroregeneration (SSNN), Romania (HSS); Ebewe Pharma, Austria (HSS); Astra-Zeneca, Mölndal, Sweden (HSS); StressGen Research Foundation, Canada (HSS); Ministry of Science & Technology, Govt. of India, New Delhi (HSS); Indian Council of Medical Research (ICMR), New Delhi (HSS). The skillful technical assistance of Kärstin Flink, Kerstin Rystedt (Uppsala); Franziska Drum, Angela Ludwig (Berlin) and secretarial assistance of Ulla Lindholm is highly appreciated.

Conflicts of interest

The authors have no conflict of interest with any of the organizations listed above.

References

1. Westman, J. & H.S. Sharma. 1998. Heat shock protein response in the central nervous system following hyperthermia. *Prog. Brain Res.* **115:** 207–239. Review.
2. Sharma, H.S. & J. Westman. 2004. *The Heat Shock Proteins and Hemeoxygenase Response in Central Nervous System Injuries, Blood-Spinal Cord and Brain Barriers in Health and Disease.* H.S. Sharma & J. Westman, Eds.: 329–360. Elsevier Inc. North Holland. San Diego, CA.
3. Tissières, A., H.K. Mitchell & U.M. Tracy. 1974. Protein synthesis in salivary glands of *Drosophila melanogaster*: relation to chromosome puffs. *J. Mol. Biol.* **84:** 389–398.
4. Craig, E.A., T.D. Ingolia & L.J. Manseau. 1983. Expression of *Drosophila* heat-shock cognate genes during heat shock and development. *Dev. Biol.* **99:** 418–426.
5. Welch, W.J. 1993. Heat shock proteins functioning as molecular chaperones: their roles in normal and stressed cells. *Philos. Trans. R Soc. Lond. B Biol. Sci.* **339:** 327–333. Review.
6. Marcuccilli, C.J. & R.J. Miller. 1994. CNS stress response: too hot to handle? *Trends Neurosci.* **17:** 135–138. Review.
7. Calabrese, V., C. Cornelius, C. Mancuso, *et al.* 2008. Cellular stress response: a novel target for chemoprevention and nutritional neuroprotection in aging, neurodegenerative disorders and longevity. *Neurochem. Res.* **33:** 2444–2471. Review.
8. Sharma, H.S. 1999. Pathophysiology of blood-brain barrier, brain edema and cell injury following hyperthermia: new role of heat shock protein, nitric oxide and carbon monoxide. An experimental study in the rat using light and electron microscopy. *Acta Universitatis Upsaliensis* **830:** 1–94.
9. Giffard, R.G., R.Q. Han, J.F. Emery, *et al.* 2008. Regulation of apoptotic and inflammatory cell signaling in cerebral ischemia: the complex roles of heat shock protein 70. *Anesthesiology.* **109:** 339–348. Review.
10. Riabowol, K.T., L.A. Mizzen & W.J. Welch. 1988. Heat shock is lethal to fibroblasts microinjected with antibodies against hsp70. *Science* **242:** 433–436.
11. Manzerra, P., S.J. Rush & I.R. Brown. 1993. Temporal and spatial distribution of heat shock mRNA and protein

(hsp70) in the rabbit cerebellum in response to hyperthermia. *J. Neurosci. Res.* **36:** 480–490.
12. Sharma, H.S. & P.J. Hoopes. 2003. Hyperthermia induced pathophysiology of the central nervous system. *Int. J. Hypertherm.* **19:** 325–354.
13. Sharma, H.S., T. Gordh, L. Wiklund, *et al.* 2006. Spinal cord injury induced heat shock protein expression is reduced by an antioxidant compound H-290/51. An experimental study using light and electron microscopy in the rat. *J. Neural. Transm.* **113:** 521–536.
14. Sharma, H.S. 2000. Neurodegeneration and regeneration in the CNS. New roles of heat shock proteins, nitric oxide and carbon monoxide. *Amino Acids* **19:** 335–337.
15. Sharma, H.S. 2007. Methods to produce hyperthermia-induced brain dysfunction. *Prog. Brain Res.* **162:** 173–199. Review.
16. Sharma, H.S. 2006. Hyperthermia influences excitatory and inhibitory amino acid neurotransmitters in the central nervous system. An experimental study in the rat using behavioural, biochemical, pharmacological, and morphological approaches. *J. Neural. Transm.* **113:** 497–519.
17. Sharma, H.S., Y. Olsson & J. Westman. 1995. A serotonin synthesis inhibitor, p-chlorophenylalanine reduces the heat shock protein response following trauma to the spinal cord: an immunohistochemical and ultrastructural study in the rat. *Neurosci. Res.* **21:** 241–249.
18. Sharma, H.S. & P.O. Sjöquist. 2002. A new antioxidant compound H-290/51 modulates glutamate and GABA immunoreactivity in the rat spinal cord following trauma. *Amino Acids* **23:** 261–272.
19. Doppler, E., E. Rockenstein, K. Ubhi, *et al.* 2008. Neurotrophic effects of Cerebrolysin in the Mecp2(308/Y) transgenic model of Rett syndrome. *Acta. Neuropathol.* **116:** 425–437.
20. Calderón Guzmán, D., N. Osnaya Brizuela, R. García Álvarez, *et al.* 2008. Cerebrolysin and morphine decrease glutathione and 5-hydroxyindole acetic acid levels in fasted rat brain. *Biomed. Pharmacother.* **63:** 517–521.
21. Sharma, H.S. & S.F. Ali. 2008. Acute administration of 3,4-methylenedioxymethamphetamine induces profound hyperthermia, blood-brain barrier disruption, brain edema formation, and cell injury. *Ann. N.Y. Acad. Sci.* **1139:** 242–258.
22. Muresanu, D.F. & H.S. Sharma. 2007. Chronic hypertension aggravates heat stress induced cognitive dysfunction and brain pathology: an experimental study in the rat, using growth hormone therapy for possible neuroprotection. *Ann. N.Y. Acad. Sci.* **1122:** 1–22.
23. Sharma, H.S. & E.A. Kiyatkin. 2009. Rapid morphological brain abnormalities during acute methamphetamine intoxication in the rat: an experimental study using light and electron microscopy. *J. Chem. Neuroanat.* **37:** 18–32.
24. Sharma, H.S. & J. Westman. 2003. Depletion of endogenous serotonin synthesis with p-CPA attenuates upregulation of constitutive isoform of heme oxygenase-2 expression, edema formation and cell injury following a focal trauma to the rat spinal cord. *Acta. Neurochir. Suppl.* **86:** 389–394.
25. Sharma, H.S., F. Nyberg, T. Gordh, *et al.* 2000. Neurotrophic factors influence upregulation of constitutive isoform of heme oxygenase and cellular stress response in the spinal cord following trauma. An experimental study using immunohistochemistry in the rat. *Amino Acids* **19:** 351–361.
26. Sherman, M.Y. & A.L. Goldberg. 2001. Cellular defenses against unfolded proteins: a cell biologist thinks about neurodegenerative diseases. *Neuron.* **29:** 15–32. Review.

Ann. N.Y. Acad. Sci. ISSN 0077-8923

ANNALS OF THE NEW YORK ACADEMY OF SCIENCES
Issue: *Neuroprotective Agents*

The proposed role of optical sensing in translational stroke research

Shailendra Joshi[1] and Sachin Agarwal[2]

[1]Department of Anesthesiology, Columbia University. [2]Department of Neurology, Columbia University

Address for correspondence: Shailendra Joshi, M.D., Department of Anesthesiology, PH 505, 622 West 165th St., New York, NY 10032. sj121@columbia.edu

The past three decades of clinical disappointments in treating stroke must compel us to rethink our strategy. Given the enormous complexity of the clinical disease, the "one size fits all" approach to stroke treatment is unlikely to succeed. The effective treatment of stroke aimed at reversing ischemic injury will require monitoring of tissue injury and response to therapeutic interventions, perhaps the use of multiple drugs, sequentially administered in a timely manner. The proposed sequential intra-arterial therapy for stroke (SITS) relies on the development of novel intra-arterial treatments of ischemic brain injury in the magnetic resonance imaging environment. However, translating SITS protocol from bench to bedside could greatly benefit from the advances in optical technologies. Compared to magnetic resonance imaging, optical sensing technology promises to be quicker, cheaper, simpler, and more versatile, and thus is ideally suited for investigating the fast kinetics and monitoring the pharmacological effects of intra-arterial drugs.

Keywords: stroke; optical imaging; reperfusion injury

Introduction

It is projected that between the years of 2005–2050 the care of stroke patients will cost an estimated 1.52 trillion dollars.[1] Ischemic stroke is therefore a major health concern and the subject of intensive research. Considerable advances have been made in understanding the pathology of ischemic stroke. Although interrupting key pathogenic mechanisms has significantly improved outcome in animal stroke models, translating those into effective clinical treatments has been challenging. The only success in improving the neurological outcome has been with early intravenous thrombolysis.[2–4] Recent studies have also shown that combining intravenous (IV) tissue plasminogen activator (tPA) pretreatment with intra-arterial (IA) thrombolysis achieves a high arterial recannalization rate with some improvement in outcome.[5–7]

Observations suggest that combination therapy for stroke is more likely to succeed compared to single drug therapy.[5] Interrupting multiple pathogenic pathways of stroke can be achieved either by multifunction of drugs or by using a combination of drugs.[6–8] Conventional systemic administration of drugs, either by intravenous or oral administration, lacks the speed of onset and the flexibility needed to contain the rapidly evolving neurological injury.[9] In contrast to IV, IA injections can instantaneously achieve therapeutic concentrations at a target site.[10] We therefore propose, sequential IA therapy for stroke (SITS), which is a series of IA interventions, guided by optical sensing or magnetic resonance imaging (MRI),[8] aimed at arresting and reversing ischemic injury and eventually to recover neurological function. Predictable, timely, and effective delivery of drug and gene therapies can create the matrix that can eventually lead to the "recovery of neural function."

The eventual goal of SITS protocol is to use MRI to guide IA therapy for human stroke. However, preclinical protocol development will be facilitated by novel optical sensing and imaging techniques which can permit a rigorous interrogation of the proposed therapeutic paradigms.[11] Currently, optical tools have been used to measure blood flow,[12,13] track redox state,[14,15] assess drug concentrations,[16,17] and determine reduced and oxyhemoglobin content of

doi: 10.1111/j.1749-6632.2009.05381.x

Table 1. Comparison of optical tools and magnetic resonance imaging (MRI) technology when applied to ischemic brain injury

Parameter	Optical technology	MRI
Cerebral blood flow*	Laser Doppler, and microsphere tracking	Feasible with tracers
Tissue O_2 delivery*	DRS: Tissue Hb, HbO_2 content NIRS: Hb, HBO_2 measurements	Paramagnetic signal shift
Tissue metabolic needs*	NAD^+/NADH ratio NIRS: Cytochrome A3 level	1H and 31P spectral analysis
Tissue edema*	Tissue fluorescence and DRS	DWI imaging
Blood-brain barrier*	Possible by tracking transfer of molecules like Evan's blue, indocarmine green	DWI imaging
Tissue activation*	NIRS and cerebral topographic mapping	FMRI
Drug delivery*	DRS (direct measurements) Optically tagged of drugs, and liposomes	Limited to specific molecules
Brain imaging*	PAT, Functional PAT	High resolution imaging possible
Tissue histology*	Optical coherence tomography, DRS	High resolution imaging possible
Cerebral angiography*	Fluorescein tagged polyethylene PAT Two photon angiography#	MRA
Molecular tracking	Tagged fluoroprobes	After magnetic tagging
Gene activation	Luciferase technique	?

DRS = diffuse reflectance spectroscopy; NIRS = near infrared spectroscopy; DWI = diffusion weighted imaging; FMRI = functional magnetic resonance imaging; PAT = photoacoustic tomography; MRA = magnetic resonance angiography; *: technologies available; #: invasive.

the brain tissue.[18,19] Compared to MRI, optical sensing and imaging technologies promise to be quicker, simpler, cheaper, and more versatile, and thus they are ideally suited for investigating the fast kinetics and pharmacological effects of IA drugs. Optical technologies are highly cost effective and devoid of the risks inherent in MR and positron emission tomography (PET) imaging. Low recurrent costs of optical devices may permit high volume investigations that will require studies with sufficient power to investigate the plethora of mechanisms and drug intervention that have been proposed for the treatment of clinical stroke (Table 1).

Pathology of ischemic stroke

Figure 1 shows some of the major pathogenic mechanisms that operate in ischemic stroke. Interrupting these pathogenic mechanisms, while successful in animal models, has failed in human trials of neuroprotective drugs.[20] The failure in part has been due to the improper selection of the neuroprotective drugs, or the conduct of trials, for example, inadequate sample size, histological rather than functional end-point or short duration of follow-up.[21] Conversely, there are several examples of clinical human trials designed using drug dosing vastly lower than the levels shown to protect the brain of animals. For some agents (e.g., *N*-methyl-D-aspartate (NMDA) antagonists), dose-limiting adverse events not fully anticipated in preclinical studies, emerged during human trials.[15] We believe that the failure could also be due to the inability of a single drug to interrupt the multiple pathogenic pathways of ischemic stroke.[22] Ischemic stroke triggers pathological changes in blood, microcirculation, and the brain tissue. Unless these pathogenic processes are effectively contained it is unlikely that full functional recovery will be feasible after ischemic stroke. Furthermore, compared to experimental stroke, clinical

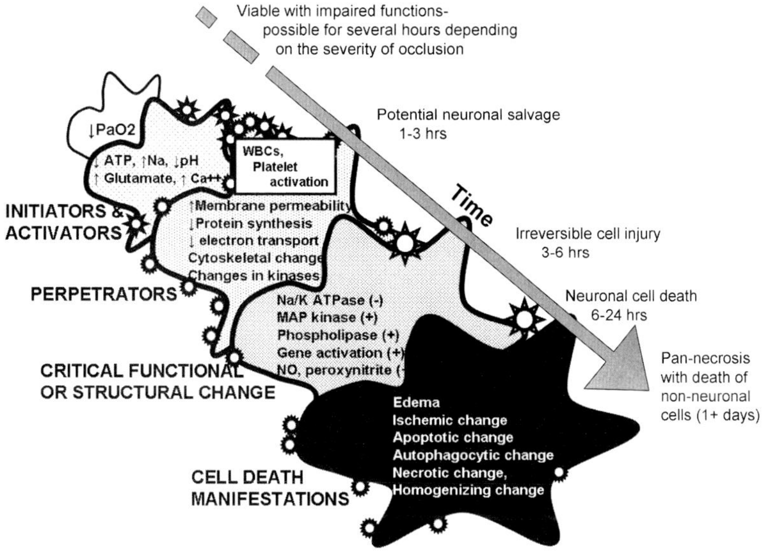

Figure 1. Ischemic brain injury: Mechanisms of ischemic neuronal injury follow a general pattern, but the pathogenic pathways are neither time-locked nor perfectly synchronized. Given the enormous complexity of ischemic brain injury, we need a more dynamic approach to stroke treatment. In this application we propose to improve the outcome of neurological injury by precisely controlling drug delivery, monitoring tissue drug concentrations, assessing injury parameters, and using specific drugs to interrupt pathogenic processes.

stroke has a far more complex paradigm. The interactions between diverse injury mechanisms become more critical in clinical stroke than in the well-controlled experimental injury models. Patient characteristics, such as age, gender, comorbidities, concurrent treatments, indeterminable time of onset of symptoms, etc., that can be controlled in animal models, are some of the additional variables that amplify the complexity of clinical stroke. Given these variables, treatment of clinical stroke might require drug interventions tailored to an individual patient. The treatment process will first require pathological characterization of injury, employing specific interventions and then follow-up monitoring of tissue response to therapeutic interventions.[23] Advances in MR imaging and endovascular surgery make it possible for us to observe thrombolysis by MR guided IA interventions. The recent emergence of IA thrombolysis offers new avenues for intervening in stroke, while interventional MR technology, MR imaging and spectroscopy, could help in delivering and monitoring the effects of drugs.[24]

Single versus multidrug therapy for stroke

Traditional approach to clinical stroke treatment relies on the delivery of a single agent usually systemically via the IV route. In animal models, systemic delivery of multiple neuroprotective drugs seems to be effective. However, in these models stroke outcome is often judged by histology, over a short time period and relatively simple functional parameters. It can be argued that the neuroprotective effects of the drug could be overestimated in relatively simple animal models. However, across the board failure of over a hundred neuroprotective drugs in clinical trials suggests other problems with the conventional experimental approach.[2] For instance, most animal and clinical studies do not emphasize the importance of determining drug concentrations in ischemic tissues. Changes in microcirculation after stroke could prevent effective delivery of neuroprotective drugs in sufficient concentrations and in a timely manner (Fig. 2). Most stroke treatment related clinical trials rely on drug delivery protocols based on pharmacokinetic data generated from healthy volunteers. The kinetics of drug delivery to the brain are complex especially after ischemic brain injury. After such an injury the capillary surface area may decrease due to the "no-reflow phenomena," drug transport could be altered due to changes in the blood-brain barrier, blood-brain drug partition may be affected by an increase in brain tissue water content due to edema, etc., and such

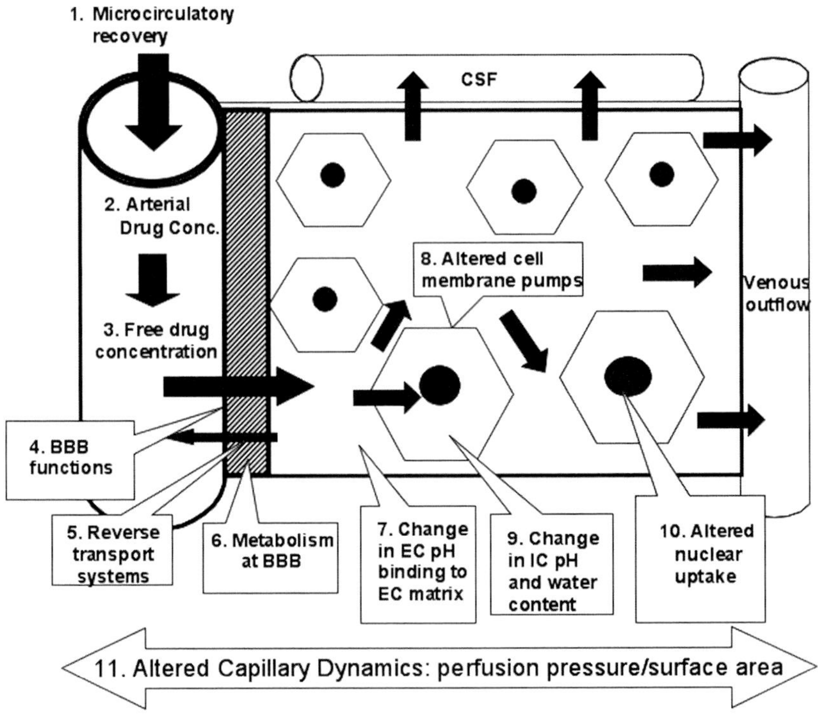

Figure 2. Changes in microcirculation that could affect drug delivery during reperfusion after ischemic stroke.

factors could have a profound effect on regional drug delivery.[25–27] Unless the drug concentrations in ischemic tissues are monitored, the failure of neuroprotective drugs could be due to inadequate delivery.

Furthermore, as mentioned earlier, it is unlikely that a single drug can reverse all the pathogenic processes shown in Figure 1. Attempts at developing multifunction drugs have so far been disappointing. Nitrones, for example, can vasodilate and scavenge free radicals, however they were not proven to be effective in clinical trials.[28] Barbiturates are another example of multifunction drugs that decrease synaptic transmission, increase seizure threshold, decrease metabolism, decrease intracranial pressure (ICP), and scavenge free radicals, yet despite decades of clinical use the evidence for their neuroprotective role is still unclear.[29] There are certain problems with developing multifunction drugs. First, it may not be possible to have the correct ratio of the desired effects. The relative importance of various pathogenic mechanisms may be different across patients and with time. Due to the dynamic nature of ischemic brain injury the relative nature of therapeutic interventions might change with time. Multifunction drugs offer a means to interrupt several pathogenic pathways in stroke but they may lack the versatility and flexibility required to treat clinical strokes.[28]

An alternate approach is to employ systemic cocktails of drugs for the treatment of stroke. The critical issue with simultaneous administration of multiple drugs is the possibility of drug interactions and synergistic side-effects that could limit their use. For example, hypothermia, calcium channel blockers, sedatives, and free radical scavengers can all result in cardiovascular depression. Therefore, simultaneous administration of multiple drugs systemically may not be feasible for the treatment of ischemic brain injury.

Sequential intra-arterial delivery of drugs

Recent advances in microcatheter technology and improvements in drug delivery protocols could significantly improve IA drug delivery.[30] IA drug delivery instantaneously results in high concentrations of drug in the arterial blood at the tissue site. Effective drug concentrations can be achieved using a

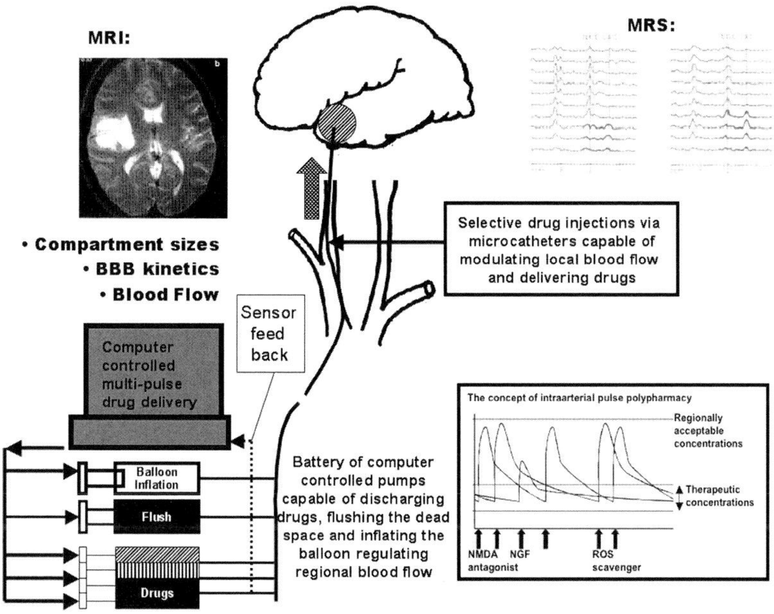

Figure 3. The proposed use of multiple IA drugs to treat stroke.

fraction of the doses administered systemically. There is still a significant dose advantage of IA drugs over systemic administration, even if repeated injections are used to maintain extended tissue drug concentrations.[10,31] Finally, as shown in Figure 3, IA drug delivery could permit delivery of multiple pharmaceutical agents to the target site relatively independent of each other. Side effects of the drugs could be mitigated by concurrently administered antidotes and nonspecific drug sequestering agents, such as cyclodextrins, that are presently in development.

IA thrombolysis provides a unique opportunity to treat ischemic brain injury because the catheter for drug delivery is already in place when the perfusion is restored. Based on the previous studies,[19] It seems that the widow of intervention in clinical stroke can be widened from 3 to 6 h, with the IA delivery of thrombolytic drugs. Therefore, IA drugs could play a significant role in the management of cerebral reperfusion injury after thrombolysis.

The ability to deliver multiple pharmaceutical agents almost instantaneously to the reperfusion zone could make phased interventions possible in the treatment of ischemic strokes. We visualize a four-stage reperfusion injury management strategy (Fig. 4). In a monitored situation how long each intervention will last will depend of the evolution of brain injury and the response to treatment.

1. *Thrombolysis*: Either by mechanical clot retraction (faster) or by thrombolytic drugs (urokinase or streptokinase) as is necessary. The goal will be restoration of adequate perfusion.
2. *Controlled reperfusion*: For example, in the very early stages of reperfusion IA interventions will be aimed to restore the milieu, such as, pH correction, calcium chelation, and IV anesthetics. We also hypothesize controlled reperfusion with hypothermia, leukocyte or platelet depleted blood with low hematocrit or use of perfluorocarbons and blood substitutes with low viscosity. Reperfusion will also lead to the release of free radicals and neurotransmitters, therefore we propose an early use of free radical scavengers and excitatory neurotransmitter antagonists. End point will be containment of reperfusion injury.
3. *Reversal phase*: Having stabilized the injury, the next stage will be to arrest the ongoing injury, prevent secondary injury by reversal of cell edema, and then anti-inflammatory and anti-apoptotic measures. The end point will be to arrest evolving neurological injury.

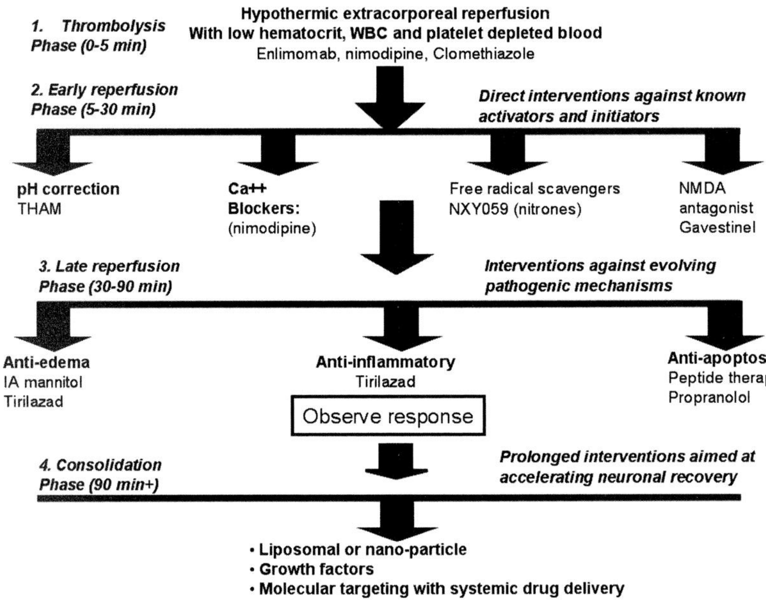

Figure 4. Sequential IA therapy of stroke.

4. *Consolidation phase*: The two aims of the consolidation phase are to ensure sustained benefits of IA interventions and to promote neurological recovery. The strategy will be to use sustained release formulation of drugs, such as liposomes or nanoparticles, as well as the delivery of growth factors and stem cells. In this phase, the end-point is to recover neurological functions.

The role of optical technology in improving IA drug delivery

The major thrust for IA drug delivery was in the treatment of brain tumors. However, due to the inability to precisely control drug concentrations, there were significant complications with IA chemotherapy. In the past, understanding the kinetics of IA drugs was difficult without rapid measurement of tissue drug concentrations (Fig. 5). There were few studies using conventional tissue sampling, MR and PET tracers were undertaken to understand IA drug kinetics, and it became clear that the pharmacokinetic models grossly failed to predict tissue drug concentrations. Optical measurements have been used to measure real time tissue concentrations of chemotherapeutic drugs.[32] High-speed tissue noninvasive optical measurements could greatly improve the understanding and delivery of IA drugs.

Optical technology in stroke research

Pulse oximetery, familiar to most physicians by now, illustrates the ease of use of optical technologies and the robustness of the equipment. Relevant to stroke research, the optical methods, such as laser Doppler flow measurement and blood flow scanning techniques, are already widely used in the laboratory. Some of the optical technology has been

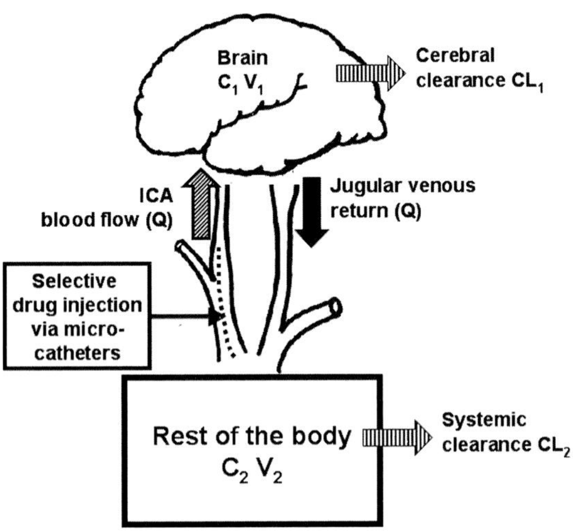

Figure 5. Basic principles of IA drug delivery. IA drug delivery is useful when there is a high regional uptake, low regional blood flow, and high systemic clearance.

incorporated in multifunction probes. Multifunction probes, in part dependent on optical technologies, have already been developed that are capable of monitoring brain ICP, blood flow, NADH concentration, cortical Ca^{++} and K^{+} currents, and cortical electrical activity.[14] Fluorescent imaging NADH concentrations of whole organs could be useful in monitoring brain ischemia and reperfusion.[33] Optical spectroscopy that tracks the rapid changes in brain tissue oxyhemoglobin concentrations and can localize cortical functions, could also be applied to monitor tissue perfusion or even investigate flow-metabolism coupling.[34] Fluorescent dyes, when topically applied to the brain cortex, can track changes in tissue Ca^{++} concentrations and tissue acidosis.[11] Tissue concentrations of drugs that have an absorption spectrum distinct from hemoglobin and de-oxyhemoglobin can be measured in virtual real time by diffuse reflectance spectroscopy.[17] Optically determined concentration of markers, such as Evan's Blue and indocarmine green, could look at the state of the blood-brain barrier. Beyond these immediate applications, optical technologies promise many other potential applications in stroke research. Optical sensing techniques, such as diffuse reflectance spectroscopy, being developed for identifying potentially malignant cells could be used to track tissue characteristics after ischemic injury. Clumping of DNA that alters light scattering properties of apoptotic cells could be used to monitor apoptosis. The incorporation of photosensitive ion channels in genetically engineered animals may provide the means to assess changes in animal behavior without the need for conditioned response training that is used to assess neurological outcomes.

Optical imaging

The current optical sensing technology that is largely based on changes in the light signal back-scattered by brain tissue is unlikely to permit tissue imaging. The light scattering properties of the skull create a significant barrier for optical imaging of brain tissue. The ability of near infrared light to penetrate 10–15 cm of human brain tissue has enabled crude 3-dimensional mapping of neonatal brain tissue. In adults, near infrared spectroscopy (NIRS) can only be used for functional cortical topography.[34] Time-gated NIRS that is currently in development could provide depth resolved functional mapping of brain tissues. In the treatment of stroke, NIRS could be used to monitor brain injury, or based on the indigocyanine clearance, could be used for measuring the regional blood flow.

The major thrust in optical imaging of brain tissue of laboratory animals comes from two techniques: photo-acoustic brain imaging and optical coherence tomography. Photo-acoustic brain imaging is based on ultrasonic 3-dimensional reconstruction of images after the brain tissue vibrates on exposure to a very short burst of laser. The technique permits imaging of brain tissue through an intact head of a small animal and has recently been used in primates.[35–37] On the other hand, optical coherence tomography permits *in vivo* imaging of tissue with the resolution of a low power microscope.[38] Because it requires exposure of neural tissues, clinically it can only be applied to the retina.[39] It is being considered for the evaluation of neuroprotective drugs in models of multiple sclerosis.[40] Although optical coherence tomography requires exposure of brain tissue, it can permit 3-D reconstruction of tissue histology at the sub-millimeter level.[41,42]

For a person not involved in optical research, the recent advances in optical technology are best highlighted by the achievements in astronomy, for example, in the quest for extrasolar planets. Deep space telescope observations can be processed with signal: noise extraction ratio that has surpassed $1{:}10^9$. Some of these techniques of data extraction could be applied to neuroscience research. There are equally rapid advances in development of light sources and detectors that could further improve signal acquisition. The concurrent development of new dyes that can be applied topically or injected intravenously might help in visualization of the cellular processes *in vivo* by optical means and could also help in optical sensing of brain functions. Collectively, advances in science in general and optical technology in particular, could have an immense impact on translational stroke research.

Conclusions

The past three decades of clinical disappointments in treating stroke must compel us to rethink our strategy. There is probably no magic bullet in the treatment of ischemic stroke, except for thrombolysis in early stroke. Given the enormous complexity of the clinical disease, the "one size fits all" approach to stroke treatment is unlikely to succeed. The effective treatment of stroke aimed at reversing ischemic injury will require monitoring of tissue injury and response to therapeutic interventions, perhaps the use of multiple drugs, sequentially administered in a timely manner. The proposed SITS relies on the development of novel IA treatments of ischemic brain injury in the MR environment. However, translating SITS protocol from bench to bedside could greatly benefit from the advances in optical technologies. Compared to MRI, optical sensing and imaging technologies promise to be quicker, simpler, and more versatile, and thus are ideally suited for investigating the fast kinetics and monitoring the pharmacological effects of IA drugs. Low recurrent cost of optical technologies could permit large studies that are sufficiently powered to address complexities of future stroke models and eventually to improve the outcome of clinical stroke.

Acknowledgment

Funding: The authors acknowledge the support of National Institute of Health Grant NCI R01 CA 1275000 (SJ).

Conflicts of interest

The authors declare no conflicts of interest.

References

1. Brown, D.L., B. Boden-Albala, K.M. Langa, *et al.* 2006. Projected costs of ischemic stroke in the United States. *Neurology* **67:** 1390–1395.
2. Editorial. 2006. Neuroprotection: the end of an era? *Lancet* **368:** 1548.
3. del Zoppo, G.J. 1995. Why do all drugs work in animals but none in stroke patients? 1. Drugs promoting cerebral blood flow [Review]. *J. Intern. Med.* **237:** 79–88.
4. del Zoppo, G.J. 1998. Clinical trials in acute stroke: Why have they not been successful? *Neurology*. **51**(3 Suppl 3): S59–S61.
5. Chen, J., Y. Li, R. Zhang, *et al.* 2004. Combination therapy of stroke in rats with a nitric oxide donor and human bone marrow stromal cells enhances angiogenesis and neurogenesis. *Brain Res.* **1005:** 21–28.
6. Floyd, R.A., R.D. Kopke, C.H. Choi, *et al.* 2008. Nitrones as therapeutics. *Free Radic. Biol. Med.* **45:** 1361–1374.
7. Sun, Y., J. Jiang, Z. Zhang, *et al.* 2008. Antioxidative and thrombolytic TMP nitrone for treatment of ischemic stroke. *Bioorg. Med. Chem.* **16:** 8868–8874.
8. Fong, J.J. & D.H. Rhoney. 2006. NXY-059: Review of neuroprotective potential for acute stroke. *Ann. Pharmacother.* **40:** 461–471.
9. Joshi, S., P.M. Meyers & E. Ornstein. 2008. Intracarotid delivery of drugs: the potential and the pitfalls. *Anesthesiology* **109:** 543–564.
10. Dedrick, R.L. 1988. Arterial drug infusion: pharmacokinetic problems and pitfalls. *J. Natl. Cancer Inst.* **80:** 84–89.
11. Hillman, E.M. 2007. Optical brain imaging *in vivo*: techniques and applications from animal to man. *J. Biomed. Opt.* **12:** 051402.
12. Schiszler, I., M. Tomita, Y. Fukuuchi, *et al.* 2000. New optical method for analyzing cortical blood flow heterogeneity in small animals: validation of the method. *Am. J. Physiol Heart. Circ. Physiol.* **279:** H1291–H1298.
13. Bolognese, P., J.I. Miller, I.M. Heger, *et al.* 1993. Laser-Doppler flowmetry in neurosurgery. *J. Neurosurg. Anesthesiol.* **5:** 151–158.
14. Mayevsky, A., T. Manor, E. Pevzner, *et al.* 2004. Tissue spectroscope: a novel *in vivo* approach to real time monitoring of tissue vitality. *J. Biomed. Opt.* **9:** 1028–1045.
15. Chance, B., S. Nioka, W. Warren, *et al.* 2005. Mitochondrial NADH as the bellwether of tissue O2 delivery. *Adv. Exp. Med. Biol.* **566:** 231–242.
16. Bigio, I.J. & S.G. Bown. 2004. Spectroscopic sensing of cancer and cancer therapy: current status of translational research. *Cancer Biol. Ther.* **3:** 259–267.
17. Mourant, J.R., T.M. Johnson, G. Los, *et al.* 1999. Non-invasive measurement of chemotherapy drug concentrations in tissue: preliminary demonstrations of *in vivo* measurements. *Phys. Med. Biol.* **44:** 1397–1417.
18. Nicklin, S.E., I.A. Hassan, Y.A. Wickramasinghe, *et al.* 2003. The light still shines, but not that brightly? The current status of perinatal near infrared spectroscopy. *Arch. Dis. Child Fetal Neonatal. Ed.* **88:** F263–F268.
19. Brown, D.W., P.A. Picot, J.G. Naeini, *et al.* 2002. Quantitative near infrared spectroscopy measurement of cerebral hemodynamics in newborn piglets. *Pediatr. Res.* **51:** 564–570.
20. Zador, Z., Z. Benyo, Z. Lacza, *et al.* 2004. [Neuroprotection in brain ischemia—doubts and hopes]. *Ideggyogy Sz.* **57:** 81–93.
21. Gladstone, D.J., S.E. Black & A.M. Hakim. 2002. Toward wisdom from failure: lessons from neuroprotective stroke trials and new therapeutic directions. *Stroke* **33:** 2123–2136.

22. Graham, S.M., L.D. McCullough & S.J. Murphy. 2004. Animal models of ischemic stroke: balancing experimental aims and animal care. *Comp. Med.* **54:** 486–496.
23. Perlman, J.M. 2006. Intervention strategies for neonatal hypoxic-ischemic cerebral injury. *Clin. Ther.* **28:** 1353–1365.
24. Iannetti, G.D. & R.G. Wise. 2007. BOLD functional MRI in disease and pharmacological studies: room for improvement? *Magn. Reson. Imaging* **25:** 978–988.
25. Molina, C.A. & J. Alvarez-Sabin. 2009. Recanalization and reperfusion therapies for acute ischemic stroke. *Cerebrovasc. Dis.* **27**(Suppl 1): 162–167.
26. del Zoppo, G.J. & T. Mabuchi. 2003. Cerebral microvessel responses to focal ischemia. *J. Cereb. Blood Flow Metab.* **23:** 879–894.
27. de la Torre, J.C., T. Fortin, J.K. Saunders, *et al.* 1992. The no-reflow phenomenon is a post-mortem artifact. *Acta Neurochir. (Wien)* **115:** 37–42.
28. Ginsberg, M.D., D.A. Becker, R. Busto, *et al.* 2003. Stilbazulenyl nitrone, a novel antioxidant, is highly neuroprotective in focal ischemia. *Ann. Neurol.* **54:** 330–342.
29. Kawaguchi, M., H. Furuya & P.M. Patel. 2005. Neuroprotective effects of anesthetic agents. *J. Anesth.* **19:** 150–156.
30. Pile-Spellman, J. 1996. Endovascular therapeutic neuroradiology (Chapter 18). In *Neuroradiology*, 3rd edn. J.M. Taveras, Ed.: 1045–1179. Williams & Wilkins. Baltimore, MD.
31. Wang, M., S. Joshi & R.G. Emerson. 2003. Comparison of intracarotid and intravenous propofol for electrocerebral silence in rabbits. *Anesthesiology* **99:** 904–910.
32. Reif, R., M. Wang, S. Joshi, *et al.* 2007. Optical method for real-time monitoring of drug concentrations facilitates the development of novel methods for drug delivery to brain tissue. *J. Biomed. Opt.* **12:** 034036.
33. Ramanujan, V.K., J.A. Jo, G. Cantu, *et al.* 2008. Spatially resolved fluorescence lifetime mapping of enzyme kinetics in living cells. *J. Microsc.* **230**(Pt 3): 329–338.
34. Boas, D.A. & R.D. Frostig. 2005. Optics in neuroscience. *J. Biomed. Opt.* **10:** 1–2.
35. Wang, L.V. 2008. Prospects of photoacoustic tomography. *Med Phys.* **35:** 5758–5767.
36. Gamelin, J., A. Aguirre, A. Maurudis, *et al.* 2008. Curved array photoacoustic tomographic system for small animal imaging. *J. Biomed. Opt.* **13:** 024007.
37. Yang, X. & L.V. Wang. 2008. Monkey brain cortex imaging by photoacoustic tomography. *J. Biomed. Opt.* **13:** 044009.
38. Rajagopalan, U.M., K. Tsunoda & M. Tanifuji. 2009. Using the light scattering component of optical intrinsic signals to visualize *in vivo* functional structures of neural tissues. *Methods Mol. Biol.* **489:** 111–132.
39. Frohman, E.M., J.G. Fujimoto, T.C. Frohman, *et al.* 2008. Optical coherence tomography: a window into the mechanisms of multiple sclerosis. *Nat. Clin. Pract. Neurol.* **4:** 664–675.
40. Zivadinov, R. 2007. Can imaging techniques measure neuroprotection and remyelination in multiple sclerosis? *Neurology* **68**(22 Suppl 3): S72–S82. Discussion S91–S96.
41. Bizheva, K., A. Unterhuber, B. Hermann, *et al.* 2004. Imaging *ex vivo* and *in vitro* brain morphology in animal models with ultrahigh resolution optical coherence tomography. *J. Biomed. Opt.* **9:** 719–724.
42. Boppart, S.A. 2003. Optical coherence tomography: technology and applications for neuroimaging. *Psychophysiology* **40:** 529–541.

Ann. N.Y. Acad. Sci. ISSN 0077-8923

ANNALS OF THE NEW YORK ACADEMY OF SCIENCES
Issue: *Neuroprotective Agents*

Neuroprotection by hypothermia plus alkalinization of dorsal root ganglia neurons through ischemia

Damien P. Kuffler

Institute of Neurobiology, Medical Sciences Campus, University of Puerto Rico, San Juan

Address for correspondence: Damien P. Kuffler, Institute of Neurobiology, 201 Blvd. del Valle, San Juan, PR 00901. dkuffler@hotmail.com

Brain and spinal cord (CNS) trauma typically directly kill some neurons leading to permanent neurological deficits. However, they also lead to a number of triggers which in turn frequently kill a vastly larger number of neurons than were killed by the initial insult. The best mechanism for reducing the extent of neurological deficits is to minimize the number of neurons that die immediately due to the trauma, and post-trauma sequelae. Neuroprotection techniques have taken many diverse forms with a breadth too great for a short review. Therefore, this review is focused on the roles of only a small number of neuroprotective agents, with its primary focus being on neuroprotection provided by hypothermia, alone and when combined with the other methods. Included are also recent results involving a novel neuroprotective technique, tested on adult human dorsal root ganglion neurons, comparing the influences of hypothermia and alkalinization singly, providing fourfold and eightfold increases in neuroprotection, respectively, but when combined providing a 26-fold increase in neuroprotection. This combinatorial approach to neuroprotection holds great promise for enhancing the degree of neuroprotection clinically following CNS trauma, leading to the preservation of maximal neurological functions.

Keywords: adult human neurons; dorsal root ganglia; hypothermia; alkalinization; ischemia; neuroprotection

Introduction

Trauma-induced ischemia and stress lead to neurotoxicity, neuron death, and permanent neurological deficits. To reduce these neurological losses interventions are required to maintain the viability of neurons that would otherwise die. Although many interventions have been tested in many different injury models, none provides sufficient neuroprotection to reduce the death of neurons caused by the sequelae of events triggered by the initial trauma.

Trauma-induced secondary insults causing neuron death include ischemia, lipid peroxidation,[1] inflammation,[2] and the excessive release of extracellular excitatory amino acids (EAAs).[3] The EAAs lead to toxic extracellular acidification and the toxicity of an excessive stimulation of an *N*-methyl-D-aspartate (NMDA) subtype of glutamate receptor,[4] allowing a massive extracellular calcium influx,[5] and disruption of calcium homeostasis of neurons.[6] The released glutamate stimulates further glutamate release in a positive feedback loop by interacting with non-NMDA receptor subtypes,[4] while calcium-induced calcium release, accompanied by a further influx of calcium through voltage-gated calcium channels after glutamate-induced depolarization, contributes to glutamate toxicity.

Hypothermia and alkalinization separately, but to a greater extent when combined, provide neuroprotection to various populations of neurons from animal models.[7–11] Clinical studies have shown that localized and global hypothermia provide neuroprotection for the human CNS.[12–15] However, there are virtually no data for human neurons on the neuroprotection provided by alkalinization alone or when combined with hypothermia.

Following trauma to the spinal cord, dorsal root ganglia (DRG) may become ischemic due to the loss of oxygenation from disrupted blood vessels that permeate the DRG. Similarly, upon removal of adult human DRG from fresh cadavers, the densely packed neurons are surrounded with a thick

doi: 10.1111/j.1749-6632.2009.05358.x

connective tissue coat and additional tissue that blocks oxygen permeation, which causes rapid ischemia. This ischemia triggers a number of secondary events, such as massive release of excitatory amino acids from the neurons, their excessive accumulation and activation of neuron NMDA and other receptors, acidification, and loss of calcium homeostasis,[4,5,16–18] that lead to neurotoxicity. Therefore, we thought intact adult human DRG would be a good model on which to test several potential neuroprotective techniques singly and in combination for the degrees of neuroprotection against the same toxic elements to which they would be exposed *in situ*.

This paper is related to another paper in this same volume that more thoroughly examines the effectiveness of different neuroprotective interventions that have been tested singly and in combination. However, in this paper we focus on the results of a novel technique, which tests the combinatorial approach to neuroprotection (hypothermia and alkalinization) and show that they provide significant neuroprotection against severe and prolonged (up to 4 h) ischemia to adult human neurons within DRG. We show that, although both hypothermia and alkalinization singly provided neuroprotection to the ischemic neurons, the neuroprotection was significantly increased when a decreasing temperature was combined with increasing alkalinity compared to physiological conditions.[11,19]

Methods

Four thoracic intact DRG were removed from organ donors within 1.5 h of cross clamping the aorta according to previously described methods.[16] Briefly, the temperature of the operating room was approximately 68° F, and as each intact DRG was removed it was placed on a sterile cloth in ambient air. Once all the required DRG had been removed they were all placed in DMEM-F12 medium on ice, and were taken to the laboratory. By the time the DRG were in the laboratory they had been ischemic for at least 2 h. Once the DRG were in the laboratory, at 68° F, and in a laminar flow hood, the tissue surrounding the DRG was removed while leaving the connective tissue capsule intact. In the absence of blood circulation and in the presence of the connective tissue capsule the neurons within the DRG would have had little access to oxygen. However, it was important to assure that the DRG were actually in an ischemic environment.

Ischemia was accomplished by placing the intact DRG in culture medium into which 100% nitrogen had been bubbled for at least 10 min. Once the DRG were in the medium 100% nitrogen was continuously bubbled into the medium for up to 4 h.

To maintain the DRG at different desired temperatures, they were maintained in medium at room temperature (68° F), on a heating table and a cooling table. The pH of the medium was adjusted using tris buffer.

After the intact DRG had been in the ischemic medium for the desired time, and at the desired pH and temperature, they were placed in culture medium that had only been exposed to ambient air. At that time, the DRG connective tissue capsule was removed, the DRG cut into small pieces with irredectomy, and the DRG neurons dissociated with enzymes over a period of 80 min.

Once the DRG neurons were fully dissociated, they were plated individually in DMEM-F12 medium on a glass cover slip coated with poly-lysine and then laminin. The viable neurons adhered to the coated cover slips immediately. After plating, the culture dishes were placed in an O_2/CO_2 incubator at 36° C in a water saturated environment.

Results

As stated, the adult human DRG used in this study were removed from cadavers, within 1–1.5 h of cross clamping of the aorta. Subsequent to removing the DRG they were transported to the laboratory where the experiments began. Thus, our starting point for the experiments with the DRG neurons was after they had been ischemic for at least 2 h, partly in the cooling cadaver, and then in medium on ice.

Our data show that for neurons maintained ischemic within intact DRG at physiological temperature (37° C), alkalinization to pH 8.3 and to 9.3 increases the yield of viable neurons by 4.5- and 7.8-fold respectively. Further, for DRG maintained ischemic at physiological pH (7.6), decreasing the temperature at which intact DRG are maintained during 1 h from 37° C to 20° C and 15° C, increases the yield of viable neurons (4.6- and 2.2-fold respectfully) (Fig. 1). The greatest degree of neuroprotection against ischemia was provided by combined hypothermia and alkalinization.

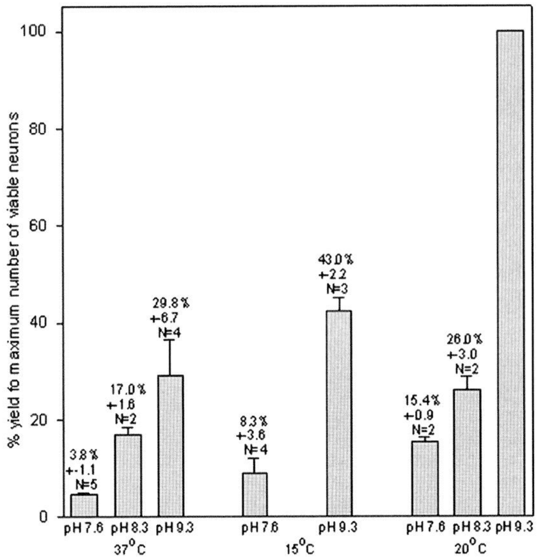

Figure 1. Graph of the yield of viable adult human neurons within intact dorsal root ganglia (DRG) when maintained for 1 h under different combinations of temperature and pH. The yields are normalized against that of DRG maintained at 20° C and pH 9.3, which provided the largest yield of viable neurons. Hypothermia and alkalinization each separately increased the yield of viable neurons, but simultaneous hypothermia and alkalinization provided greater neuroprotection than either one alone.

Compared to DRG maintained under physiological conditions (37° C/pH 7.6), DRG maintained hypothermic and alkaline (15° C/pH 9.3 and 20° C/pH 9.3) had significantly larger yields of 11.3- and 26.3-fold respectively. These results show that combined hypothermia and alkalinization provide adult human DRG neurons significant neuroprotection against ischemia, and ischemia-induced causes of neuron death.

Neuroprotection over time

Examination of neuron viability within intact ischemic DRG showed that the death of adult human neurons closely follow an exponential decay. Thus, after 0.5 h the yield of viable neurons was 15%, after 1 h 3.8%, and after 1.5 h 1.5%. However, for intact DRG maintained ischemic under hypothermic and alkaline conditions (20° C/pH 9.3), the yield of viable neurons decreased far more slowly than for DRG under physiological conditions. Compared to the maximum possible yield of viable neurons, after 0.5 h the yield of viable neurons was 82.4% (a 5.6-fold larger yield), after 1.5 h it was 39.1% (a 26-fold larger yield), and after 2 h it was 14% (a 23.3-fold larger yield) (Fig. 2). These are the first data showing neuroprotection against ischemia for adult human neurons provided by alkalinization alone, and enhanced neuroprotection for adult human neurons provided by alkalinization combined with hypothermia.

The limited number of available adult human donors restricted the number of times we could test each set of conditions, and the combinations of temperatures and pH we could test. However, the results show a dramatic and consistent increase in yield of viable neurons provided by combined hypothermia and alkalinization versus physiological conditions.

Susceptibilities of adult human versus rat dorsal root ganglia neurons to ischemia

Adult rat and human DRG neurons show a strikingly different susceptibility to death due to ischemia. Ischemic adult human neurons die much more rapidly than adult rat DRG neurons. Over 4 h of ischemia, the number of viable adult rat DRG neurons decreased in a linear manner under both physiological versus hypothermic and alkaline conditions, while for adult human neurons, the death rate was nearly exponential under physiological conditions of temperature and pH. Virtually all adult human DRG neurons were dead after 3 h of ischemia, while after 4 h of ischemia the yield of viable adult rat DRG neurons from DRG maintained under physiological condition was 18%, and 76% from DRG maintained hypothermic and alkaline.

The differences in tolerance to ischemia by adult rat neurons may be an evolutionary adaptation. Such an adaptation would have allowed rats to survive in hostile, low oxygen-content, underground environments, where they would be relatively safe from predation from other mammals. However, these differences in results indicate that caution must be used when attempting to extrapolate results from animal models to humans.

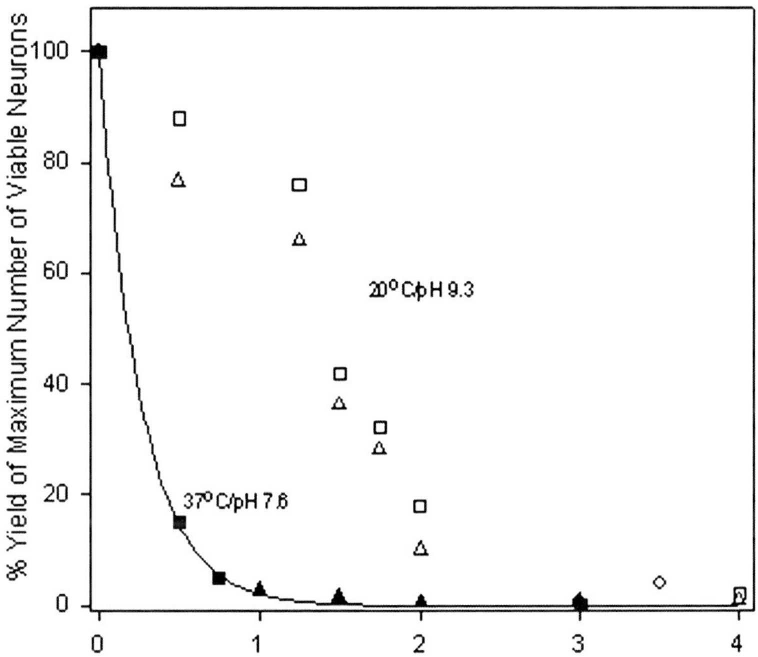

Figure 2. Plot of the decreasing yield of viable neurons dissociated from intact adult human dorsal root ganglia (DRG) maintained ischemic up to 4 h under physiological conditions (37° C/pH 7.4) (*filled circles, triangles,* and *squares*), versus hypothermia and alkaline (20° C/pH 9.3) (*open circles, triangles,* and *squares*). The data for the physiological conditions closely fit a single exponential, three parameter regression curve.

Possible mechanisms by which hypothermia and alkalinization provide neuroprotection

These experiments did not allow a determination of the mechanisms by which hypothermia and alkalinization provided protection against ischemia. However, based on what is known about ischemia-triggered secondary causes of neuron death, it is possible to speculate on the mechanisms underlying the observed protection.

Ischemia leads to the excessive release of extracellular EAAs.[3–5,17,18,20–22] DRG neurons contain and release EAAs, such as glutamate and aspartate,[23,24,29] and possess receptors to these amino acids.[4] Following isolation of intact DRG, the large and densely packed neurons, surrounded by tissue and a connective tissue coat, become ischemic and therefore exposed to an ischemia-induced excessive accumulation of EAAs and prolonged acidification (pH 7.3 to 6.5)[4,25,26] because the EAAs cannot diffuse away. Acidification due to the accumulation of EAAs induces both necrotic and apoptotic neuron loss.[27] The accumulation of EAAs also leads to excessive activation of NMDA receptors,[4] that induces a massive influx of extracellular calcium[5] which in turn leads to a disruption of calcium homeostasis,[6,28] lipid peroxidation,[26] and neuron death. Further, the released glutamate stimulates its own release in a positive feedback loop by its interaction with non-NMDA receptor subtypes.[4] Calcium-induced calcium release, and a further influx of calcium through voltage-gated calcium channels after glutamate-induced depolarization, contributes to glutamate toxicity.

Mild hypothermia (30–35° C) provides neuroprotection from ischemia-induced excitotoxicity by markedly inhibiting the cellular release of excitatory amino acids, reducing their excessive accumulation, excessive NMDA receptor activation, and development of extracellular acidification. Hypothermia may play a similar role in the present experiments.

If the observed neuron death was triggered by EAA-induced acidification, extracellular alkalinization would prevent the development of acidification, which in turn would reduce the extent of neuron death. Therefore, it may have been anticipated that simultaneous hypothermia and alkalinization would provide greater neuroprotection than either one alone, by reducing the release and accumulation of EAA release, extracellular acidification, excessive activation of NMDA receptors, and by reducing the loss of calcium homeostasis.

However, it is still important to separate the potential excitotoxic components of EEAs from the acidosis brought about by their massive release. Thus, neuroprotection by hypothermia is not merely explained by blocking or reducing the release of glutamate or other EAAs during ischemia, because hypothermia itself appears to play a pivotal role in neuroprotection.

With increasing alkalinization, calcium solubility decreases rapidly, so as the extracellular pH approaches 9.3, most calcium has precipitated into calcium bicarbonate, and there is little if any free calcium to enter neurons, thus creating a neuroprotective environment free from calcium toxicity.

The present results demonstrate that, consistent with data from experiments on other neuron models, hypothermia and alkalinization separately provide protection against prolonged ischemia to adult human DRG neurons within intact DRG, and ischemic-triggered secondary causes of death. However, the data also show that hypothermia and alkalinization combined provide significantly greater neuroprotection than either one alone. This demonstration is similar to that for neurons within intact adult rat DRG.[11] No previous studies have examined mechanisms for neuroprotection of isolated adult human neurons.

Clinical implications

Under physiological conditions, 1 h of ischemia causes the yield of viable neurons from within intact adult human DRG to decrease to 3.8%. However, under combined hypothermic and alkaline conditions for 1 h of ischemia, the yield of viable neurons increased by 23-fold. These results indicate that clinically to preserve neuron viability and neurological functions through a period of ischemia the cellular environment of the ischemic neurons must be changed as soon as possible after the onset of ischemia to a neuronal environment that is neuroprotective. One approach to accomplish this is to create a focal change in the cellular environment in the region of the trauma and ischemia as rapidly as possible to one that is hypothermic (20° C) and alkaline (pH 9.3).

To accomplish a change in the neuronal environmental immediately following a spinal cord trauma may be difficult or impossible if an individual must be transported from the site of the accident to a hospital. However, it is possible to immediately make the region of trauma hypothermic by application of an ice pack or other external cooling device to the region of trauma. This should be done even without a neurological exam because the cooling will give rise to no deleterious effects. Then upon arrival at a hospital a more focused change in the neuronal environment can be accomplished by reverse venous perfusion of the region of spinal cord trauma with hypothermic and alkaline saline.

Conflicts of interest

The author declares no conflicts of interest.

References

1. McDonald, E.S. & A.J. Windebank. 2000. Mechanisms of neurotoxic injury and cell death. *Neurol Clin.* **18:** 525–540.
2. Schnell, L. *et al.* 1999. Acute inflammatory responses to mechanical lesions in the CNS: differences between brain and spinal cord. *Eur. J. Neurosci.* **11:** 3648–3658.
3. Follis, F. *et al.* 2000. Competitive NMDA receptor antagonists and spinal-cord ischemia. *J. Invest. Surg.* **13:** 117–121; discussion 123–114.
4. Sucher, N.J., S.A. Lipton & E.B. Dreyer. 1997. Molecular basis of glutamate toxicity in retinal ganglion cells. *Vision Res.* **37:** 3483–3493.
5. Frandsen, A. & A. Schousboe. 1991. Dantrolene prevents glutamate cytotoxicity and Ca2+ release from intracellular stores in cultured cerebral cortical neurons. *J. Neurochem.* **56:** 1075–1078.
6. Leist, M. & P. Nicotera. 1998. Calcium and neuronal death. *Rev. Physiol. Biochem. Pharmacol.* **132:** 79–125.
7. Parrino, P.E. *et al.* 1999. Spinal cord protection during aortic cross-clamping using retrograde venous perfusion. *Ann. Thorac. Surg.* **67:** 1589–1594; discussion 1594–1585.
8. Lucas, J.H. *et al.* 1994. *In vitro* investigations of the effects of nonfreezing low temperatures on lesioned and uninjured mammalian spinal neurons. *J. Neurotrauma.* **11:** 35–61.

9. Ross, S.D. *et al.* 2000. Hypothermic retrograde venous perfusion with adenosine cools the spinal cord and reduces the risk of paraplegia after thoracic aortic clamping. *J. Thorac. Cardiovasc. Surg.* **119:** 588–595.
10. Herold, J.A. *et al.* 1994. Complete prevention of postischemic spinal cord injury by means of regional infusion with hypothermic saline and adenosine. *J. Thorac. Cardiovasc. Surg.* **107:** 536–541; discussion 541–532.
11. Cruz, O. & D.P. Kuffler. 2005. Neuroprotection of adult rat dorsal root ganglion neurons by combined hypothermia and alkalinization against prolonged ischemia. *Neuroscience* **132:** 115–122.
12. Hartemink, K.J. *et al.* 2004. Novel applications of therapeutic hypothermia: report of three cases. *Crit. Care* **8:** R343–R346.
13. Hammer, M.D. & D.W. Krieger. 2003. Hypothermia for acute ischemic stroke: not just another neuroprotectant. *Neurologist* **9:** 280–289.
14. Ovbiagele, B. *et al.* 2003. Potential role of neuroprotective agents in the treatment of patients with acute ischemic stroke. *Curr. Treat. Options Neurol.* **5:** 367–375.
15. Debillon, T. *et al.* 2003. Whole-body cooling after perinatal asphyxia: a pilot study in term neonates. *Dev. Med. Child Neurol.* **45:** 17–23.
16. Sosa, I.J. *et al.* 1998. Isolation and long-term survival of adult human sensory neurons *in vitro*. *Neurosurgery* **42:** 681–685; discussion 685–686.
17. Garthwaite, J. & G. Garthwaite. 1990. Mechanisms of excitatory amino acid neurotoxicity in rat brain slices. *Adv. Exp. Med. Biol.* **268:** 505–518.
18. Siesjo, B.K., C.D. Agardh & F. Bengtsson. 1989. Free radicals and brain damage. *Cerebrovasc. Brain Metab. Rev.* **1:** 165–211.
19. Reyes, O., I. Sosa & D.P. Kuffler. 2006. Neuroprotection of adult human neurons against ischemia by hypothermia and alkalinization. *P.R. Health Sci. J.* **25:** 43–50.
20. Siesjo, B.K. *et al.* 1989. Calcium, excitotoxins, and neuronal death in the brain. *Ann. N.Y. Acad. Sci.* **568:** 234–251.
21. Meldrum, B. & J. Garthwaite. 1990. Excitatory amino acid neurotoxicity and neurodegenerative disease. *Trends Pharmacol. Sci.* **11:** 379–387.
22. Loikkanen, J.J., J. Naarala & K.M. Savolainen. 1998. Modification of glutamate-induced oxidative stress by lead: the role of extracellular calcium. *Free Radic. Biol. Med.* **24:** 377–384.
23. Otori, Y., J.Y. Wei & C.J. Barnstable. 1998. Neurotoxic effects of low doses of glutamate on purified rat retinal ganglion cells. *Invest Ophthalmol. Vis. Sci.* **39:** 972–981.
24. Harry, G.J. *et al.* 1998. *In vitro* techniques for the assessment of neurotoxicity. *Environ. Health Perspect.* **106**(Suppl 1): 131–158.
25. Li, Y., C.L. Schlamp & R.W. Nickells. 1999. Experimental induction of retinal ganglion cell death in adult mice. *Invest. Ophthalmol. Vis. Sci.* **40:** 1004–1008.
26. Torp, R. *et al.* 1993. Effect of ischaemia and reperfusion on the extra- and intracellular distribution of glutamate, glutamine, aspartate and GABA in the rat hippocampus, with a note on the effect of the sodium channel blocker BW1003C87. *Exp. Brain Res.* **96:** 365–376.
27. Ding, D. *et al.* 2000. Acidosis induces necrosis and apoptosis of cultured hippocampal neurons. *Exp. Neurol.* **162:** 1–12.
28. Cebers, G., A. Cebere & S. Liljequist. 1998. Metabolic inhibition potentiates AMPA-induced Ca2+ fluxes and neurotoxicity in rat cerebellar granule cells. *Brain Res.* **779:** 194–204.
29. Mattson, M.P. & K. Furukawa. 1998. Signaling events regulating the neurodevelopmental triad. Glutamate and secreted forms of beta-amyloid precursor protein as examples. *Perspect. Dev. Neurobiol.* **5:** 337–352.

Ann. N.Y. Acad. Sci. ISSN 0077-8923

ANNALS OF THE NEW YORK ACADEMY OF SCIENCES
Issue: *Neuroprotective Agents*

Combinatorial techniques for enhancing neuroprotection

Hypothermia and alkalinization

Damien P. Kuffler
Institute of Neurobiology, Medical Sciences Campus, University of Puerto Rico, San Juan
Address for correspondence: Damien P. Kuffler, Institute of Neurobiology, 201 Blvd. del Valle, San Juan, PR 00901. dkuffler@hotmail.com

Brain and spinal cord (CNS) trauma typically kill a number of neurons, but even more neurons are killed by secondary causes triggered by the initial trauma. Thus, a minor insult may rapidly cause the death of a vastly larger number of neurons and complete paralysis. The best mechanism for reducing the extent of neurological deficits is to minimize the number of neurons killed by post-trauma sequelae. Neuroprotection techniques take many diverse forms with a breadth too great for a short review. Therefore, this review focuses on the neuroprotection provided by hypothermia and a number of other neuroprotective techniques, when administered singly or in combination, because it is generally found that combinations of applications lead to significantly better neuroprotection than is achieved by any one alone. The combinatorial approach to neuroprotection holds great promise for enhancing the degree of neuroprotection following trauma, leading to maximum maintenance of neurological function.

Keywords: adult human neurons; dorsal root ganglia; hypothermia; alkalinization; ischemia; neuroprotection

Introduction

Trauma and its sequelae

Trauma and stress lead to neurotoxicity and neurological deficits, with interventions required to provide neuroprotection and prevent the loss of neurological function. Although many interventions have been tested in many different injury models, none provides sufficient neuroprotection. This article discusses different neuroprotective interventions, and concludes that effective neuroprotection is only possible when several neuroprotective techniques are administered simultaneously. In another paper in this volume, the author discusses a novel technique that significantly provides neuroprotection against severe ischemia of adult human dorsal root ganglion (DRG) neurons using techniques simultaneously.

Trauma-induced secondary insults causing neuron death include ischemia, lipid peroxidation,[1] inflammation,[2] and the excessive release of extracellular excitatory amino acids (EAAs).[3] The EAAs lead to toxic extracellular acidification and the toxicity of an excessive stimulation of a *N*-methyl-D-aspartate (NMDA) subtype of glutamate receptor,[4] allowing a massive extracellular calcium influx,[5] and disruption of calcium homeostasis of neurons.[6] The released glutamate stimulates further glutamate release in a positive feedback loop by interacting with non-NMDA receptor subtypes,[4] while calcium-induced calcium release, accompanied by a further influx of calcium through voltage-gated calcium channels after glutamate-induced depolarization, contributes to glutamate toxicity.

Electrophysiological and other studies on adult rat DRG neurons have shown that small changes in the cellular environment (predominantly increases in temperature and decreases in pH), result in dramatic changes in membrane properties that kill neurons.[7] Neuron death is also triggered by excitotoxins,[8] and trauma-induced inflammation.[9] Whole body hypothermia[10] and increasing pH provide neuroprotection to adult rat CNS neurons against infarct-induced ischemia.[11] However, clinically there are few data on how to provide neuroprotection against ischemia and trauma induced secondary events.

Clinically whole body hypothermia provides limited neuroprotection, probably because it requires

doi: 10.1111/j.1749-6632.2009.05353.x

interactions with additional environmental conditions. The temperature that provides neuroprotection varies from mild (33–35° C)[12] to moderate (30–32° C),[13] severe (27–29° C),[13] and extreme (20° C).[14] However, localized hypothermia (32° C) provides good neuroprotection during periods of compromised cerebral blood flow and oxygen delivery.[15]

Neuroprotection by one mechanism is enhanced when combined with another. Neuroprotection provided by regional hypothermia against 45 min of ischemia is increased by the simultaneous infusion with adenosine.[16] Adenosine provides neuroprotection by suppressing the neurotoxic GABA-activated current (IGADA) in a majority of the neurons (77%).[17] Similarly, regional hypothermia together with the simultaneous infusion of an NMDA receptor antagonist enhances the neuroprotection provided by hypothermia.[18] It has also been reported that hypothermia and alkalinization combined provided greater neuroprotection to ischemic adult rat DRG neurons than either one applied alone.[19]

Alkalinization also provides neuroprotection ischemia,[20] with alkalinization to pH 8.2 protecting adult rat CNS neurons against ischemic effects of infarct,[11] and primary culture mouse neocortical neurons from azide-induced chemical anoxia.[21]

Stressors leading to neuron death

Some studied stressors include stroke, surgically required ischemia, stress-related hyperthermia, drug-induced hyperthermia, and various drugs and diseases. A good example for a trigger of neurotoxicity is ischemia essential during neonatal, pediatric, and adult cardiac and cardiopulmonary bypass surgery, for which deep hypothermia is still the most important method for providing neuroprotection.

Hyperthermia

Trauma induced heat stress leads to hyperthermia, which leads to neurotoxicity.[22] The neurotoxicity primarily results from the increased permeability of the blood-brain barrier (BBB), allowing serum proteins to enter causing edema, inducing neuron stress and neurotoxicity and a significant decrease in cerebral blood flow.[22,23] A number of diseases and drugs, such as bradykinin, physiological states, including pain, hypoxic and aglycemic stress, and stroke also cause increased BBB permeability.[24] Thus, factors that decrease BBB permeability and edema, such as the administration of growth hormone, pretreatment with the potent antioxidant H-290/51,[25] or Cerebrolysin (Cere), a commercial mixture of neurotrophic factors, inhibit hyperthermia-induced neurotoxicity.[26]

Hypothermia

Hypothermia has been extensively used in various forms as a neuroprotective technique during such situations as required surgery-induced ischemia, following stroke, and following consumption of drugs or diseases that cause hyperthermia. Hypothermia also appears to be an ideal neuroprotective intervention against hypoxic-ischemic encephalopathy after perinatal asphyxia. In addition, hypothermia prolongs the therapeutic time window, for optimal neuroprotection following transient perinatal hypoxia-ischemia (HI), when the therapy starts before overt secondary energy failure and its irreversible neurotoxic cascade.[27] However, the manner in which hypothermia is applied, focally or systemically, the extent of hypothermia that is optimal for different tissues, the duration of hypothermia, and when it is applied, must be optimized.

Hypothermia to <28° C is rarely compatible with life, with few cases describing individuals surviving such low temperatures. However, individuals have survived with a core body temperature below 21.0° C without neurological deficits.[28] Mild hypothermia significantly reduces hepatic injury in a warm ischemia model in lean and obese rats and significantly improved 24 h survival in obese rats.[29]

Although severe hypoxia ischemia may not cause immediate neurotoxicity and death, it can trigger complex biochemical cascades leading to the delayed neuronal loss. Clinically and experimentally, the times during which hypothermia are required are the latent phase after reperfusion, with initial recovery of cerebral energy metabolism, and a secondary phase characterized by the accumulation of cytotoxins, seizures, cytotoxic edema, and failure of cerebral oxidative metabolism starting 6 to 15 h post insult. Moderate cerebral hypothermia, initiated as early as possible before the onset of secondary deterioration, and continued for a sufficient duration in relation to the severity of the cerebral injury, is associated with potent, long-lasting neuroprotection in both adult and perinatal species. Clinical trials using head cooling with mild hypothermia, and moderate whole body cooling show that post-resuscitation cooling is generally safe in intensive care, and reduces death or disability at 18 months of age after neonatal encephalopathy.[30]

Immediately up to 3 h after reperfusion hypothermic reperfusion of rabbits undergoing 15 min of abdominal aortic occlusion for 15 min to induce spinal cord ischemia, significantly reduced ischemia-induced spinal cord neuronal damage.[31] In adults, resuscitation from cardiac arrest results in reperfusion injury that leads to increased postresuscitation mortality and delayed neuronal death. Delivery of adenosine following 12 min of rat brain ischemia following cardiac arrest and resuscitation increases the proportion of animals surviving to 4 days and significantly delays hippocampal CA1 neuronal loss. Adenosine treatment provides its neuroprotective effects via significantly lowering brain temperature during recovery.[32] Moderate hypothermic circulatory arrest, without any adjunctive cerebral protection, at 26 to 28° C for patients with ascending aortic aneurysms extending into the proximal aortic arch, provides cerebral neuroprotection in selected patients.[33] However, this approach is only advisable for patients for whom the surgery can be performed within 10 min.[33] Hypothermia to 35 to 33° C after resuscitation from cardiac arrest equally improves neuronal survival and neurologic recovery in rats.[34]

Hyperbaric oxygenation is more effective than normobaric oxygenation in providing neuroprotection, reducing infarct volume and improving clinical outcomes, during transient focal cerebral ischemia/reperfusion when applied early and at high doses.[35] Therefore, combining hypothermia with hyperbaric oxygenation should lead to enhanced neuroprotection than is provided by either approach alone.

Neuroprotection: whole body versus focal hypothermia

Whole body hypothermia

The use of whole-body surface cooling for stroke therapy is limited primarily because of management problems and severe side effects (e.g., pneumonia),[36] although whole body hypothermia of adult cardiac arrest patients leads to significantly improved survival rates and neurologic outcomes.[37,38] Hypothermia following transient (2 h) middle cerebral artery occlusion of the rat significantly postpones neuronal injury and reduces ischemic cell death.[39]

The survival rates and neurologic outcomes of adult cardiac arrest patients are significantly improved by whole body hypothermia.[37] Twenty-six hours of mild to moderate resuscitative hypothermia (30° C rectal temperature) started 2 h after hypoxic-ischemic injury protects CNS neurons, and provides long-lasting behavioral improvements throughout brain maturation despite the severity of the injury and the delayed onset of cooling,[40] and hypothermia after transient (2 h) middle cerebral artery occlusion significantly postpones neuronal injury and reduces ischemic neuron death.[39]

What has not been determined is the time frame in which hypothermia should be applied following cerebral challenge, the degree of hypothermia, and the duration of its application to provide optimal neuroprotection. The management of hypothermia and adverse events that accompany it has reduced the interest in the widespread application of whole-body surface cooling especially in elderly stroke patients. However, in the case of newborn infants, optimizing hypothermic treatment requires a means for inducing uniform systemic hypothermia.[41] In the case of neurons within adult human and rat DRG, hypothermia is neuroprotective against up to four hours of ischemia, with maximum neuroprotection provided at 20° C versus 36° C.[42] This neuroprotective effect is similar to that for cerebral neurons of newborn humans.[43]

Focal hypothermia

Focal hypothermic perfusion of the region of neurotrauma via venous or arterial hypothermic perfusion is an alternative to whole body hypothermia and externally locally applied hypothermia (a solid ice cap), for example following hypoxic events in neonates.[41] Similarly retrograde cerebral perfusion for 90 min at 20° C, improves cerebral neuroprotection after prolonged hypothermic circulatory arrest, compared to reperfusion with normothermic perfusion.[44]

Although whole body hypothermia is therapeutic following neonatal hypoxic-ischemic brain injury, 45 min of global hypoxic-ischemic insult, selective head cooling combined with mild total-body hypothermia during anesthesia enhances local neuroprotection and minimizes the occurrence of systemic side effects and stress associated with unsedated whole-body cooling.[45] Selective brain hypothermia decreases the production of hydroxyl radicals (−OH) induced by hypoxia-ischemia and hypothermic reperfusion and decreases neuronal damage in neonatal rat brain.[46]

These results indicate that hypothermia by itself provides neuroprotection, and that focal hypothermia provides safer and more effective neuroprotection than whole body hypothermia. Other experiments show that focal hypothermia is even more effective when combined with different factors.

Enhancing neuroprotection by combining hypothermia with additional components

Thoracic aortic surgery, occluding specific spinal cord arteries, can lead to postoperative paraplegia in up to 40% of high-risk patients. However, the neurotoxicity due to ischemic injury caused by thoracic aortic occlusion (30 min) can be significantly reduced by retrograde venous perfusion-cooling (4° C) of the spinal cord alone, but to a greater extent when combined with adenosine and infused into the accessory hemiazygous vein.[47] Retrograde venous perfusion of the spinal cord with phenytoin, a voltage-sensitive sodium channel blocker, provides significant protection during prolonged spinal cord ischemia and focal and global cerebral ischemic models.[16]

Neurotrophins

Additional factors enhancing neuroprotection come from two groups of molecules. One is the polypeptide growth factors (e.g., basic fibroblast growth factor (bFGF), epidermal growth factor (EGF) and brain-derived neurotrophic facter (BDNF)). The second are extensively complex multiple forms of molecules, consisting of sialic acid-containing glycosphingolipids or gangliosides (e.g., the ganglioside (GM1)), neurotrophic factors, which are involved in virtually all stages of neuron development, differentiation, growth, and functioning, which provide neuroprotection against toxic levels of glutamate or its non-physiological agonist kainate *in vitro*. Therefore, both groups of molecules should be beneficial following ischemia.[48] The administration of neurotrophic factors, singly or simultaneously, provide neuroprotection but the optimal approach for their application has not been determined.

There is extensive literature on the influences and mechanisms of action of specific neurotrophic factors which cannot be covered here. However, it is important to state that BDNF protects neurons against ischemia-induced neuron death in infants[49] by protecting neurons against glutamate excitoxicity,[50] and a single topical application of BDNF or insulin-like growth factor 1 (IGF-1) within 5 to 30 min of a focal trauma to the rat spinal cord attenuates spinal cord injury (SCI)-induced breakdown of the blood-spinal cord barrier (BSCB), edema formation, motor dysfunction, and cell injury.[51] However, a combination of BDNF and glial cell-derived neurotrophic factor (GDNF) (but not with neurotrophic-3 or nerve growth factor) given 60 or 90 min after SCI significantly reduces motor dysfunction and spinal cord pathology at 5 h, suggesting a potential therapeutic approach for the treatment of SCI in clinical situations.[51] In the case of BDNF and ciliary neurotrophic factor, each rescue photoreceptors from collateral retinal damage caused by photodynamic therapy, but their combined effects are greater than either one alone.[52]

Erythropoietin (Epo), a cytokine, induces direct and indirect effects on neurons by enhancing antioxidotic enzyme production, antagonizing glutamate's cytotoxic action, metabolizing free radicals, normalizing cerebral blood flow, reducing inflammatory responses, affecting neurotransmitters release, stimulating neoangiogenesis, and having anti-apoptotic actions post peripheral nervous system (PNS) and CNS trauma. Therefore, Epo's administration contributes to the recovery of mechanical allodynia and may be effective in peripheral nerve regeneration after neurorrhaphy.[53] Another effective neuroprotective neurotrophic factor is activity-dependent neurotrophic factor.[54] Knowing that all these factors provide neuroprotection, it is critical to determine their effects on neuroprotection when combined with hypothermia.

Deep hypothermia induces substantial cytotoxicity in brain cells, while simultaneously playing an important role in neuroprotection by increasing the release of the pro-inflammatory cytokine interleukin-6 (IL-6), and increasing the levels of the astrocytic protein S100B in the serum and cerebrospinal fluid of patients.[55] Under hypothermic conditions, nanomolar concentrations of S100B increase IL-6 release from brain cells, which modulates pro-inflammatory cytokines and stimulates neurite outgrowth. Thus, S100B differentially influences cytokine release and cytotoxicity from distinct brain cells while inhibiting neuroregeneration by suppressing hypothermia-induced axonal outgrowth.[55] Hypertonic saline dextran has neuroprotective properties, and when combined with hypothermia, both neuroprotection and neurological recovery are enhanced following circulatory arrest.[56]

Neuronal pentraxins (NPs) define a family of novel proteins, called "long pentraxins," that are exclusively expressed in central neurons, and are homologous to the C-reactive and acute-phase proteins in the immune system. They are neuroprotective against hypoxia-induced neuronal death.[57]

During cardiac surgery, neuroprotection is crucial, and the major protective methods are the administration of steroids and deep hypothermia. Methylprednisolone (MP) significantly increases cell survival after deep hypothermia, while also suppressing important neuroprotective and regenerative processes induced by IL-6. Therefore, more specific immune modulation than that provided by MP is needed to protect the brain during cardiac surgery.[58]

Progesterone is neuroprotective against glutamate-induced toxicity, partially by its induction of the expression of BDNF. However, additional data indicate that progesterone is protective via multiple and potentially related mechanisms.[59]

Anti-inflammatory agents

The adenosine A2A agonist ATL-146e ameliorates reperfusion inflammation, reducing subsequent paralysis and neuronal apoptosis after spinal cord ischemia via the adenosine A2A agonist binding to inducible neuronal A2A-R, which is upregulated on lumbar spinal cord motor neurons after ischemia and during spinal cord reperfusion.[60] Other approaches providing neuroprotection and neurological recovery following surgical decompression after acute SCI include the administration of the semisynthetic second generation tetracycline derivative, minocycline, potassium channel blockers, neuroregeneration and neuroprotective approaches using the Rho antagonist, Cethrin, the use of anti-NOGO monoclonal antibodies to augment plasticity and regeneration, and cell-mediated repair using stem cells, bone marrow stromal cells, and olfactory ensheathing cells.[61] Aprotinin is used in cardiac surgery for its anti-inflammatory and hemostatic benefits, is neuroprotective of other serine protease inhibitors via reducing excitotoxic cell death, and directly protects against glutamatergic excitotoxicity.[27]

Activation of the nicotinic acetylcholine receptor (nAChR), a neurotrophic gene-regulating factor, has neuroprotective/trophic actions and involves the fibroblast growth factor (FGF-2) gene as a target of nAChR signaling. Thus, FGF-2 could be involved in nAChR mechanisms mediating the neuronal survival, trophism, and plasticity.[62]

The Bcl-2 protein is neuroprotective as an antiapoptotic agent acting via an anti-inflammatory mechanism, and its gene expression is upregulated by statins, and, and not by cholesterol regulation.[63] The neuroprotection by Bcl-2 is further enhanced by mild hypothermia by further inducing the expression of Bcl-2 mRNA.[64]

Immunotherapy

The immune system is involved in the pathogenic processes and protection against neurodegenerative processes caused by microbes, trauma, toxic metabolites, autoimmunity, and a wide variety of degenerative processes. Therapeutic modalities may take advantage of CNS immune responses leading to research toward understanding the optimal mechanisms by which advantages can be taken of the immune system to fight neurodegenerative attacks.[65]

Multiple sclerosis (MS), a chronic inflammatory disease of the CNS, is a predominantly CD^{4+} T cell mediated autoimmune disorder, but also involves other immune cells and factors (even non-immune) including CNS antigen-driven clonally expanded B cells, auto-antibodies, complement, mediators of the innate immune responses in MS lesions, oligodendroglial cell (OGC) loss, attenuated remyelination, axonopathy, and gliosis. Treatment of the pathogenesis of MS will probably require a multifaceted spectrum of immune activity, involving their specific and/or multiple pathogenic steps including initiation, peripheral activation, molecular co-stimulation and immune effector responses during early, transitional, and late phases of disease, and enhancement of neuroprotection and reparative mechanisms.[66]

The discovery that small molecule ligands for peptidyl-prolyl isomerase (PPIase) possess powerful neuroprotective and neuroregenerative properties *in vitro* and *in vivo* suggests therapeutic utility for such compounds in neurodegenerative disease.[67] The neurotrophic effects of these compounds are independent of the immunosuppressive pathways by which drugs such as FK506 and rapamycin operate.[68]

FK506 acts as a powerful neuroprotective agent providing protection *in vivo* against focal cerebral ischemia, even when administered up to 60 min post-occlusion,[69] and at a concentration comparable with the immunosuppressant dose used in humans.[70] However, although neurons are maintained viable during the period of the ischemic insult, many neurons die during the period of reperfusion and warming.[71] Administration of FK506 during perperfusion provides neuroprotection to neurons that die during the reperfusion.[71] It is possible that the administration and maintenance of alkalinization, combined with administration of FK506, will provide even greater neuroprotection through the period of reperfusion.

The mechanism by which FK506 prevents ischemic brain damage remains unknown, but may depend on de novo protein synthesis, rather than on the inhibition of calcineurin. But, beside the widespread therapeutic use of ligands of immunophilins as immunosuppressants, FK506 and V-10,367 mediate neuroprotection of retinal ganglion neurons against optic nerve crush-induced cell death that occurs when the optic nerve is crushed within 2 mm of the eye,[72] but they do not enhance the rate of retinal ganglion cell axon outgrowth.[73]

Alkalinization

Hypothermia provides neuroprotection to spinal neurons against ischemia.[15,74–76] Similarly, alkalinization provides neuroprotection against ischemia of adult rat and adult human DRG neurons.[19,77] However, the neuroprotection against ischemia provided by hypothermia and alkalinization of adult rat and adult human DRG neurons is significantly enhanced (up to 23-fold) when hypothermia and alkalinization are combined.

High levels of NO generated by NOS isoforms are partially responsible for exacerbating the neuronal damage induced by middle cerebral artery occlusion (MCAo) by intraluminal filament.[78,79] Endothelial nitric oxide synthase (eNOS) overexpression occurs in several pathological conditions, and is activated by tumor necrosis factor-alpha (TNF-alpha), a proinflammatory cytokine that plays important roles in several neurodegenerative diseases. eNOS activation by TNF-alpha confers cytoprotection from excitotoxicity and neurotoxic triggers, such as reactive oxygen species, endoplasmic reticulum stress, DNA damage, and mutated alsin itself.[78] Thus, neuron overexpression of eNOS provides a broad-range damage-activated neuroprotective mechanism, and establishes a link of pathophysiological relevance between this enzyme and inflammation accompanying neurodegenerative diseases.[79]

Role of pH on calcium ion neurotoxicity

At a normal extracellular Ca^{2+} concentration, large activation of neuronal calcium channels leads to massive entry of extracellular calcium ions, causing excessive intracellular Ca^{2+} accumulation, which is neurotoxic. The relative concentration of Ca^{2+} depends on pH, with calcium requiring a pH of less than 6 to enter solution as Ca^{2+}. At physiological pH (7.6) Ca^{2+} solubility is 160 mg/L, and increases to 6,390 mg/L at pH 7.0, but decreasing 40-fold to 10.1 at pH 8.4.[80] As the pH approaches 9.3, most Ca^{2+} has precipitated from solution into calcium bicarbonate, thus decreasing the concentration of soluble extracellular calcium that could enter neurons, and therefore, alkalinization will provide a neuroprotection against calcium toxicity.

Conclusions and clinical implications

The present data demonstrate that among the most effective neuroprotective agents against many types of CNS insults is hypothermia and alkalinization. However, the neuroprotection provided by hypothermia is significantly augmented when it is combined with other neuroprotective techniques, especially alkalinization. These conclusions are summarized in Table 1, which is far from comprehensive. Therefore, to provide optimal neuroprotection in the immediate aftermath of CNS trauma, hypothermia must be combined with other techniques that assist in maintaining the viability of the largest possible number of neurons in the immediate post-trauma neurotoxic environment caused by secondary sequelae of spinal trauma. The maintenance of the largest number of viable neurons

Table 1. Neuroprotection provided by hypothermia is significantly augmented when combined with other neuroprotective techniques, especially alkalinization

Neuronal insult	Neuroprotective factors acting singly				Enhanced neuroprotection by combined factors
ischemia	hypothermia/ epidermal growth factor (EGF)/steroids	immunosuppressants (FK506 and V-10,367)/ hyperbaric oxygenation/ polypeptide growth factors (e.g., bFGF)	gangliosides/ neurotrophic factors/neuronal pentraxins	BDNF/nAChR/ FGF-2/sialic acid-containing glycosphingolipids/ voltage-sensitive sodium channel blocker	hypothermia + alkalinization/hypothermia + hyperbaric oxygenation/selective head cooling combined + mild total-body hypothermia/combined neurotrophic factors/ hypertonic saline dextran + hypothermia
acidification	alkalinization	carbon dioxide	alpha2-adrenergic agonists	voltage-dependent C-type gating acceleration	alkalinization + hypothermia/ glyoxal and H(2)O(2)
excessive amino acid transmitter accumulation	hypothermia deferoxamine (DFO), a chelator of non-protein-bound iron	GPI-1046 (non-immunosuppressant)/ tea polyphenol (an antioxidant) and anti-inflammatory agent	alkalinization glutamate transporters, GLT-1 and GLAST/ magnesium-induced block NMDA receptors	thyroid hormone (T(3)) memantine (an NMDA receptor antagonist)/ antiepileptic drugs	hypothermia + alkalinization memantine + tea polyphenol
excessive extracellular calcium concentrations	hypothermia	alkalinization	inhibition of cGMP formation	inhibition of nitric oxide synthase (NOS)	hypothermia + alkalinization
hyperthemia	hypothermia	postsynaptic density-95 inhibitors	minoxidil by opening mitochondrial KATP channels	arimoclomol, a coinducer of heat shock proteins	hypothermia + alkalinization
lipid peroxidation	hypothermia	ApoE	anti-alpha4beta1 treatment	inhibition of mitogen-activated protein kinase pathway with PD98096 or U0126	
excessive intracellular calcium	alkalinization	hypothermia	memantine	tea polyphenol	hypothermia + alkalinization memantine + tea polyphenol
nitric oxide	eNOS activation by TNF-alpha	volatile anesthetic agents	neurotransmitters/ ischemic postconditioning	ischemic preconditioning	ischemic preconditioning and ischemic postconditioning
pathogenic immune system	activation of immune effector responses	peptidyl-prolyl isomerase	activation of Toll-like receptors	enhanced autoimmunity	activation of Toll-like receptors + recruitment of neuroprotective T lymphocytes.

Continued.

Table 1. *Continued*

Neuronal insult	Neuroprotective factors acting singly				Enhanced neuroprotection by combined factors
apoptosis	Bcl-2	alpha2 adrenoceptor signaling	progesterone/ inhibition of isoflurane-induced caspase-3 expression	enhance neuroprotective autoimmunity	Bcl-2 + hypothermia
inflammation	adenosine A2A agonist	serine protease inhibitors	aprotinin	blocking CD47 ligand thrombospondin 1	
excessive stimulation of NMDA-R	hypothermia	alkalinization/ MK-801/nicotinic cholinergic receptor stimulation	adenosine/ downregulation of NMDA receptor surface expression	preservation of mitochondrial membrane potential/glutathione	hypothermia + alkalinization
increased BBB permeability	growth hormone	cerebrolysin	melatonin, a powerful antioxidant	inhibition of mitochondrial permeability transition (mPT)	
reperfusion	hypothermia	adenosine	FK506	preconditioning with moderate oxidative stress	hypothermia + adenosine/alkalinization + FK506
hydroxyl radicals	hypothermia	erythropoietin/peptidic metal chelators	IL-6/halogenated derivatives of aromatic amino acids	activity-dependent neurotrophic factor	
GABA receptor activation	adenosine	GluR5 agonist	ATPA	GABA(A) receptor agonist muscimol/GABA(B) receptor agonist baclofen	GABA(A) receptor agonist muscimol + GABA(B) receptor agonist baclofen
glutamate toxicity	polypeptide growth factors	gangliosides/ erythropoietin	EGF/ApoE	ILF/BDNF	

BBB: blood-brain barrier; EGF: epidermal growth factor; bFGF: basic fibroblast growth factor; BDNF: brain derived nerve factor; nAChR: nicotinic acetylcholine receptor; ATPA: propanoic acid ((RS)-2-amino-3-(3-hydroxy-5-tert-butylisoxazol-4-yl)); NMDA: *N*-methyl-D-aspartate; ApoE: apolipoprotein E; ILF: interleukin-2 enhancer binding factor.

means the least amount of neurological losses and a significantly reduced need to attempt to induce axon regeneration to reestablish lost neurological function.

Conflicts of interest

The author declares no conflicts of interest.

References

1. McDonald, E.S. & A.J. Windebank. 2000. Mechanisms of neurotoxic injury and cell death. *Neurol. Clin.* **18:** 525–540.
2. Schnell, L. *et al.* 1999. Acute inflammatory responses to mechanical lesions in the CNS: differences between brain and spinal cord. *Eur. J. Neurosci.* **11:** 3648–3658.
3. Follis, F. *et al.* 2000. Competitive NMDA receptor antagonists and spinal-cord ischemia. *J. Invest. Surg.* **13:** 117–121; discussion 123–114.
4. Sucher, N.J., S.A. Lipton & E.B. Dreyer. 1997. Molecular basis of glutamate toxicity in retinal ganglion cells. *Vision Res.* **37:** 3483–3493.
5. Frandsen, A. & A. Schousboe. 1991. Dantrolene prevents glutamate cytotoxicity and Ca^{2+} release from intracellular stores in cultured cerebral cortical neurons. *J. Neurochem.* **56:** 1075–1078.
6. Leist, M. & P. Nicotera. 1998. Calcium and neuronal death. *Rev. Physiol. Biochem. Pharmacol.* **132:** 79–125.
7. Amorim, P., J.E. Cottrell & I.S. Kass. 1999. Effect of small changes in temperature on CA1 pyramidal cells from rat hippocampal slices during hypoxia: implications about the mechanism of hypothermic protection against neuronal damage. *Brain Res.* **844:** 143–149.

8. Adachi, K. *et al.* 1998. Mechanism of the pathogenesis of glutamate neurotoxicity in retinal ischemia. *Graefes Arch. Clin. Exp. Ophthalmol.* **236:** 766–774.
9. Schnell, L. *et al.* 1999. Cytokine-induced acute inflammation in the brain and spinal cord. *J. Neuropathol. Exp. Neurol.* **58:** 245–254.
10. Debillon, T. *et al.* 2003. Whole-body cooling after perinatal asphyxia: a pilot study in term neonates. *Dev. Med. Child Neurol.* **45:** 17–23.
11. Dietrich, W.D. *et al.* 1993. Intraischemic but not postischemic brain hypothermia protects chronically following global forebrain ischemia in rats. *J. Cereb. Blood Flow Metab.* **13:** 541–549.
12. Mori, K. *et al.* 2001. Effects of hypothermia on blood flow and neural activity in rabbit spinal cord during postischemic reperfusion. *Jpn. J. Physiol.* **51:** 71–79.
13. Mori, K. *et al.* 1998. Effects of mild (33 degrees C) and moderate (29 degrees C) hypothermia on cerebral blood flow and metabolism, lactate, and extracellular glutamate in experimental head injury. *Neurol. Res.* **20:** 719–726.
14. Sosa, I.J. *et al.* 1998. Isolation and long-term survival of adult human sensory neurons *in vitro. Neurosurgery* **42:** 681–685; discussion 685–686.
15. Parrino, P.E. *et al.* 1999. Spinal cord protection during aortic cross-clamping using retrograde venous perfusion. *Ann. Thorac. Surg.* **67:** 1589–1594; discussion 1594–1585.
16. Ross, S.D. *et al.* 2000. Hypothermic retrograde venous perfusion with adenosine cools the spinal cord and reduces the risk of paraplegia after thoracic aortic clamping. *J. Thorac. Cardiovasc. Surg.* **119:** 588–595.
17. Hu, H.Z. & Z.W. Li. 1997. Modulation by adenosine of GABA-activated current in rat dorsal root ganglion neurons. *J. Physiol.* **501**(Pt 1): 67–75.
18. Lucas, J.H. *et al.* 1994. *In vitro* investigations of the effects of nonfreezing low temperatures on lesioned and uninjured mammalian spinal neurons. *J. Neurotrauma.* **11:** 35–61.
19. Cruz, O. & D.P. Kuffler. 2005. Neuroprotection of adult rat dorsal root ganglion neurons by combined hypothermia and alkalinization against prolonged ischemia. *Neuroscience* **132:** 115–122.
20. Ishikawa, T. & M. Marsala. 1999. Hypothermia prevents biphasic glutamate release and corresponding neuronal degeneration after transient spinal cord ischemia in the rat. *Cell Mol. Neurobiol.* **19:** 199–208.
21. Jorgensen, N.K. *et al.* 1999. Increases in $[Ca^{2+}]i$ and changes in intracellular pH during chemical anoxia in mouse neocortical neurons in primary culture. *J. Neurosci. Res.* **56:** 358–370.
22. Sharma, H.S. & C.E. Johanson. 2007. Blood-cerebrospinal fluid barrier in hyperthermia. *Prog. Brain Res.* **162:** 459–478.
23. Sharma, H.S. *et al.* 2007. Antibodies to serotonin attenuate closed head injury induced blood brain barrier disruption and brain pathology. *Ann. N.Y. Acad. Sci.* **1122:** 295–312.
24. McCaffrey, G. *et al.* 2008. Occludin oligomeric assembly at tight junctions of the blood-brain barrier is disrupted by peripheral inflammatory hyperalgesia. *J. Neurochem.* **106:** 2395–2409.
25. Sharma, H.S., P.O. Sjoquist & S.F. Ali. 2007. Drugs of abuse-induced hyperthermia, blood-brain barrier dysfunction and neurotoxicity: neuroprotective effects of a new antioxidant compound H-290/51. *Curr. Pharm. Des.* **13:** 1903–1923.
26. Muresanu, D.F. 2007. Neuroprotection and neuroplasticity—a holistic approach and future perspectives. *J. Neurol. Sci.* **257:** 38–43.
27. Iwata, Y. *et al.* 2008. Aprotinin confers neuroprotection by reducing excitotoxic cell death. *J. Thorac. Cardiovasc. Surg.* **135:** 573–578; discussion 578.
28. Moser, B. *et al.* 2005. One night in a snowbank: a case report of severe hypothermia and cardiac arrest. *Resuscitation* **65:** 365–368.
29. Choi, S. *et al.* 2005. Mild hypothermia provides significant protection against ischemia/reperfusion injury in livers of obese and lean rats. *Ann. Surg.* **241:** 470–476.
30. Bennet, L. *et al.* 2007. The effect of cerebral hypothermia on white and grey matter injury induced by severe hypoxia in preterm fetal sheep. *J. Physiol.* **578:** 491–506.
31. Tsutsumi, K. *et al.* 2004. Effect of delayed induction of postischemic hypothermia on spinal cord damage induced by transient ischemic insult in rabbits. *Jpn. J. Thorac. Cardiovasc. Surg.* **52:** 411–418.
32. Xu, K. *et al.* 2006. Adenosine treatment delays postischemic hippocampal CA1 loss after cardiac arrest and resuscitation in rats. *Brain Res.* **1071:** 208–217.
33. Kamiya, H. *et al.* 2006. Short moderate hypothermic circulatory arrest without any adjunctive cerebral protection for surgical repair of the ascending aorta extending into the proximal aortic arch: is it safe? *Heart Surg Forum.* **9:** E759–E761.
34. Logue, E.S., M.J. McMichael & C.W. Callaway. 2007. Comparison of the effects of hypothermia at 33 degrees C or 35 degrees C after cardiac arrest in rats. *Acad. Emerg. Med.* **14:** 293–300.

35. Eschenfelder, C.C. *et al.* 2008. Neuroprotection by oxygen in acute transient focal cerebral ischemia is dose dependent and shows superiority of hyperbaric oxygenation. *Cerebrovasc. Dis.* **25:** 193–201.
36. Wagner, K.R. & M. Zuccarello. 2005. Local brain hypothermia for neuroprotection in stroke treatment and aneurysm repair. *Neurol. Res.* **27:** 238–245.
37. Florian, B. *et al.* 2008. Long-term hypothermia reduces infarct volume in aged rats after focal ischemia. *Neurosci. Lett.* **438:** 180–185.
38. Gressens, P. *et al.* 2008. Analysis of neuronal, glial, endothelial, axonal and apoptotic markers following moderate therapeutic hypothermia and anesthesia in the developing piglet brain. *Brain Pathol.* **18:** 10–20.
39. Zhang, Z.G., M. Chopp & H. Chen. 1993. Duration dependent post-ischemic hypothermia alleviates cortical damage after transient middle cerebral artery occlusion in the rat. *J. Neurol. Sci.* **117:** 240–244.
40. Wagner, B.P., J. Nedelcu & E. Martin. 2002. Delayed postischemic hypothermia improves long-term behavioral outcome after cerebral hypoxia-ischemia in neonatal rats. *Pediatr. Res.* **51:** 354–360.
41. Horn, A.R. *et al.* 2006. Selective cerebral hypothermia for post-hypoxic neuroprotection in neonates using a solid ice cap. *S. Afr. Med. J.* **96:** 976–981.
42. Reyes, O., I. Sosa & D.P. Kuffler. 2003. Neuroprotection of spinal neurons against blunt trauma and ischemia. *P.R. Health Sci. J.* **22:** 277–286.
43. Mujsce, D.J. *et al.* 1994. Differences in intraischemic temperature influence neurological outcome after deep hypothermic circulatory arrest in newborn dogs. *Stroke* **25:** 1433–1441; discussion 1442.
44. Ding, Y. *et al.* 2004. Local saline infusion into ischemic territory induces regional brain cooling and neuroprotection in rats with transient middle cerebral artery occlusion. *Neurosurgery* **54:** 956–964; discussion 964–955.
45. Tooley, J.R. *et al.* 2003. Head cooling with mild systemic hypothermia in anesthetized piglets is neuroprotective. *Ann. Neurol.* **53:** 65–72.
46. Hashimoto, T., M. Yonetani & H. Nakamura. 2003. Selective brain hypothermia protects against hypoxic-ischemic injury in newborn rats by reducing hydroxyl radical production. *Kobe J. Med. Sci.* **49:** 83–91.
47. Parrino, P.E. *et al.* 2000. Retrograde venous perfusion with hypothermic saline and adenosine for protection of the ischemic spinal cord. *J. Vasc. Surg.* **32:** 171–178.
48. Hicks, D. *et al.* 1998. Growth factors and gangliosides as neuroprotective agents in excitotoxicity and ischemia. *Gen. Pharmacol.* **30:** 265–273.
49. Cheng, Y. *et al.* 1997. Marked age-dependent neuroprotection by brain-derived neurotrophic factor against neonatal hypoxic-ischemic brain injury. *Ann. Neurol.* **41:** 521–529.
50. Marini, A.M. *et al.* 2007. Preconditioning and neurotrophins: a model for brain adaptation to seizures, ischemia and other stressful stimuli. *Amino Acids* **32:** 299–304.
51. Sharma, H.S. 2007. A select combination of neurotrophins enhances neuroprotection and functional recovery following spinal cord injury. *Ann. N.Y. Acad. Sci.* **1122:** 95–111.
52. Paskowitz, D.M. *et al.* 2007. Neurotrophic factors minimize the retinal toxicity of verteporfin photodynamic therapy. *Invest. Ophthalmol. Vis. Sci.* **48:** 430–437.
53. Lykissas, M.G. *et al.* 2007. Axonal regeneration stimulated by erythropoietin: an experimental study in rats. *J. Neurosci. Methods.* **164:** 107–115.
54. Gozes, I. *et al.* 1997. Antiserum to activity-dependent neurotrophic factor produces neuronal cell death in CNS cultures: Immunological and biological specificity. *Brain Res. Dev. Brain Res.* **99:** 167–175.
55. Schmitt, K.R. *et al.* 2007. S100B modulates IL-6 release and cytotoxicity from hypothermic brain cells and inhibits hypothermia-induced axonal outgrowth. *Neurosci. Res.* **59:** 68–73.
56. Kaakinen, T. *et al.* 2006. Hypertonic saline dextran improves outcome after hypothermic circulatory arrest: a study in a surviving porcine model. *Ann. Thorac. Surg.* **81:** 183–190.
57. Hossain, M.A. 2008. Hypoxic-ischemic injury in neonatal brain: involvement of a novel neuronal molecule in neuronal cell death and potential target for neuroprotection. *Int. J. Dev. Neurosci.* **26:** 93–101.
58. Schmitt, K.R. *et al.* 2006. Methylprednisolone attenuates hypothermia- and rewarming-induced cytotoxicity and IL-6 release in isolated primary astrocytes, neurons and BV-2 microglia cells. *Neurosci. Lett.* **404:** 309–314.
59. Kaur, P. *et al.* 2007. Progesterone increases brain-derived neuroptrophic factor expression and protects against glutamate toxicity in a mitogen-activated protein kinase- and phosphoinositide-3 kinase-dependent manner in cerebral cortical explants. *J. Neurosci. Res.* **85:** 2441–2449.
60. Cassada, D.C. *et al.* 2002. Adenosine A2A agonist reduces paralysis after spinal cord ischemia: correlation with A2A receptor expression on motor neurons. *Ann. Thorac. Surg.* **74:** 846–849; discussion 849–850.

61. Baptiste, D.C. & M.G. Fehlings. 2007. Update on the treatment of spinal cord injury. *Prog. Brain Res.* **161:** 217–233.
62. Belluardo, N. *et al.* 2000. Central nicotinic receptors, neurotrophic factors and neuroprotection. *Behav. Brain Res.* **113:** 21–34.
63. Johnson-Anuna, L.N. *et al.* 2007. Simvastatin protects neurons from cytotoxicity by up-regulating Bcl-2 mRNA and protein. *J. Neurochem.* **101:** 77–86.
64. Franke, C. *et al.* 2007. Bcl-2 upregulation and neuroprotection in guinea pig brain following chronic simvastatin treatment. *Neurobiol. Dis.* **25:** 438–445.
65. Gendelman, H.E. 2002. Neural immunity: friend or foe? *J. Neurovirol.* **8:** 474–479.
66. Bauman, T.M. & L.H. Kasper. 2004. Novel approaches and cutting edge immunotherapies in multiple sclerosis. *Front. Biosci.* **9:** 2302–2322.
67. Guo, X. *et al.* 2001. Neuroimmunophilins: novel neuroprotective and neuroregenerative targets. *Ann. Neurol.* **50:** 6–16.
68. Hamilton, G.S. *et al.* 2002. Synthesis of N-glyoxyl prolyl and pipecolyl amides and thioesters and evaluation of their *in vitro* and *in vivo* nerve regenerative effects. *J. Med. Chem.* **45:** 3549–3557.
69. Giordani, F. *et al.* 2003. Tacrolimus (FK506) reduces ischemia-induced hippocampal damage in rats: a 7- and 30-day study. *Braz. J. Med. Biol. Res.* **36:** 495–502.
70. Sharkey, J. & S.P. Butcher. 1994. Immunophilins mediate the neuroprotective effects of FK506 in focal cerebral ischaemia. *Nature* **371:** 336–339.
71. Suehiro, E. *et al.* 2001. The immunophilin ligand FK506 attenuates the axonal damage associated with rapid rewarming following posttraumatic hypothermia. *Exp. Neurol.* **172:** 199–210.
72. Rosenstiel, P. *et al.* 2003. Differential effects of immunophilin-ligands (FK506 and V-10,367) on survival and regeneration of rat retinal ganglion cells *in vitro* and after optic nerve crush *in vivo*. *J. Neurotrauma.* **20:** 297–307.
73. Campbell, G. *et al.* 1999. Spontaneous axonal regeneration after optic nerve injury in adult rat. *Neuroreport* **10:** 3955–3960.
74. Cambria, R.P. & J.S. Giglia. 1998. Prevention of spinal cord ischaemic complications after thoracoabdominal aortic surgery. *Eur. J. Vasc. Endovasc. Surg.* **15:** 96–109.
75. Meldrum, B. *et al.* 1985. Ischaemic brain damage: the role of excitatory activity and of calcium entry. *Br. J. Anaesth.* **57:** 44–46.
76. Svensson, L.G. & E.S. Crawford. 1993. Aortic dissection and aortic aneurysm surgery: clinical observations, experimental investigations, and statistical analyses. Part III. *Curr. Probl. Surg.* **30:** 1–163.
77. Reyes, O., I. Sosa & D.P. Kuffler. 2006. Neuroprotection of adult human neurons against ischemia by hypothermia and alkalinization. *P. R. Health Sci. J.* **25:** 43–50.
78. Dohare, P. *et al.* 2008. Neuroprotective efficacy and therapeutic window of curcuma oil: in rat embolic stroke model. *BMC Complement Altern. Med.* **8:** 55.
79. Dohare, P., S. Varma & M. Ray. 2008. Curcuma oil modulates the nitric oxide system response to cerebral ischemia/reperfusion injury. *Nitric Oxide* **19:** 1–11.
80. Goss, S.L. *et al.* 2007. Determination of calcium salt solubility with changes in pH and P(CO(2)), simulating varying gastrointestinal environments. *J. Pharm. Pharmacol.* **59:** 1485–1492.

Ann. N.Y. Acad. Sci. ISSN 0077-8923

ANNALS OF THE NEW YORK ACADEMY OF SCIENCES
Issue: *Neuroprotective Agents*

A combination of tumor necrosis factor-α and neuronal nitric oxide synthase antibodies applied topically over the traumatized spinal cord enhances neuroprotection and functional recovery in the rat

Hari Shanker Sharma

Laboratory of Cerebrovascular Research, Department of Surgical Sciences, Anesthesiology and Intensive Care Medicine, University Hospital, Uppsala University, Uppsala, Sweden

Address for correspondence: Hari Shanker Sharma, PhD (BHU), Dr. Med Sci (UU), Professor of Neurobiology (MRC), Docent in Neuroanatomy (UU); Frödingsgatan 12:28, SE-75421 Uppsala, Sweden. Sharma@surgsci.uu.se

The possibility that neutralization of nitric oxide synthase and tumor necrosis factor alpha (TNF-α) in the cord using their antiserum will induce neuroprotection and improve functional outcome following spinal cord injury (SCI) was examined in a rat model. The SCI was induced in rats by a unilateral incision of the right dorsal horn at the T10–11 segments under equithesin anesthesia. TNF-α and/or neuronal nitric oxide synthase (nNOS) antibodies were applied over the traumatized spinal cord at 10–90 minutes after injury and functional recovery and cord pathophysiology were examined at five hours. Topical application of TNF-α antiserum at 10 min followed by NOS antiserum at 20 min after SCI significantly improved functional recovery and attenuated blood-spinal cord barrier (BSCB) disturbances, edema formation, and cord pathology. These neuroprotective effects were also seen when the NOS antiserum was applied 10 min after injury followed by TNF-α antiserum at 30 min after trauma. However, when TNF-α antiserum was applied 1 h after injury and NOS antiserum was given either before or after TNF-α antiserum, no neuroprotective effects were observed. Interestingly, neuronal injury was tightly correlated with nNOS expression in the cord in antibody treated groups. These novel observations suggest that early blockade of TNF-α and nNOS expression within 20–30 min after SCI is beneficial in nature. This indicates that TNF-α and nitric oxide play synergistic roles in the pathophysiology of SCI and combined antibodies therapy has added neuroprotective values in spinal trauma.

Keywords: spinal cord injury; nitric oxide synthase; tumor necrosis factor alpha; functional outcome; spinal cord pathology; motor disturbances

Introduction

Spinal cord injury (SCI) is a serious clinical situation for which development of suitable therapeutic strategies has still not been worked out in detail (see Refs. 1–3). One of the main reasons for our failure to achieve neuroprotection following SCI is largely due to an inability to arrest or restrict the functions of so many neurodestructive agents that are released following trauma using one therapy in a comprehensive manner (see Refs. 1, 3, 4). Thus, the need of the hour is to find a suitable combination of neurotherapeutic agents that could neutralize the neurodestructive elements in the cord after injury in a timely fashion to achieve good neuroprotection.

Recently, nitric oxide and tumor necrosis factor alpha (TNF-α) have been suggested to play major roles in the spinal cord pathophysiology after trauma.[5–8] Thus, an upregulation of neuronal nitric oxide synthase (nNOS) is seen in experimental models of SCI within 5 h.[9] An increased production of TNF-α is also reported in SCI during the early phase of cord pathology.[10,11] Although, few studies indicate a neuroprotective role of TNF-α and NOS expression in SCI, several investigations support a

doi: 10.1111/j.1749-6632.2009.05327.x

neurodestructive role of these agents in spinal cord pathology.[1–3,12–15,24]

Previous experiments from our laboratory suggest that blockade of nNOS expression in the spinal cord within 5 min after trauma using topical application of nNOS antibodies is quite effective in reducing spinal cord cell and tissue injuries.[6–9,16,17,24] However, late application of nNOS antiserum on the traumatized spinal cord (e.g., 10 min after) was ineffective.[9,16,17] On the other hand, topical application of TNF-α given 10 min after SCI was most effective in reducing spinal cord cell and tissue damage,[17] whereas, pretreatment (10 or 30 min before) or post injury application (30 or 60 min after) of TNF-α antiserum resulted in very minimal or no effects on cord pathology (see Ref. 8). This indicates that the timing of blockade of nNOS and TNF-α are essential factors in inducing neuroprotection in SCI. Our results further show that application of TNF-α antiserum was also able to effectively reduce nNOS expression in the cord that was closely associated with attenuation in cord pathology.[18,19] This indicates that TNF-α and nitric oxide are contributing to spinal cord pathology probably through nitric oxide mediated mechanisms.

Because antibodies are most powerful agents in neutralizing their tissue antigens *in vivo*, it appears that antisera raised against specific neurodestructive elements could have potential therapeutic values in SCI (see Refs. 20–23). Thus, a possibility exists that a suitable combination of antibodies may enhance neuroprotection if administered either at different time intervals after injury or given in combination at suitable times after SCI.

Keeping these views in consideration, in this investigation we applied nNOS and TNF-α antiserum either subsequently at different time intervals after SCI or given in combination at various time periods after trauma and examined functional outcome and cord pathology in our rat model. Furthermore, expression of nNOS in the spinal cord was also investigated during the combined treatment of nNOS and TNF-α antibodies following SCI.

Materials and methods

Animals

Experiments were carried out on male Wistar rats (body weight 250–350 g) housed at a controlled ambient temperature 21 ± 1° C with 12-h light and 12-h dark schedule. Food and tap water were supplied *ad libitum* before the experiment.

All experiments were conducted according to National Institute of Health (NIH) guidelines for handling of experimental animals and approved by a local Instructional Ethics Committee.

Spinal cord injury

Under equithesin anesthesia (3 ml/kg, i.p.) one segment laminectomy was done at the T10–11 segments. Spinal cord injury (SCI) was inflicted in animals over the right dorsal horn of the T10–11 segments (1.5 mm deep and 4.5 mm long) using a sterile scalpel blade under stereotaxic guidance. The deepest part of the lesion largely remained within the Rexed's lamina VII.[25] The wound was covered with cotton soaked in saline to avoid direct contact of the spinal cord with air.

Antiserum treatment

A separate group of animals were treated with nNOS and/or TNF-α antisera using a microliter syringe as described earlier.[8] The monoclonal nNOS antiserum (1:20) and monoclonal TNF-α antiserum (1:20) diluted in phosphate buffer saline (01 M, pH 7.0) was used (see Refs. 9, 20). About 20 μl of antisera was topically applied over the traumatized spinal cord following 10 min to 90 min after injury (see detail in Table 1).

Parameters measured

The treated and untreated spinal cord traumatized rats were evaluated for functional outcome and cord pathology using standard procedures as described earlier (see Refs. 2, 26).

Functional outcome was measured using Tarlov scale and inclined plane angle tests (see below).

Tarlov scale

The Tarlov scale for hind limb function was assessed as 0 = total paraplegia; 1 = no spontaneous movement but responds to pinch; 2 = spontaneous movement; 3 = able to support weight but unable to walk; 4 = walk with gross deficits; 5 = walks with mild deficits; 6 = normal walk.[26]

Inclined plane angle test

For inclined plane angle test, the animals were placed on an inclined plane platform and the angle of the plane was adjusted as such that animals can stay

Table 1. Effects of nNOS and TNF-α antibody treatment in spinal cord injury

Experiment type	Treatment with antibodies: Spinal cord injury 0 min	10 min	20 min	30 min	60 min	90 min	Functional outcome 300 min	Results (300 min): BSCB breakdown	Edema	Cell injury/ nNOS
Control	–	–	–	–	–	–	nil	nil	nil	nil
Untreated SCI	–	–	–	–	–	–	Worsened	Increased	Present	Present
Treatment	SCI	nNOS abs	TNF-α abs				Improved	Reduced	Reduced	Reduced
	SCI	nNOS abs		TNF-α abs			Improved	Reduced	Reduced	Reduced
	SCI			nNOS abs	TNF-α abs		NE	NE	NE	NE
	SCI				TNF-α abs	nNOS abs	NE	NE	NE	NE
	SCI	TNF-α abs	nNOS abs				Improved	Reduced	Reduced	Reduced
	SCI		TNF-α abs	nNOS abs			Improved	Reduced	Reduced	Reduced
	SCI			TNF-α abs	nNOS abs		NE	NE	NE	NE
	SCI				TNF-α abs	nNOS abs	NE	NE	NE	NE
	SCI		TNF-α abs + nNOS abs				Improved	Reduced	Reduced	Reduced
	SCI			TNF-α abs + nNOS abs			NE	NE	NE	NE
	SCI				TNF-α abs + nNOS abs		NE	NE	NE	NE

SCI = spinal cord injury; nil = absent; NE = no effect as compared to untreated injured group; TNF-α = Tumor necrosis factor alpha; nNOS = neuronal nitric oxide synthase; BSCB = blood-spinal cord barrier. Monoclonal mouse TNF-α antiserum (1:20) and monoclonal nNOS antiserum (1:20) were used in this investigation. For details see text. The antibodies were applied over the traumatized spinal cord (20 μL in 10 s) at various time intervals after injury (see above). For combination therapy 20 μL of each antibody were applied subsequently over the traumatized spinal cord (for details see Sharma and Sharma, 2008).

on the platform for 5 s without falling.[2,26] Normal animals can stay 5 sec at an angle of 60° without any problem.[26] Spinal cord injured animals will not stay on the inclined plane test beyond the angle of 30° or higher.[16,17] Thus, treatment with drugs will allow animals to stay between 30° and higher plane angles depending on the magnitude and duration of the neuroprotection (see Ref. 26).

Blood-spinal cord barrier permeability

The blood-spinal cord barrier (BSCB) permeability was examined using Evans blue albumin (EBA) and radioiodine ($^{[131]}$I).[2,20–22] These tracers (EBA 2% of a 0.3 mL/100 g solution; radioiodine 10 μCi/100 g) were administered together into the right femoral vein and allowed to circulate for 5 min. The intravascular tracer was washed out with 0.9% NaCl perfusion through the heart followed by 4% buffered paraformaldehyde solution.[25,26] After perfusion, the spinal cord tissues were removed and samples from T9, T10–11, and T12 segments were dissected out and weighed and measured for radioactivity in a 3-inch well type Gamma counter (Packard, Meriden, CT). Immediately before perfusion, a sample of whole blood (about 1 mL) was withdrawn after cardiac puncture for determination of blood radioactivity. Leakage of tracers across the spinal cord was expressed as percentage increase over the blood radioactivity.[27]

After measurement of radioactivity, the cord samples were homogenized in a mixture of sodium sulphate (0.5%, pH 7.4) and acetone to extract Evans blue dye entered into the cord. After centrifugation of the homogenate (900 *g*) for 10 min, the supernatant was discarded and the dye entered into the solution was measured in a spectrophotometer (Carl Zeiss, Jena, Germany) at 620 nm. Calculation of EBA dye entered into the cord was done using standard EBA solution.[27]

Spinal cord edema

In separate groups, animals after SCI were decapitated and their spinal cord was removed immediately. The major blood clots and superficial vessels seen over the spinal cord were removed and the cord segments T9, T10–11, and T12 were dissected out.[25] These spinal cord tissues samples (sizes 65 to 85 mg) were weighed immediately and placed into an oven maintained at 90° C to obtain their dry weights. After 96 h of drying their dry weights were determined. The water content was calculated from the differences between dry and wet weights of the samples as described earlier.[25]

Spinal cord pathology

Spinal cord neuronal damage and expression of nNOS were examined using morphological approaches employing standard histopathological and immunohistochemical techniques.[9,16] For this purpose, after the experiments animals were perfused *in situ* with 4% buffered paraformaldehyde and the spinal cord was dissected out. The spinal cord samples were placed in the same fixative for 1 week at 4° C.[8,9] Some tissue pieces from T9 and T12 were processed for paraffin embedding and some tissue sections were cut (40 μm thick) from these segments using Vibratome (Oxford Instruments, Oxford, United Kingdom). For paraffin embedded materials, about 3 μm thick sections were cut and processed for Nissl and Haematoxylin and Eosin staining using histological techniques. A few paraffin sections from the identical segments were processed for nNOS immunostaining using monoclonal nNOS antibodies (supplied by Professor Per Alm of Lund University as gift) in dilutions of 1:500 as described earlier.[9] The immunostaining was finally developed using peroxidase and antiperoxidase reaction. The free floating Vibratome sections were also processed for nNOS immunostaining using the same antibodies and identical technical procedures (see Refs. 8, 9, 16, 28).

Statistical analyses

Quantitative data obtained from this study were analyzed for statistical significance using ANOVA followed by Dunnet's test for multiple group comparison. Semiquantitative data obtained from morphological analyses were evaluated for statistical significance using Chi Square test. A P-value less than 0.05 was considered significant.

Results

Pathophysiology of spinal cord injury

A focal incision of the right dorsal horn results in massive pathological changes in the cord associated with prominent functional disability at 5 h (see Tables 1 and 2). Thus, functional outcome in terms of hind limb function and inclined plane angle test were deteriorated in these animals (Tables 1 and 2). Marked increase in the BSCB permeability to EBA and radioiodine was seen at 5 h in the spinal cord traumatized animals (Tables 1 and 2). At this time profound edema development occurred in these cord segments (Table 2). In general, the pathological changes were most marked in caudal segments (T12) as compared to the rostral cord (T9).

Histopathological studies revealed marked neuronal damage, sponginess and edema in the spinal cord (Table 2). Profound upregulation of nNOS expression was also seen in these spinal cord segments (Fig. 1; Table 2). These cellular changes and nNOS expression were most prominent in the T12 segment as compared to the T9 segment of the cord (Table 2).

Effect of neuronal nitric oxide synthase or tumor necrosis factor alpha antiserum applied alone on spinal cord pathology

Topical application of nNOS antiserum (1:20) alone either 5 min before of 5 min after SCI markedly attenuated spinal cord edema formation, cell injury and upregulation of nNOS expression (Fig. 1). Whereas, topical application of TNF-α antiserum (1:20) alone at 10 min after SCI resulted in the most marked neuroprotection that was also associated with a significant reduction in nNOS expression in the spinal cord segments (Fig. 1). However, pretreatment with TNF-α antiserum, for example, 30 min before or after SCI, was not that effective in reducing cord pathology or nNOS expression in the spinal cord (Fig. 1).

Effect of nNOS and TNF-α antiserum applied at different time intervals on spinal cord pathology

When nNOS antiserum was applied over the traumatized spinal cord and followed by TNF-α antiserum or vice versa at different time intervals after injury, neuroprotection was achieved only during early phases of these antisera applications

Table 2. Effects of nNOS and TNF-α antibodies treatment on functional outcome and pathophysiology of spinal cord injury

Type of experiment	Parameters measured (5 h): Functional Outcome: Tarlov Scale Score	Functional Outcome: Inclined plane test (°)	BSCB permeability: Evans blue mg %: T9	Evans blue mg %: T12	BSCB permeability: [131]Iodine %: T9	[131]Iodine %: T12	Edema formation: Water content %: T9	Water content %: T12	Cell injury: Neuronal injury (nr): T9	Neuronal injury (nr): T12	nNOS+ cells (nr): T9	nNOS+ cells (nr): T12
Control $n = 6$												
	6	60	0.21 ± 0.08	0.23 ± 0.05	0.26 ± 0.04	0.28 ± 0.03	65.34 ± 0.12	66.04 ± 0.08	0	0	1 ± 2	1 ± 1
Untreated SCI $n = 8$							**Neurodestructive**					
	3 ± 1*	33 ± 4*	1.35 ± 0.10**	1.98 ± 0.23**	2.07 ± 0.22**	2.38 ± 0.17**	67.78 ± 0.34**	68.15 ± 0.23**	25 ± 8**	32 ± 6**	18 ± 6**	24 ± 4**
Antibodies Treatment after SCI												
nNOS 10 min+TNF-α 20 min $n = 6$							**Neuroprotective**					
	4 ± 1*a	42 ± 4*a	0.56 ± 0.14**a	0.67 ± 0.21**a	0.76 ± 0.10**a	0.89 ± 0.24**a	66.03 ± 0.34*a	66.89 ± 0.41**a	12 ± 3*a	18 ± 4*a	8 ± 4*a	10 ± 3*a
nNOS 10 min+TNF-α 30 min $n = 5$							**Neuroprotective**					
	4 ± 2*a	40 ± 2*a	0.64 ± 0.08**a	0.73 ± 0.08*a	0.81 ± 0.10*a	0.94 ± 0.12*a	66.56 ± 0.10*a	67.15 ± 0.16*a	18 ± 6*a	22 ± 5*a	12 ± 4*a	14 ± 5*a
nNOS 30 min+TNF-α 60 min $n = 8$							**No protective effects**					
	3 ± 1	35 ± 4	1.30 ± 0.32	1.78 ± 0.34	1.98 ± 0.44	2.08 ± 0.56	66.98 ± 1.04	67.56 ± 0.67	23 ± 8	30 ± 7	18 ± 8	22≈9
TNF-α 60 min+nNOS 90 min $n = 6$							**No protective effects**					
	2 ± 1	30 ± 3	1.45 ± 0.21	1.89 ± 0.43	2.12 ± 0.12	2.44 ± 0.33	67.34 ± 0.21	67.88 ± 0.51	24 ± 6	28 ± 8	20 ± 6	22 ± 8
TNF-α 10 min+nNOS 20 min $n = 8$							**Neuroprotection**					
	4 ± 1*a	45 ± 4**a	0.48 ± 0.08**a	0.56 ± 0.06**a	0.64 ± 0.12**a	0.68 ± 0.10**a	66.04 ± 0.11*a	66.23 ± 0.23**a	9 ± 2*a	10 ± 5*a	6 ± 3*a	8 ± 4*a
TNF-α 20 min+nNOS 30 min $n = 6$							**Neuroprotection**					
	4 ± 2*a	43 ± 6*a	0.58 ± 0.21*a	0.67 ± 0.21*a	0.70 ± 0.10*a	0.74 ± 0.11*a	66.37 ± 0.13*a	66.89 ± 0.21*a	10 ± 2*a	14 ± 3*a	9 ± 2*a	12 ± 4*a
TNF-α 30 min+nNOS 60 min $n = 6$							**Neuroprotective?**					
	3 ± 1	38 ± 5	0.96 ± 0.12a	0.98 ± 23a	1.23 ± 0.12a	1.43 ± 0.22a	66.56 ± 0.21a	66.88 ± 0.21a	15 ± 5a	20 ± 4a	10 ± 6a	14 ± 4a
TNF-α 60 min+nNOS 90 min $n = 6$							**No protective effects**					
	3 ± 1	30 ± 5	1.45 ± 0.23	1.65 ± 0.12	2.05 ± 0.32	2.34 ± 0.21	68.04 ± 0.21	68.23 ± 0.28	20 ± 6	25 ± 5	16 ± 6	22 ± 6
TNF-α+nNOS 20 min $n = 5$							**Neuroprotective**					
	4 ± 1*a	42 ± 3*a	0.54 ± 0.10*a	0.67 ± 0.21*a	0.74 ± 0.11*a	0.81 ± 0.22*a	66.56 ± 0.23*a	66.94 ± 0.18*a	10 ± 6*a	15 ± 4*a	16 ± 5*a	18 ± 4*a
TNF-α+nNOS 30 min $n = 6$							**Neuroprotective?**					
	3 ± 2	30 ± 4	0.95 ± 0.10	1.24 ± 0.21	1.89 ± 0.23	2.13 ± 0.18	66.89 ± 0.32	67.34 ± 0.23	22 ± 6	28 ± 4	20 ± 6	22 ± 5
TNF-α+nNOS 60 min $n = 6$							**No protective effects**					
	2 ± 2	30 ± 5	1.58 ± 0.12	1.89 ± 0.21	2.34 ± 0.21a	2.67 ± 0.21a	68.03 ± 0.21	68.34 ± 0.28	24 ± 6	26 ± 7	18 ± 8	22 ± 6

* = $P < 0.05$, ** $P < 0.01$, compared from control; a = $P < 0.05$, compared from SCI; ANOVA followed by Dunnet's test (for all quantitative data); Chi-square test (for morphology data). SCI = spinal cord injury; TNF-α = Tumor necrosis factor alpha, nNOS = neuronal nitric oxide synthase. Monoclonal mouse TNF-α antiserum (1:20) and monoclonal nNOS antiserum (1:20) were used in this investigation. For details see text. The antibodies were applied over the traumatized spinal cord (20 μL in 10 s) at various time intervals after injury (see above). For combination therapy 20 μL of each antibody were applied subsequently over the traumatized spinal cord (for details see Sharma and Sharma, 2008).

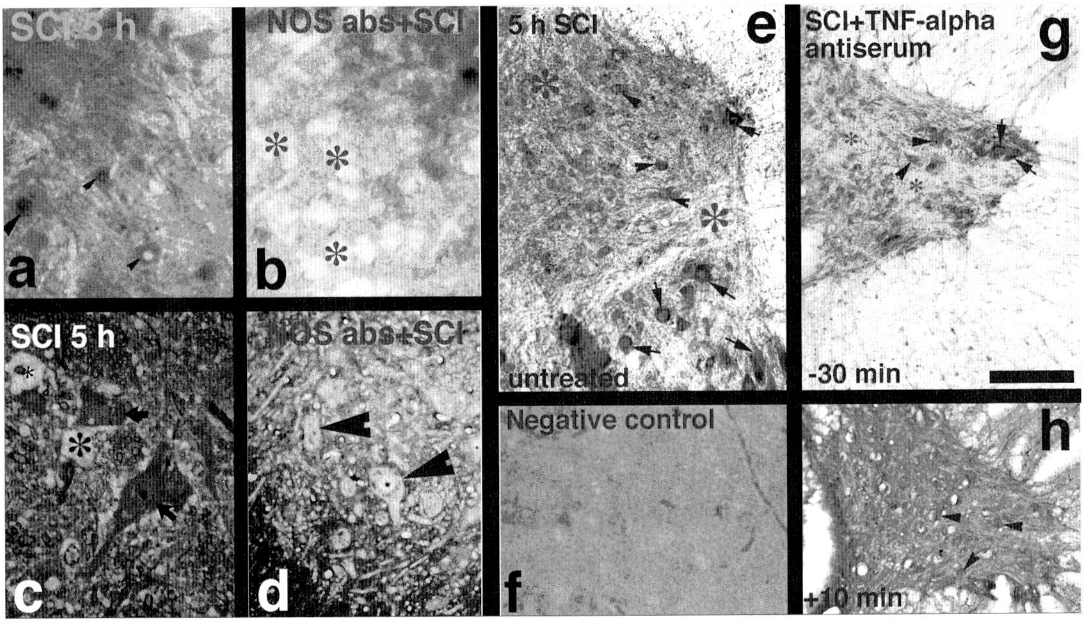

Figure 1. Upregulation of neuronal nitric oxide synthase (nNOS) expression (**a,e**) and cell injury (**c**) after spinal cord injury and their modification with nNOS antiserum (**b,d**) or tumor necrosis factor alpha (TNF-**α**) antiserum (**g,h**) treatment. nNOS antiserum markedly attenuated nNOS expression and cell injury in the cord at 5 h if applied 5 min after injury (**b,d**). On the other hand, TNF-**α** antiserum was most effective in attenuating nNOS expression and edema when given 10 min after (**h**) but not 30 min (**g**) before spinal cord injury. **f** = negative control for nNOS expression on Vibratome sections (see Refs. 8, 9). Bar: 25 **μ**m.

(Tables 1 and 2). Thus application of nNOS antiserum at 10 min followed by TNF-α antiserum either at 20 min or 30 min after injury resulted in a marked improvement in functional outcome and significant reduction in spinal cord pathology, for example, BSCB breakdown, edema formation and cell injury at 5 h (Table 2). However, nNOS antisera applied 30 min after SCI followed by TNF-α antiserum applied 60 min after SCI did not result in any neuroprotection or improvement in functional outcome in these animals (Tables 1 and 2). Likewise, application of TNF-α antiserum at 60 min followed by nNOS antiserum 90 min after injury also did not influence the functional outcome or spinal cord pathology (Tables 1 and 2).

Interestingly, when TNF-α antiserum was given first at 10 or 20 min followed by nNOS antiserum treatments at 20 or 30 min after injury, respectively, significant improvements in functional outcome and marked reduction in spinal cord pathophysiology were observed (Tables 1 and 2). However, application of TNF-α antiserum at 30 min or 60 min followed by nNOS antiserum given at 60 min or 90 min after SCI respectively did not induce any neuroprotection or improved functional outcome following injury (Tables 1 and 2).

In these animals, a close parallelism was observed between neuronal damage and nNOS expression in the spinal cord. Thus, when nNOS or TNF-α given at different time intervals after injury was able to attenuate cord pathology. These treatments also reduced neuronal injury and nNOS expression in the cord (Table 2).

Effect of nNOS and TNF-α antiserum applied in combination on spinal cord pathology

A combination of TNF-α antiserum with nNOS antiserum when applied over the traumatized cord was also able to attenuate cord pathology and improved functional outcome, if given 20 min after SCI (Tables 1 and 2). However, this effect was not seen when these antisera in combination were given at 30 or 60 min after injury (Tables 1 and 2). In these animals, a reduction in neuronal injury and nNOS expression was evident when nNOS and TNF-α antisera were applied in combination 20 min after SCI.

However, this effect was not seen when the antibodies in combination were given at 30 or 60 min after trauma.

Correlation between nNOS expression and neuronal injury

It appears that nNOS has a very tight correlation with neuronal injury in this SCI model (see Fig. 2). Thus a reduction in nNOS expression was always associated with pronounced neuroprotection in the spinal cord (Table 2). A close correlation was obtained between neuronal injury and nNOS expression in the spinal cord following application of TNF-α and/or nNOS antiserum at various time intervals after injury, either alone or in combination (see Fig. 2). Interestingly, this correlation between nNOS and neuronal damage appears to be tighter in the rostral T9 segment as compared to the caudal T12 segment of the injured cord (Fig. 2).

Discussion

The salient new finding of this study is that antibodies to neurodestructive elements, for example, nNOS and TNF-α, when applied over the traumatized spinal cord within 30 min following injury are capable of inducing profound neuroprotection in the cord. This effect was not seen when these antibodies were applied within 30 min after SCI. This indicates that early production of nitric oxide and TNF-α in the cord following trauma are involved in the pathophysiology of SCI. Thus, neutralization of these neurodestructive factors using their antisera could be one of the important tools to achieve neuroprotection in the cord following trauma (see Ref. 20).

In this investigation, our observations are limited to 5 h duration after SCI. Thus, it is unclear from this investigation whether these nNOS and TNF-α antisera are only able to delay the development of cord pathology or could also be able to induce sustained long-term neuroprotection. However, our findings have potential clinical applications for SCI in humans. Thus, it is quite possible to treat human cases of SCI with these antisera locally at the site of accidents while transporting victims to the specialized clinics of advanced healthcare centers. A delay of a few hours in development of spinal cord pathology in human cases using these antisera may tremendously improve the functional outcome and dramatically enhance the quality of patient care as early destruction of the cord cells and tissues following SCI are crucial for long-term disability.[16,17]

Our observations further show that a suitable combination of these antibodies markedly improved the functional outcome in rats. These results suggest that neuroprotection in the cord induced by the combination of nNOS and TNF-α antibodies are also capable in improving the

Regression Coefficients
T9 Cell injury vs. T9 NOS+cells

	Coefficient	Std. Error	Std. Coeff.	t-Value	P-Value
Intercept	3,683	1,575	3,683	2,338	,0248
T9 NOS+cells	1,064	,107	,849	9,919	<,0001

Regression Coefficients
T12 cell injury vs. T12 NOS+ cells

	Coefficient	Std. Error	Std. Coeff.	t-Value	P-Value
Intercept	4,583	2,129	4,583	2,153	,0378
T12 NOS+ cells	1,010	,115	,818	8,770	<,0001

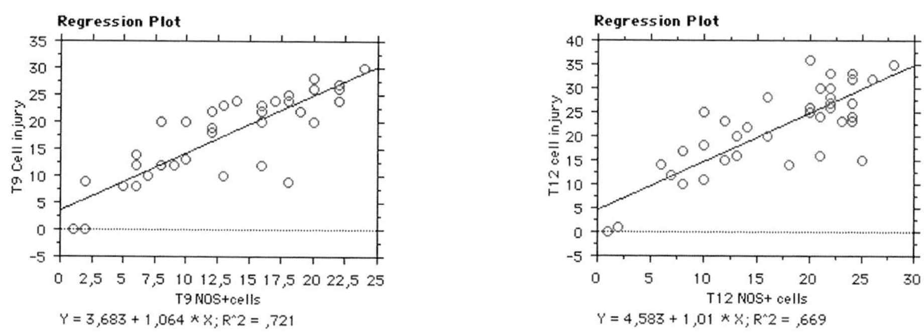

Figure 2. Correlation between neuronal injury and neuronal nitric oxide synthase (nNOS) expression in the T9 and T12 segment of the cord after spinal cord injury and their modification with nNOS and tumor necrosis factor alpha (TNF-α) antiserum treatments. A close correlation between nNOS expression and neuronal damage is seen that was most tight in the rostral spinal cord segment (T9) compared to caudal segment (T12).

functional outcome following SCI. This observation is in line with the idea that a reduction in cord pathology is instrumental in functional improvement in SCI.[26] Thus, an early treatment with antisera of nNOS and TNF-α in human cases may not only delay spinal cord pathology but will also improve functional outcome of the victims. However, this is a subject that requires additional investigations.

We observed that late application of these antisera, that is, 30 min and beyond injury, did not improve the functional outcome or the spinal cord pathology. This indicates that neutralization of nNOS and TNF-α during early phases of SCI is crucial in inducing neuroprotection. It is quite likely that after the first 30 min of SCI these neurodestructive elements may be able to induce a cascade of events leading to the release of several other neurodestructive factors that could play important roles in sustaining spinal cord cell and further tissue injury.[1,16,17,20,26] Thus neutralization of nNOS and TNF-α in the spinal cord after 30 min or more after injury remains ineffective.

Interestingly, there were no appreciable differences in neuroprotection observed in SCI when NOS antisera were applied first followed by TNF-α or vice versa in this investigation. This suggests that nitric oxide and TNF-α could contribute to cord pathology in synergy.[16] Alternatively, TNF-α induced cord pathology is mediated through increased nitric oxide production.[8,9] Blockade of nNOS expression by application of TNF-α antiserum in SCI is in line with this idea see (Refs. 8, 17).

We observed a close correlation between nNOS expression and cell injury in the spinal cord following treatment with nNOS and TNF-α antibodies. Thus, antibodies to nNOS and TNF-α when applied either subsequently or in combination within 30 min of insult are capable of significantly reducing nNOS expression. However, later application of these antibodies did not attenuate effectively the number of nNOS positive neurons in the spinal cord (see Fig. 2). This suggests that overproduction of nitric oxide from activated nNOS neurons is instrumental in spinal cord cell and tissue injuries.[16,18,20–23]

Overproduction of nitric oxide (NO) contributes to neurotoxicity through the generation of oxidant compounds, such as peroxynitrite and superoxide anion.[29–31] Thus the NO generated from activated NOS will react with the superoxide anion to produce the potent oxidant, peroxynitrite (ONOO-).[32,33] Peroxynitrite could then inhibit DNA synthesis, liberate iron from the iron storage protein ferritin, and influence iron metabolism at the post-transcription level (see Refs. 29–31). Damage to DNA by NO and ONOO- induced activation of the nuclear enzyme poly (ADP ribose) synthetase (PARS) is also quite likely.[34–36] Activation of PARS causes cell death by rapid depletion of cell energy.[37]

It is quite likely that overproduction of NO will induce endothelial cell membrane damage directly and thus cause BSCB disruption (see Refs. 9, 16, 17). Alternatively, the NO will bind to the heme-iron protein in guanylyl cyclase to elicit cGMP.[34–36,38,39] An increased cGMP or cAMP formation within the endothelial cells contributes to microvascular permeability changes (see Ref. 16).

Breakdown of the BSCB to proteins or large molecules will also allow many other serum factors or vasoactive compounds to enter into the spinal cord microenvironment.[1–3,16,17] Profound alterations in the extracellular fluid microenvironment and the cellular compartments in the cord by altered ionic, chemical, immunological, and metabolic balances will then contribute to vasogenic edema formation leading to spinal cord cell and tissue injuries.[3,5–8,10,17,19,20] These macro- and micromolecular events lead to profound cellular stress resulting in abnormal expression of several proteins and enzymes including free radicals and activation of NOS.[34–36,38,39] Reduction in nNOS expression by TNF-α and nNOS antibodies in this investigation associated with neuroprotection in the cord further supports this hypothesis.[8,9]

The precise mechanism by which TNF-α antiserum attenuates nNOS activation is unclear from this investigation. It appears that various neurodestructive elements that are upregulated in SCI may damage cell and tissues through mechanisms involving NOS expression.[10–14] Previously, Lee *et al.*[40] showed that SCI is able to induce an upregulation of TNF-α 1 h after trauma. In these experiments, an increased level of NO is detected at 4 h after SCI. Administration of TNF-α antiserum into the center of the crushed spinal cords several minutes after lesion resulted in attenuation of NO level in the spinal cord. This treatment also reduced the number of cells undergoing apoptotic death 24 h after injury.[40] Thus, our results further show that endogenous TNF-α could be one of the important neurodestructive factors for SCI induced NOS upregulation (see Ref. 8). Obviously, topical application of TNF-α antiserum is able to neutralize endogenous TNF-α, which results in a marked downregulation of NOS expression as well as cell and tissue injuries in the cord (see Ref. 20).

The ability of nNOS antiserum to neutralize NOS expression suggests that topical application of antibodies are able to penetrate spinal cord tissues rapidly and could bind to *in vivo* tissue antigens.[8,16] As a result, increased nNOS activity could not be detected in the injured spinal cord after nNOS antiserum application. Blockade of nNOS expression by nNOS antiserum thus resulted in marked neuroprotection. Failure of nNOS antibodies to reduce nNOS expression in the cord when applied 30 min after injury indicates that the antiserum was not able to neutralize already activated nNOS before antiserum application (see Ref. 20). Thus, no neuroprotection was seen in animals by either TNF-α or nNOS antibodies when they were applied during the later periods of SCI.

Conclusion

In conclusion, our results show that both TNF-α and nitric oxide are potential neurodestructive agents in the spinal cord following injury. Both these neurodestructive elements are working together in inducing cell and tissue injuries in the cord through nitric oxide mediated mechanisms. Suitable neutralization of these harmful agents by a combination of antibodies enhanced the neuroprotection and functional recovery. Taken together our observations are the first to demonstrate that a combination of TNF-α and nNOS antibodies have profound neuroprotective effects in SCI when applied within 30 min after trauma. This suggests the possible therapeutic potential of these antibodies in combination for the treatment of human cases of SCI in clinical situations.

Acknowledgments

This investigation is supported by grants from Swedish Medical Research Council Nrs. 2710 (HSS); 11205 (HSS); Astra-Zeneca, Mölndal, Sweden, Acure Pharma, Uppsala, Sweden; Alexander Humboldt Foundation, Bonn, Germany; The University Grants Commission, New Delhi, India and The Indian Council of Medical Research, New Delhi, India. The skillful technical assistance of Kärstin Flink and Kerstin Rystedt and the secretarial assistance of Aruna Sharma is acknowledged with thanks.

Conflicts of interest

The author has no conflict of interest with any granting agencies mentioned above.

References

1. Sharma, H.S. 2008. New perspectives for the treatment options in spinal cord injury. *Expert Opin. Pharmacother.* **9:** 2773–800. Review.
2. Sharma, H.S. 2007. A select combination of neurotrophins enhances neuroprotection and functional recovery following spinal cord injury. *Ann. N.Y. Acad. Sci.* **1122:** 95–111.
3. Stålberg, E., H.S. Sharma & Y. Olsson. 1998. *Spinal Cord Monitoring. Basic Principles, Regeneration, Pathophysiology and Clinical Aspects.* 1–527. Springer. Wien, New York.
4. Sharma, H.S. 2009. Blood–central nervous system barriers: the gateway to neurodegeneration, neuroprotection and neuroregeneration. In *Handbook of Neurochemistry and Molecular Neurobiology*. A. Lajtha, N. Banik & S.K. Ray, Eds.: 363–457. Springer, U.S. 10.1007/978-0-387-30375-8.
5. Sharma, H.S., F. Nyberg, T. Gordh, *et al.* 2006. Topical application of dynorphin A (1–17) antibodies attenuates neuronal nitric oxide synthase up-regulation, edema formation, and cell injury following focal trauma to the rat spinal cord. *Acta. Neurochir. Suppl.* **96:** 309–315.
6. Sharma, H.S., L. Wiklund, R.D. Badgaiyan, *et al.* 2006. Intracerebral administration of neuronal nitric oxide synthase antiserum attenuates traumatic brain injury-induced blood-brain barrier permeability, brain edema formation, and sensory motor disturbances in the rat. *Acta. Neurochir. Suppl.* **96:** 288–294.
7. Sharma, H.S., R.D. Badgaiyan, P. Alm, *et al.* 2005. Neuroprotective effects of nitric oxide synthase inhibitors in spinal cord injury-induced pathophysiology and motor functions: an experimental study in the rat. *Ann. N.Y. Acad. Sci.* **1053:** 422–434.
8. Sharma, H.S., T. Winkler, E. Stålberg, *et al.* 2003. Topical application of TNF-alpha antiserum attenuates spinal cord trauma induced edema formation, microvascular

permeability disturbances and cell injury in the rat. *Acta. Neurochir. Suppl.* **86:** 407–413.

9. Sharma, H.S., J. Westman, Y. Olsson & P. Alm. 1996. Involvement of nitric oxide in acute spinal cord injury: an immunocytochemical study using light and electron microscopy in the rat. *Neurosci. Res.* **24:** 373–384.
10. Pan, W. & A.J. Kastin. 2008. Cytokine transport across the injured blood-spinal cord barrier. *Curr. Pharm. Des.* **14:** 1620–1624. Review.
11. Pan, W., L. Zhang, J. Liao, *et al.* 2003. Selective increase in TNF alpha permeation across the blood-spinal cord barrier after SCI. *J. Neuroimmunol.* **134:** 111–117.
12. Bethea, J.R. & W.D. Dietrich. 2002. Targeting the host inflammatory response in traumatic spinal cord injury. *Curr. Opin. Neurol.* **15:** 355–360. Review.
13. González Deniselle, M.C., S.L. González & A.F. De Nicola. 2001. Cellular basis of steroid neuroprotection in the wobbler mouse, a genetic model of motoneuron disease. *Cell Mol. Neurobiol.* **21:** 237–254. Review.
14. Bethea, J.R., H. Nagashima, M.C. Acosta, *et al.* 1999. Systemically administered interleukin-10 reduces tumor necrosis factor-alpha production and significantly improves functional recovery following traumatic spinal cord injury in rats. *J. Neurotrauma.* **16:** 851–863.
15. Dolga, A.M., I. Granic, T. Blank, *et al.* 2008. TNF-alpha-mediates neuroprotection against glutamate-induced excitotoxicity via NF-kappaB-dependent up-regulation of K2.2 channels. *J. Neurochem.***107:** 1158–1167.
16. Sharma, H.S. & P. Alm. 2004. Role of nitric oxide on the blood-brain and the spinal cord barriers. In *The Blood-Spinal Cord and Brain Barriers in Health and Disease.* H.S. Sharma & J. Westman, Eds.: 191–230. Elsevier Academic Press. San Diego.
17. Sharma, H.S. 2004. Pathophysiology of the blood-spinal cord barrier in traumatic injury. In *The Blood-Spinal Cord and Brain Barriers in Health and Disease.* H.S. Sharma & J. Westman, Eds.: 437–518. Elsevier Academic Press. San Diego.
18. Sharma, H.S. 2007. Neurotrophic factors in combination: a possible new therapeutic strategy to influence pathophysiology of spinal cord injury and repair mechanisms. *Curr. Pharm. Des.* **13:** 1841–1874. Review.
19. Sharma, H.S. 2005. Pathophysiology of blood-spinal cord barrier in traumatic injury and repair. *Curr. Pharm. Des.* **11:** 1353–1389. Review.
20. Sharma, H.S. & A. Sharma. 2008. Antibodies as promising novel neuroprotective agents in the central nervous system injuries. *Central Nervous System Agents in Medicinal Chemistry.* **8:** 143–169. Review. DOI: 10.2174/187152408785699640.
21. Sharma, H.S., F. Nyberg, T. Gordh, *et al.* 2006. Topical application of dynorphin A (1–17) antibodies attenuates neuronal nitric oxide synthase up-regulation, edema formation, and cell injury following focal trauma to the rat spinal cord. *Acta. Neurochir. Suppl.* **96:** 309–315.
22. Winkler, T., H.S. Sharma, T. Gordh, *et al.* 2002. Topical application of dynorphin A (1–17) antiserum attenuates trauma induced alterations in spinal cord evoked potentials, microvascular permeability disturbances, edema formation and cell injury: an experimental study in the rat using electrophysiological and morphological approaches. *Amino Acids* **23:** 273–281.
23. Sharma, H.S., J. Westman & F. Nyberg. 1997. Topical application of 5-HT antibodies reduces edema and cell changes following trauma of the rat spinal cord. *Acta. Neurochir. Suppl.* **70:** 155–158.
24. Sharma, H.S., Y. Olsson & F. Nyberg. 1995. Influence of dynorphin A antibodies on the formation of edema and cell changes in spinal cord trauma. *Prog. Brain Res.* **104:** 401–416. Review.
25. Sharma, H.S. & Y. Olsson. 1990. Edema formation and cellular alterations following spinal cord injury in the rat and their modification with p-chlorophenylalanine. *Acta. Neuropathol.* **79:** 604–610.
26. Sharma, H.S., S.F. Ali, W. Dong, *et al.* 2007. Drug delivery to the spinal cord tagged with nanowire enhances neuroprotective efficacy and functional recovery following trauma to the rat spinal cord. *Ann. N.Y. Acad. Sci.* **1122:** 197–218.
27. Sharma, H.S. & P.K. Dey. 1986. Influence of long-term immobilization stress on regional blood-brain barrier permeability, cerebral blood flow and 5-HT level in conscious normotensive young rats. *J. Neurol. Sci.* **72:** 61–76.
28. Sharma, H.S. & E.A. Kiyatkin. 2009. Rapid morphological brain abnormalities during acute methamphetamine intoxication in the rat: an experimental study using light and electron microscopy. *J. Chem. Neuroanat.* **37:** 18–32.
29. Oury, T.D., Y.-S. Ho, C.A. Piantadosi, *et al.* 1992. Extracellular superoxide dismutase, nitric oxide and central nervous system O2 toxicity. *Proc. Natl. Acad. Sci. USA* **89:** 9715–9719.
30. Lipton, S.A., D.J. Singel & J.S. Stamler. 1994. Neuroprotective and neurodestructive effects of nitric oxide and redox congeners. *Ann. N.Y. Acad. Sci.* **738:** 382–387.
31. Stamler, J.S. 1994. Redox signalling: nitrosylation and related target interactions of nitric oxide. *Cell* **78:** 931–936.
32. Radi, R., J.S. Beckman, K.M. Bush, *et al.* 1991. Peroxynitrite oxidation of sulfhydryls. The cytotoxic potential of

superoxide and nitric oxide. *J. Biol. Chem.* **266:** 4244–4250.

33. Koppenol, W.H., J.J. Moreno, W.A. Pryor, *et al.* 1992. Peroxynitrite, a cloaked oxidant formed by nitric oxide and superoxide. *Chem. Res. Toxicol.* **5:** 834–842.
34. Lautier, D., J. Lagueux, J. Thibodeau, *et al.* 1993. Molecular and biochemical features of poly (ADP-ribose) metabolism. *Mol. Cell Biochem.* **122:** 171–193.
35. Beckman, J.S. 1994. The double-edged role of nitric oxide in brain function and superoxide-mediated injury. *J. Dev. Physiol.* **15:** 53–59.
36. Bolanos, J.P., S.J.R. Heales, J.M. Land, *et al.* 1995. Effect of peroxynitrite on the mitochondrial respiratory chain: differential susceptibility of neurones and astrocytes in primary culture. *J. Neurochem.* **64:** 1965–1972.
37. Zhang, Z.G., M. Chopp, S. Gautam, *et al.* 1994. Upregulation of neuronal nitric oxide synthase and mRNA, and selective sparing of nitric oxide synthase-containing neurons after focal cerebral ischemia in rat. *Brain Res.* **654:** 85–95.
38. Kubes, P. & D.N. Granger. 1992. Nitric oxide modulates microvascular permeability. *Am. J. Physiol.* **262:** H611–H615.
39. Ochoa, L.F., J.M.B. Pinheiro, A. Siflinger-Birnboim, *et al.* 1993. Effects of nitric oxide (NO) on endothelial barrier function. *FASEB J.* **7:** A770.
40. Lee, Y.B., T.Y. Yune, S.Y. Baik, *et al.* 2000. Role of tumor necrosis factor-alpha in neuronal and glial apoptosis after spinal cord injury. *Exp. Neurol.* **166:** 190–195.

Ann. N.Y. Acad. Sci. ISSN 0077-8923

ANNALS OF THE NEW YORK ACADEMY OF SCIENCES
Issue: *Neuroprotective Agents*

Effects of histone deacetylase inhibitor Trichostatin A on epigenetic changes and transcriptional activation of *Bdnf* promoter 1 by rat hippocampal neurons

Feng Tian,[1] Ann M. Marini,[2] and Robert H. Lipsky[3]

[1]Section on Cancer Genetics, Genetics Branch, National Cancer Institute, NIH, Bethesda, Maryland. [2]Department of Neurology and Program in Neuroscience, Uniformed Services University of the Health Sciences, Bethesda, Maryland. [3]Department of Neurosciences, Inova Health System, Inova Fairfax Hospital, Falls Church, Virginia

Address for correspondence: Robert H. Lipsky, 3300 Gallows Road, Falls Church, VA 22042. robert.lipsky@inova.org

Histone acetylation/deacetylation is a central mechanism for regulating transcription through chromatin remodeling. The brain-derived neurotrophic factor gene (*Bdnf*) is regulated in part through chromatin remodeling. An inhibitor of histone deacetylase (HDAC) activity, Trichostatin A (TSA), has differential effects on two activation dependent regions of the *Bdnf* gene physically linked to transcription sites for exons 1 and 4. We determined that TSA treatment of cultures of hippocampal neurons produced a stronger response at promoter 1. Transcriptional activation of promoter 1 correlated with increased occupancy of the promoter by acetylated histones (H3AcK9/K14). TSA treatment also produced a time-dependent increase in the level of H3AcK9 and H3AcK14 protein and *Hdac1* mRNA levels and HDAC1 protein levels. Taken together, these findings suggest that inhibition of HDAC activity by TSA activates *Bdnf* transcription and a compensatory change in HDAC1 expression in neurons. This response may reflect a genome-wide change in gene expression.

Keywords: brain-derived neurotrophic factor; chromatin remodeling; epigenetic modification; histone; HDAC; TSA

Introduction

Modifications in chromatin structure, a process termed chromatin remodeling, are critical determinants of gene expression. This process involves numerous types of posttranslational modifications on amino-terminal "core" histone tails that comprise the nucleosome. These modifications include acetylation, methylation, phosphorylation, ubiquitinylation, and ADP-ribosylation, all of which alter DNA-histone interactions.

The acetylation state of histones is a general mechanism for regulating chromatin and is associated with transcriptional activation. Transcriptional activation involves not only the recruitment of transcription factors and RNA polymerase, but also the removal of repressor proteins, among them, histone deacetylases (HDACs). Deacetylation is linked with silencing of transcription by chromatin condensation.[1,2] These processes offer targets for altering both short-term and long-acting forms of transcriptional activity. HDAC inhibitors, such as valproic acid and Trichostatin A (TSA), have been used in a variety of experimental conditions to alter gene expression,[3–5] producing changes in phenotype at the molecular, cellular, and behavioral levels.[6,7]

One gene whose expression is critical to long-acting changes in brain function as well as response to injury is brain-derived neurotrophic factor (BDNF). Among its primary functions, BDNF modulates the strength of existing synaptic connections and acts in the formation of new synaptic contacts.[8–11] While transcriptional regulation of the *Bdnf* gene (rodent nomenclature, which will be used thereafter) has been extensively studied over the past decade, much remains to be understood in how separate signal transduction events converge on a complex array of regulatory sequences that determine transcriptional strength. This complexity is underscored by the structural organization of

doi: 10.1111/j.1749-6632.2009.05175.x

the *Bdnf* gene, which occupies more than 70 kb of the human genome and is composed of ten 5′ exons that are differentially spliced to a single 3′ terminal exon. The *Bdnf* gene is transcribed from unique promoters whose pre-mRNAs undergo alternative splicing. This complex transcriptional regulation gives rise to at least three pre-pro-BDNF isoforms in humans,[12–14] whose functions are just beginning to be understood.[15] The overall structural organization of *Bdnf* is highly conserved in mammals. In rat and mouse, eight exons with separate promoters have been characterized.[16]

Activation of *Bdnf* transcription involves changes in chromatin structure through changes in DNA methylation and posttranslational histone modification.[17–20] Here, we sought to characterize changes in histone-associated processes at promoter 1 of the *Bdnf* gene when rat hippocampal neurons maintained in culture are treated with TSA.

Materials and methods

Preparation of hippocampal neurons

Hippocampal cultures were prepared from embryonic day 19 (E19) Sprague–Dawley embryos essentially as described previously.[21–23] The hippocampi were dissected and placed into ice-cold Hank's solution with 1 mmol/L HEPES and 1 μL/mL penicillin-streptomycin (10,000 units penicillin and 10,000 μg/mL streptomycin). The tissue was then incubated with 1.25% trypsin (Invitrogen, Carlsbad, CA) in 10 mL Hank's solution and incubated at 37° C for 15 min and then rinsed with 10 mL Hank's solution. Soybean trypsin inhibitor (2 mg/mL) in 10 mL Hank's solution was then added and the mixture incubated at 37° C for 5 min. The cell preparation was then washed with 10 mL of minimum essential medium (MEM, Invitrogen) containing: 10 mmol/L sodium bicarbonate, 1 mmol/L pyruvate (pyruvic acid, sodium salt), 20 mmol/L potassium chloride, 1 mmol/L HEPES plus 10% fetal bovine serum, and 2 mmol/L L-glutamine, pH 7.2. The cell suspension was then diluted with MEM to achieve a seeding density of 2.5×10^5–5.0×10^5 cells/mL and distributed into 10 cm dishes or 6 well plates that were pre-coated with poly D-lysine (50 μg/mL). The cells were incubated for 5 h at 37° C in a humidified incubator containing 95% air/5% CO_2. The cell media was then aspirated and replaced with the identical volume of neurobasal media containing 2% B27 supplement, 1 mol/L HEPES, 2 mmol/L L-glutamine, and 50 mg/mL gentamicin, which is preheated to 37° C. On day *in vitro* (DIV) 3, and every other day thereafter, one-fifth of the culture medium was removed and replaced with fresh media to replenish vital nutrients. Cultures were used between DIV 8–11. Procedures using animals were conducted according to the principles set forth in the National Institutes of Health (NIH) Publication no. 85-23, Guide for the Care & Use of Laboratory Animals & the Animal Welfare Act of 1986, as amended. Every effort was made to minimize the number of animals.

Drug treatments

TSA (Sigma, St. Louis, MO) was prepared in dimethyl sulfoxide (DMSO) (Sigma). Hippocampal neurons were plated into six-well plates grown in Neurobasal medium with B27 supplement. Neurons were treated with a final concentration of 250 nmol/L TSA up to 16 h or with DMSO (vehicle control). Hippocampal neurons were maintained in six-well plates for real time reverse-transcribed polymerase chain reaction or 10 cm dishes for protein extraction, or chromatin immunoprecipitation (ChIP) and incubated for 5 h at 37° C in a humidified incubator assay.

Chromatin immunoprecipitation detection primers within *Bdnf* promoter 1

To determine if specific sites within the promoter respond to chromatin remodeling following TSA treatment, we designed two sets of PCR primers: one site was proximal to the transcription start site of exon 1 (pm51): forward, 5′-AACTTTTCTAAGAA GTTTCC TTTTTACCA-3′; reverse, 5′-TGAGCC AGTTACGTGACCAACT-3′. The second site, termed the distal site, is located approximately 4 kb 5′ of the transcription start site (pm9): forward, 5′-AGCTCTTGCAGACTAAATCGTGAGTTT-3′; reverse, 5′-CAAGAACCTGGTGTTGAGCTCATAT-TT-3′.

ChIP

The ChIP assay was modified from the EZ- ChIP kit protocol (Upstate Biotechnology, Lake Placid, NY). Rat hippocampal neurons in 10 cm dishes (E19, DIV 9, 0.5×10^7 cells per dish) were treated with 250 nmol/L TSA for 8 h or treated with vehicle for the same time period. Crosslinking was performed at room temperature by adding 37% formaldehyde to the cell culture medium at 1% final concentration and incubated for 10 min. The reaction was stopped by the addition of 2.5 mol/L glycine to a final concentration of 125 mmol/L, followed by 5 min incubation at room temperature. Cells were washed twice with 8 mL cold phosphate-buffered saline (PBS) containing a protease inhibitor cocktail (Roche, Nutley, NJ), then removed to 15 mL tube in 1 mL PBS with protease inhibitor. Samples were centrifuged at 700 *g* for 10 min at 4° C. The cell pellet from four dishes was pooled and suspended in 1 mL SDS lysis buffer with protease inhibitor cocktail. The lysate was snap frozen in the ethanol-dry ice bath and then thawed in a 37° C water bath. This process was repeated four times. The final lysate was sonicated on ice using a Misonix sonicator 3000, MicrotipTM 419 (Farmingdale, NY) at a power setting of 6, 12 pulses (12 s on, 2.5 min off). Samples were centrifuged at 12,000 *g*, at 4° C for 10 min to remove insoluble material, and the supernatant containing DNA-protein complexes was collected. To test for reproducibility, 5 μL of the sonicated chromatin was retained and 90 μL ddH_2O were added, followed by 4 μL 5 mol/L NaCl. The solution was then incubated 4–5 h at 65° C to reverse the DNA-protein crosslinks. RNase A (1 μL from 1 U stock) was added and the mixture incubated for 30 min at 37° C, followed by incubation with 2 μL 0.5 mol/L EDTA, 4 μL 1 mol/L Tris-HCl and 1 μL Proteinase K at 45° C for 1–2 h. A sample of 5–20 μL was fractionated on a 1.5% native agarose gel with a 100 bp DNA marker. The sonicated DNA produced fragments from 150 to 1000 bp. The cell supernatant from three different cultures was pooled. The pooled cell supernatant was precleared with salmon sperm DNA/protein A or G agarose 50% slurry for 1 h at 4° C with agitation, and centrifuged at 1500 rpm for 2 min to recover the beads. The beads were then resuspended in dilution buffer for subsequent immunoprecipitation. An aliquot (20 μL) of the precleared DNA preparation served as an input control and was reserved for later use. Antibodies for ChIP assays were anti-HDAC1 and anti-MeCP2. The antibodies were added to the precleared chromatin preparation, incubated on a rocking platform 16 h at 4° C. As a negative control, nonimmune rabbit or mouse IgG (Upstate Biotechnology) were used in place of specific antibodies. Immune complexes were precipitated by the addition of salmon sperm DNA/protein A or G agarose slurry for 1–2 h at 4° C and pelleted at 700 *g* for 1 min. The pellets were washed five times (1 mL each) in a low-salt wash buffer, high-salt wash buffer, and LiCl wash buffer, and twice with TE buffer. Immune complexes were treated twice in 100 μL of 1% SDS and 100 mmol/L $NaHCO_3$ at room temperature for 15 min. Protein–DNA cross links were reversed by adding 8 μL 5 mol/L NaCl and incubating the mixture at 65° C for 5 h, followed by treatment with 1 U of RNase A and 20 μg proteinase K at 37° C for 1 h. The DNA was then processed using PCR purification columns (Qiagen, Valencia, CA). Levels of specific proteins occupying *Bdnf* promoter 1 were determined by a semi-quantitative PCR assay. Conditions for PCR were: 1 cycle 94° C, 10 min; 24–40 cycles 94° C, 15 s, 50–65° C, 20 s, 72° C, 30 s, followed by an extension at 72° C, 7 min. PCR products were resolved on TBE polyacrylamide gels and the amplicon band visualized by ethidium bromide staining. Molecular size was determined using appropriate size standards (O'GeneRuler, Fermentas Inc., Hanover, MD). Input and immunoprecipitated DNA reactions were performed in triplicate. Representative ChIP results are presented in the Results section. Buffer-only "no antibody" conditions were used as negative ChIP controls and did not produce a band following PCR. In addition, immunoprecipitated chromatin with nonimmune rabbit IgG produced similar results as "no antibody" controls.

Western blot

Western blot analysis was performed as described previously (Wu *et al.*, 2004). Briefly, the culture medium was removed and the cells washed twice with ice cold Locke's buffer (154 mmol/L NaCl; 5.6 mmol/L KCl; 1 mmol/L $MgCl_2$; 2.3 mmol/L $CaCl_2$; 5.6 mmol/L D-glucose; 8.6 mmol/L HEPES; 1 mmol/L vanadate; pH 7.4). Hippocampal neurons were disrupted in 200 μL of lysis buffer (1% Nonidet P-40, 20 mmol/L Tris, pH 8.0, 137 mmol/L NaCl, 10% glycerol, 1 mmol/L phenylmethylsulphonyl fluoride, 0.15 units/ml aprotinin, 20 μmol/L leupeptin, 1 mmol/L sodium vanadate at 4° C). After removal of cellular debris by centrifugation, protein levels in the lysates were measured by the Bradford Coomassie Blue colorimetric assay (Bio-Rad Laboratories, Hercules, CA) and equalized accordingly. Samples were boiled in the presence of sample buffer (2% SDS, 100 mmol/L dithiothreitol, 10% glycerol, 0.25% bromphenol blue, pH 6.8) for 5 min. Boiled samples (20 μg/lane) were fractionated through 4–12% Bis–Tris gradient gels (Invitrogen) and proteins were transferred to Polyvinylidene Fluoride (PVDF) membranes (0.45 μm, Millipore, Billerica, MA). After blocking with 5% non-fat dry milk dissolved in Tris-buffered saline containing 0.2% Tween 20 (TBST) for 1 h at room temperature, washed three times in TBST and the immobilized proteins were incubated overnight at 4° C with specific antibodies: anti H3AcK9 1:5000, H3AcK14 1:5000 (Upstate Biotechnology). After further washing, the blots were incubated with the appropriate horse radish peroxidase (HRP)-conjugated secondary antibody for 1–2 h at room temperature. The blots were washed as described above and immunoreactive bands were visualized using the enhanced chemiluminescence system (ECL) according to the manufacturer's recommendations (Amersham-Pharmacia, Piscataway, NJ). Total histone H3 was used as the reference. Blots were stripped with Restore Western Blot Stripping Buffer (Pierce, Rockford, IL) and washed with TBST and the blot incubated with anti- H3 (Cell Signaling, Beverly, MA) overnight at 4° C. Blots were then washed with TBST for 30 min followed by incubation with the appropriate secondary antibody linked to HRP for 1 h. Immunoreactive bands were visualized by ECL.

Reverse-transcribed polymerase chain reaction

Total RNA was extracted from hippocampal neurons using RNA STAT-60 (Tel-Test, Friendswood, TX), RNeasy mini kit (QIAGEN, Valencia, CA), and DNA-free kit (Applied Biosystems/Ambion, Austin, TX). The final RNA preparation was free of DNA contamination, as determined by a reverse transcriptase-less control, was reverse transcribed using a cloned AMV first-strand cDNA synthesis kit (Invitrogen). PCR primers for *Hdac1*, *Mecp2*, and *Gapdh* were used in semi-quantitative assays. The primers were: *Hdac1*, forward 5′-CATGCCAAGTGTGTGGAGTTCGT-3′; reverse 5′-GTCCAGCACCGAGCGACATT-3′; *Mecp2*, forward 5′-CAGCTCCAACAGGATTCCATGGT-3′; reverse 5′-TGATGTCTCTGCTTTGCCTGCCT-3′. Real time PCR was performed on an ABI PRISM® 7700 sequence detector with the sequence specific PCR primers and a detection probe designed using Primer Express® software (ABI, Foster City, CA) and synthesized by the manufacturer.

Real time PCR primers and probes

The rat *Bdnf* exon 1 primers and probe sequences were: forward primer: 5′-GCGTTGAGAAAGCTGCTTCAG-3′; reverse primer: 5′-GAATGAGCGAGGTTACCAATGAC-3′. The *Bdnf* exon 1-specific probe sequence was: 5′-CGCCCGCTATATAGCAGGGCAGT-3′. The amplification primers for Rat *BDNF* exon 4: 5′-TTCCACTATCAATAATTTAACTTCTTTGC-3′ (forward primer), and 5′-CTCTTACTATATATTTCCCCTTCTCTTCAGT-3′ (reverse primer). Detection probe: 5′-TACATATCGGCCACCAAAGACTCGC-3′. Rat *Gapdh* was used as an internal reference and was purchased from ABI.

Results

Trichostatin A robustly induces *Bdnf* exon 1-specific mRNA levels relative to *Bdnf* exon 4-containing transcripts

Histone acetylation is an associated feature of transcriptionally active genes.[24] An inhibitor of HDAC activity, TSA, has differential effects on *Bdnf* promoters 1 and 4 in Neuro2A cells treated with TSA (300 nmol/L) for 48 h.[16] We wanted to determine if TSA treatment of rat hippocampal neurons maintained in culture lead to differential changes in *Bdnf* exon 1 and exon 4-specific mRNA levels. Using a TSA concentration that produced maximal levels of *Bdnf* exon 1 and exon 4 mRNAs (250 nmol/L),[25] we measured the temporal response of *Bdnf* exon 1 mRNA levels relative to exon 4-specific mRNA levels. Exon 4-specific mRNA levels increased only 2-fold at the same TSA concentration by 8 h, while exon 1 mRNA levels were enhanced more than 12-fold (Fig. 1). These results suggest that the promoters controlling exon 1 and exon 4-specific transcription respond differently to an HDAC inhibitor and that the molecular mechanisms responsible for altering chromatin structure at each of these promoters may differ.

Increased occupancy of acetylated H3 (H3AcK9/14) at promoter 1 following TSA treatment

Histone acetylation is involved in transcriptional activation. *Bdnf* promoters 1 and 4 are activated

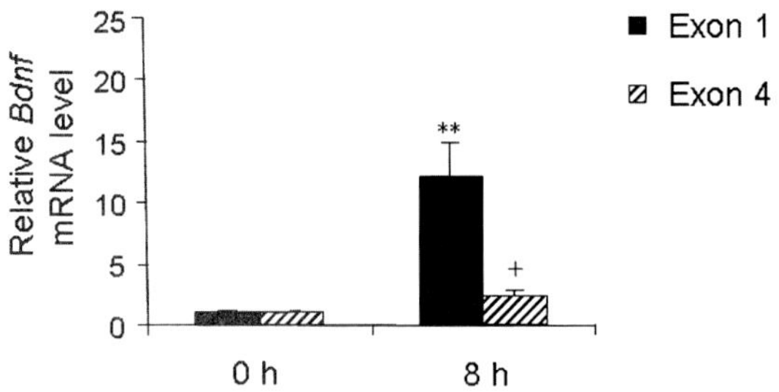

Figure 1. Induction of *Bdnf* exon 1 and exon 4-specific mRNA levels in Trichostatin A (TSA)-treated hippocampal neurons. Cultured hippocampal neurons were incubated with a 250 nmol/L for 8 h on day *in vitro* 8. Mean expression values for each *Bdnf* transcript were determined after normalization to the average expression values of the *Gapdh* gene from each template. Data are presented as fold-change relative to baseline (0 h) expression (means ± SD). Student's t test, $^{+}P < 0.05$, $^{**}P < 0.01$, compared to respective 0 h control.

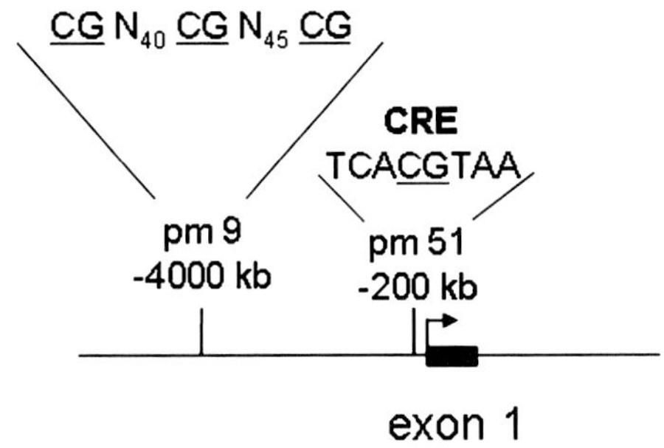

Figure 2. Schematic of genomic region of *Bdnf* promoter 1 analyzed by chromatin immunoprecipitation (ChIP) assays. Depicted are the DNA sequences from approximately −4000 to −200 relative to exon 1 and the location of ChIP PCR amplicons within the promoter are: pm9, the distal site, pm51, the proximal site. The transcription start site is indicated by the right-facing arrow. The CRE element within the proximal promoter region is labeled in bold letters. The CpG dinucleotides within promoter 1 are underlined, separated by nucleotide sequence, indicated in subscript.

when histone deacetylation is inhibited *in vivo*[20] or conversely, when acetylated histones are enhanced at promoters 1 and 4 *in vivo*.[26] Other investigators have observed histone changes associated with *Bdnf* promoter 1, being consistently hyperacetylated in the hippocampus following pilocarpine treatment *in vivo*.[17] As a first approach to characterizing histone changes taking place at *Bdnf* promoter 1 following TSA treatment, we analyzed two sites from the 5′ flanking sequence of exon 1, which also contains multiple potential transcription factor binding sites and CpGs, for presence of acetylated H3 in primary hippocampal neurons treated with TSA (250 nmol/L) or vehicle-treated neurons by ChIP assays. One site analyzed is located 200 bp 5′ from a known transcription start site mapped previously by Nakayama and colleagues[27] and is represented by the pm51 ChIP PCR amplicon (Fig. 2). This site is contained within a ChIP PCR amplicon that was characterized previously *in vivo*[26] and also contains a CRE element that responds to *N*-methyl-D-aspartate (NMDA) receptor activation through the release of HDAC1.[25] A second site, but more distal to the pm51 site was also examined. This site, defined by the pm9 PCR amplicon, is located approximately 4 kb 5′ from the transcription start site (Fig. 2) in a region rich in CpG dinucleotides. We determined occupancy of the promoter 1 sites after 1 h and 8 h TSA treatment. The transcription start site proximal region, pm51, and the distal site, pm9, showed a rapid time-dependent increase in H3AcK9/14 occupancy that was sustained up to 8 h following TSA treatment (Fig. 3). These results support the concept that region-specific alterations in histone acetylation

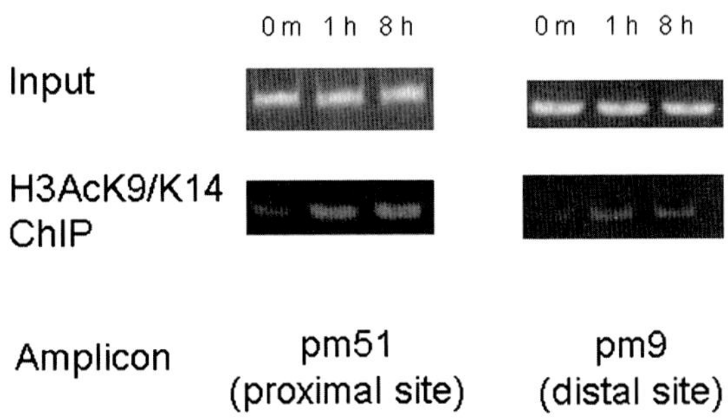

Figure 3. Histone acetylation changes by hippocampal neurons after Trichostatin A (TSA) treatment. Chromatin immunoprecipitation (ChIP) assays showing H3 acetylation (H3AcK9/14) changes within *Bdnf* promoter 1 regions after 1 h and 8 h TSA treatment. The figure shows a representative ChIP with anti-H3AcK9/14 antibody. The immunoprecipitated DNA was amplified by a semi-quantitative PCR assay (Materials and Methods). Above the antibody-specific lanes are samples from each region-specific PCR reaction, or "input" DNAs.

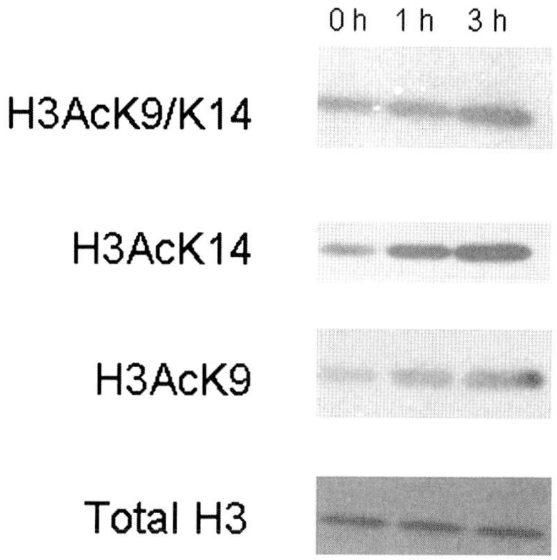

Figure 4. Trichostatin A (TSA) increases acetylated histone (H3AcK9/K14) levels by hippocampal neurons. Neuronal cultures were treated with 250 nmol/l TSA for up to 3 h. Total proteins were extracted and fractionated through polyacrylamide gels and transferred to polyvinylidene fluoride (PVDF) membranes as described in Materials and Methods. Immobilized proteins were incubated overnight at 4° C with specific antibodies: anti H3AcK9 1:5000 or H3AcK14 1:5000 or a mixture of both antibodies. After further washing, the blots were incubated with the appropriate HRP-conjugated secondary antibody and the immunoreactive bands visualized using enhanced chemiluminescence (ECL). Total histone H3 was used as the reference.

at promoter 1 are associated with transcriptional derepression.

Time-dependent increase in H3AcK9 and H3AcK14 protein levels following TSA treatment

It is known that HDAC inhibitors, including TSA, enhance levels of H3 acetylation in primary cortical neurons.[28] Because we observed that TSA treatment increased H3AcK9/K14 binding to promoter 1 *in vivo*, we wanted to determine if protein levels of H3AcK9 and H3AcK14 were modulated by cultured hippocampal neurons following TSA treatment. By Western blot, we observed a time-dependent increase in these H3-specific acetylated lysine residues, up to 3 h (Fig. 4), consistent with the idea that *Bdnf* promoter 1 region has a greater capacity for further modification. Because the higher levels of H3AcK9 and H3AcK14 protein were observed up to 3 h TSA treatment, it is likely that TSA may act on other genes besides *Bdnf*.

Time-dependent increase in *Hdac1* mRNA and HDAC1 protein levels following TSA treatment

HDAC inhibition causes, in what has been proposed to be, a compensatory increase in *Hdac* isoform mRNA levels in different cell lines.[29–31] This is part of an autoregulatory mechanism for HDAC expression, targeting the *Hdac1* promoter.[29] We sought to determine if *Hdac1*expression was altered in TSA treated hippocampal neurons. As shown in Figure 5, TSA treatment increased *Hdac1* mRNA and protein levels in a time-dependent fashion. This response appears to be specific, as another gene, *Mecp2,* which has been shown to be activated by a structurally different HDAC inhibitor, valproate, in the C6 glioma cell line,[31] was not activated by TSA treatment.

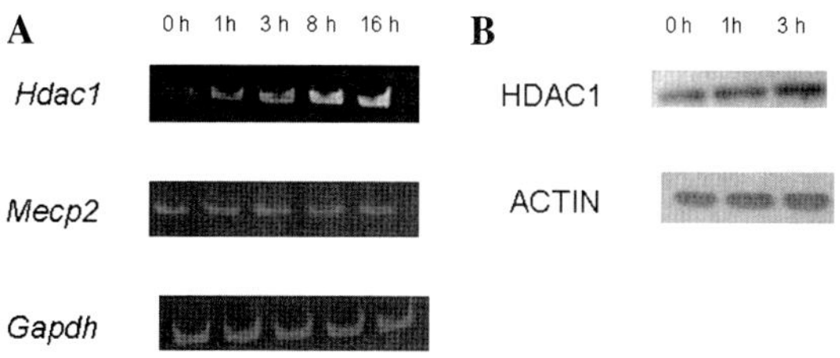

Figure 5. Time-dependent changes in *Hdac1* or *Mecp2* mRNA levels (A) and HDAC1 protein levels (B) by hippocampal neurons following Trichostatin A (TSA) treatment. *Panel A* depicts a representative reverse transcription polymerase chain reaction (RT-PCR) assay. Total RNA was extracted from TSA-treated neurons at the times indicated and reverse-transcribed for semi-quantitative RT-PCR as described in Materials and Methods. *Hdac1* mRNA levels increased with time, as seen by the increased band intensity, while intensity of the *Mecp2*, and *Gapdh*-specific bands were constant. *Panel B* shows a representative Western blot prepared from the same neuronal cultures treated with TSA (250 nmol/L) for the indicated times. The cells were lysed and immunoblotted with the specific antibody as described in Materials and Methods. The blots were incubated sequentially with anti-HDAC1 (HDAC1) and anti-actin (Actin) antibodies. Immunoreactive HDAC1 levels increased with time after TSA treatment.

Discussion

In this study, we observed differential effects of TSA on transcription from *Bdnf* promoters 1 and 4 by rat hippocampal neurons in culture. *Bdnf* exon 1 mRNA levels were strongly induced by TSA in a time-dependent fashion compared to exon 4. These results suggested that promoters 1 and 4 respond differentially to signals affecting chromatin structure and support our previous findings that examined *in vivo* occupancy of these promoters by HDACs, specifically HDAC1, under conditions of NMDA receptor activation.[25] In that previous study, we noted that HDAC1 binding of promoter 1 near the transcription start site was reduced at least 3 h following NMDA receptor activation, consistent with increased levels of exon 1-containing transcripts. No HCAC1 binding at the distal site was seen under any condition. In contrast, NMDA receptor activation produced a rapid but less pronounced increase in exon 4-specific transcripts although there were similar temporal changes in HDAC1 binding to promoter 4. In the current study, we observed that TSA treatment produced a rapid time-dependent increase in H3AcK9/14 occupancy at two sites, one proximal and one distal to the transcription start site (Fig. 3). This result suggests that TSA may support more wide-ranging changes in chromatin structure at promoter 1 that may account for the strong transcriptional response following TSA treatment.

The more widespread occupancy of promoter 1 by acetylated H3 was mirrored by increased acetylated H3 protein levels, suggesting TSA may have transcriptional effects on the entire genome rather than individual genes. This observation was supported by RT-PCR experiments performed on the same set of TSA treated neurons to determine the expression of transcriptional repressors HDAC1 and MeCP2. Under these conditions, *Hdac1* mRNA levels were increased while *Mecp2* mRNA levels remained unchanged. Additionally, HDAC1 protein levels were increased by TSA treatment (Fig. 5). Taken together, these data suggest that there is a compensatory change in HDAC1 expression with inhibition of HDAC activity in neurons. This may reflect a genome wide change in gene expression. This conclusion is supported by findings reported in different cell lines treated with valproate (C6 gliomoa cells[30,31]) or TSA (Hep 3B cells[32]; 3T3 cells[33]), or cortical neurons treated with either lithium, valporate, or TSA.[28] In fact, there is a large literature to support a role for HDAC inhibition and chromatin remodeling events leading to transcriptional activation. The signal transduction pathways mediating these changes in chromatin architecture have yet to be elucidated. Because modulation of BDNF expression has a critical role in neuroprotective pathways following brain trauma or stroke, treatments that promote neuronal rescue through activation of endogenous BDNF expression may improve functional outcome.

Acknowledgment

This study was supported by an extramural grant F-192EG-C1 from the Defense Brain and Spinal Cord Injury Program (AMM).

Conflicts of interest

The authors declare no conflicts of interest.

References

1. Strahl, B.D. & C.D. Allis. 2000. The language of covalent histone modifications. *Nature* **403:** 41–45.
2. Berger, S.L. 2007. The complex language of chromatin regulation during transcription. *Nature* **447:** 407–412.
3. Kim, Y.B., M. Yoshida & S. Horinouchi. 1995. Selective induction of cyclin-dependent kinase inhibitors and their roles in cell cycle arrest caused by trichostatin A, an inhibitor of histone deacetylase. *Ann. N.Y. Acad. Sci.* **886:** 200–203.
4. Seth, K.A. & J.A. Majzoub. 2001. Repressor element silencing transcription factor/neuron-restricitve silencing factor (REST/NRSF) can act as an enhancer as well as a repressor of corticotropin-releasing hormone gene transcription. *J. Biol. Chem.* **276:** 13917–13923.
5. Quivy, V. & C. Van Lint. 2002. Diversity of acetylation targets and roles in transcriptional regulation: the human immunodeficiency virus type 1 promoter as a model system. *Biochem. Pharmacol.* **64:** 925–934.
6. Vanhaecke, T., P. Papeleu, G. Elaut, *et al.* 2004. Trichostatin A-like hydroxamate histone deacetylase inhibitors as therapeutic agents: toxicological point of view. *Curr. Med. Chem.* **11:** 1629–1643.
7. McGowan, P.O., M.J. Meaney & M. Szyf. 2008. Diet and the epigenetic (re)programming of phenotypic differences in behavior. *Brain Res.* **1237:** 12–24.
8. Thoenen, H. 1995. Neurotrophins and neuronal plasticity. *Science* **270:** 593–598.

9. Katz, L. & C.J. Shatz. 1996. Synaptic activity and the construction of cortical circuits. *Science* **274:** 1133–1138.
10. Lu, B. & A. Figurov. 1997. Role of neurotrophins in synapse development and plasticity. *Rev. Neurosci.* **8:** 1–12.
11. Arancio, O. & M.V. Chao. 2007. Neurotrophins, synaptic plasticity and dementia. *Curr. Opin. Neurobiol.* **17:** 325–330.
12. Marini, A.M., X. Jiang, X. Wu, *et al.* 2004. Role of BDNF and NF- κB in neuronal plasticity and survival: from genes to phenotype. *Restor. Neurol. Neurosci.* **22:** 121–130.
13. Liu, Q.R., D. Walther, T. Drgon, *et al.* 2005. Human brain derived neurotrophic factor (BDNF) genes, splicing patterns, and assessments of associations with substance abuse and Parkinson's disease. *Am. J. Med. Genet. B Neuropsychiatr. Genet.* **134:** 93–103.
14. Pruunsild, P., A. Kazantseva, T. Aid, *et al.* 2007. Dissecting the human BDNF locus: bidirectional transcription, complex splicing, and multiple promoters. *Genomics* **90:** 397–406.
15. Jiang, X., J. Zhou, D.C. Mash, *et al.* 2008. Human BDNF isoforms are differentially expressed in cocaine addicts and are sorted to the regulated secretory pathway independent of the Met66 substitution. *Neuromolecular. Med.* **11:** 1559–1174.
16. Aid, T., A. Kazantseva, M. Piirsoo, *et al.* 2007. Mouse and rat BDNF gene structure and expression revisited. *J. Neurosci. Res.* **85:** 525–535.
17. Huang, Y., J.J. Doherty & R. Dingledine. 2002. Altered histone acetylation at glutamate receptor 2 and brain-derived neurotrophic factor genes is an early event triggered by status epilepticus. *J. Neurosci.* **22:** 8422–8428.
18. Chen, W.G., Q. Chang, Y. Lin, *et al.* 2003. Derepression of BDNF transcription involves calcium-dependent phosphorylation of MeCP2. *Science* **302:** 885–889.
19. Martinowich, K., D. Hattori, H. Wu, *et al.* 2003. DNA methylation-related chromatin remodeling in activity-dependent BDNF gene regulation. *Science* **302:** 890–893.
20. Tsankova, N.M., O. Berton, W. Renthal, *et al.* 2006. Sustained hippocampal chromatin regulation in a mouse model of depression and antidepressant action. *Nat. Neurosci.* **9:** 519–525.
21. Cheng, B., K. Furukawa, J. A. O'Keefe, *et al.* 1995. Basic fibroblast growth factor selectively increases AMPA-receptor subunit GluR1 protein level and differentially modulates Ca^{2+} responses to AMPA and NMDA in hippocampal neurons. *J. Neurochem.* **65:** 2525–2536.
22. Jiang, X., F. Tian, K. Mearow, *et al.* 2005. The excitoprotective effect of N-methyl-D-aspartate receptors is mediated by a brain-derived neurotrophic factor acutocrine loop in cultured hippocampal neurons. *J. Neurochem.* **94:** 713–722.
23. Wu, X., D. Zhu, X. Jiang, *et al.* 2004. AMPA protects cultured neurons against glutamate excitotoxicity through a phosphqatidylinositol 3-kinase-dependent activation in extracellular signal-regulated kinase to up-regulate BDNF gene expression. *J. Neurochem.* **90:** 807–818.
24. Mellor, J. 2006. Dynamic nucleosomes and gene transcription. *Trends Genet.* **22:** 320–329.
25. Tian, F., A.M. Marini & R.H. Lipsky. 2009. NMDA receptor activation induces differential epigenetic modification of *Bdnf* promoters in hippocampal neurons. *Amino Acids.* PMID: 19565326.
26. Bredy, T.W., H. Wu, C. Crego, *et al.* 2007. Histone modification around individual BDNF promoters in prefrontal cortex are associated with extinction of conditioned fear. *Learn Mem.* **14:** 268–276.
27. Nakayama, M., Y. Gahara, T. Kitamura, *et al.* 1994. Distinctive four promoters collectively direct expression of brain-derived neurotrophic factor gene. *Brain Res. Mol. Brain Res.* **21:** 206–218.
28. Yasuda, S., M-H. Liang, Z. Marinova, *et al.* 2009. The mood stabilizers lithium and valproate selectively activate the promoter of brain-derived neurotrophic factor in neurons. *Mol. Psychiatry* **14:** 51–59.
29. Schuettengruber, B., E. Simboeck, H. Khier, *et al.* 2003. Autoregulation of mouse histone deacetylase 1 expression. *Mol. Cell Biol.* **23:** 6993–7004.
30. Castro, L.M., M. Gallant & L.P. Niles. 2005. Novel targets for valproic acid: up-regulation of melatonin receptors and neurotrophic factors in C6 glioma cells. *J. Neurochem.* **95:** 1227–1236.
31. Kim, B., L.M.R. Castro, S. Jawed, *et al.* 2008. Clinically relevant concentrations of valproic acid modulate melatonin MT_1 receptor, HDAC and MECP2 mRNA expression in C6 glioma cells. *Eur. J. Pharmacol.* **589:** 45–48.
32. Gray, S.G. & T.J. Ekstrom. 1998. Effects of cell density and trichostatin A on the expression of HDAC1 and p57Kip2 in Hep 3B cells. *Biochem. Biophys. Res. Commun.* **245:** 423–427.
33. Hauser, C., B. Scheuttengruber, S. Bartl, *et al.* 2002. Activation of the mouse histone deacetylase 1 gene by co-operative histone phosphorylation and acetylation. *Mol. Cell Biol.* **22:** 7820–7830.

Ann. N.Y. Acad. Sci. ISSN 0077-8923

ANNALS OF THE NEW YORK ACADEMY OF SCIENCES
Issue: *Neuroprotective Agents*

Enhanced expression of glycine *N*-methyltransferase by adenovirus-mediated gene transfer in CNS culture is neuroprotective

May-Jywan Tsai,[1,2] Yi-Ming Arthur Chen,[3,4] Ching-Feng Weng,[5] Dann-Ying Liou,[1] Hsin-Chun Yang,[1] Chien-Hung Chen,[1] Roanna I-Hsin Liao,[1] Fu-Shan Kuo,[1] Chiuan-Wen Chiu,[1] Huai-Sheng Kuo,[1] Ming-Chao Huang,[1,2,6,9] Yi-Lo Lin,[1] Meng-Jen Lee,[1,7] Wen-Chun Kuo,[1] Wen-Cheng Huang,[1,2,9] and Henrich Cheng[1,2,8–10]

[1]Neural Regeneration Laboratory, [2]Center for Neural Regeneration, Department of Neurosurgery, Neurological Institute, Taipei Veterans General Hospital, Taiwan. [3]AIDS Prevention and Research Center, National Yang-Ming University, Taiwan. [4]Institute of Microbiology and Immunology, National Yang-Ming University, Taiwan. [5]Department of Biotechnology, National Dong-Hwa University, Taiwan. [6]School of Medicine, Taipei Medical University, Taiwan. [7]Institute of Biochemical Sciences and Technology, Chaoyang University of Technology, Taiwan. [8]Department of Pharmacology, [9]Faculty of Medicine, [10]Institute of Brain Science, School of Medicine, National Yang-Ming University, Taiwan

Address for correspondence: Henrich Cheng, MD, PhD, Neural Regeneration Laboratory, Department of Neurosurgery, Neurological Institute, Taipei Veterans General Hospital, No. 322, Shih-pai Road, Sec. 2, Taipei, Taiwan 11217. hc_cheng@vghtpe.gov.tw

Glycine *N*-methyltransferase (GNMT) is the most abundant hepatic methyltransferase and plays important roles in regulating methyl group metabolism. In the central nervous system, GNMT expression is low and its function has not been revealed. The present study examines the effect of GNMT overexpression by adenovirus-mediated transfer in cortical mixed neuron-glial cultures. Infection of adenovirus encoding green fluorescence protein to cultures demonstrates high preference for non-neuronal cells. Optimal GNMT overexpression in cultures by adenoviral GNMT (Ad-GNMT) infection not only induces protein kinase C phosphorylation, but also increases neuronal/oligodendroglial survival. Furthermore, these Ad-GNMT-infected cultures are significantly resistant to H_2O_2 toxicity and lipopolysaccharide stimulation. Conditioned media from Ad-GNMT-infected microglia also significantly enhance neuronal survival. Taken together, enhanced GNMT expression in mixed neuronal-glial cultures is neuroprotective, most likely mediated through non-neuronal cells.

Keywords: GNMT; adenovirus; neuron-glia interaction; lipopolysaccharide

Introduction

The inability of central nervous system (CNS) axonal regeneration to occur following injury is, at least, caused by the intrinsic properties of the neuron itself,[4] the absence of neurotrophic and attractive factors,[10] as well as the presence of inhibitory factors in the environment.[13] Many results have been reported in myelin-derived inhibitory proteins and their signaling pathways regarding blocking axon regeneration.[12] The trophic stimuli promoting survival and growth of neurons have a critical role in CNS regeneration.[5]

Methyl group and folate-dependent one-carbon metabolism play an important role in the methylation of phospholipids, neurotransmitters, proteins, and nucleic acids.[20,21] An adequate supply of methyl groups is essential in preventing associated pathologies, such as cancer, vascular disease, and neural defects. Glycine *N*-methyltransferase (GNMT) plays a key role in the regulation of hepatic methyl group metabolism by the enzymatic conversion of glycine and S-adenosylmethionine (SAM) to sarcosine and S-adenosylhomocysteine (SAH), respectively. GNMT functions to optimize the SAM/SAH ratio, an indicator of trans-methylation potential.

doi: 10.1111/j.1749-6632.2009.05169.x

The expression of GNMT is highly responsive to environmental factors and is tissue-specific, most abundant in the liver, pancreas, and prostate.[21] GNMT, participating in detoxification, is often downregulated in hepatocellular carcinoma.[3,9] In addition, GNMT has protective effects against exposure to carcinogens by decreasing DNA adduct formation.[2]

CNS expresses minute levels of GNMT compared to the liver. The function of GNMT in the brain has not been revealed. The present study attempts to explore the function of GNMT in the CNS. Adenovirus encodes GNMT or green fluorescent protein (GFP), as mock control, were prepared and purified. Adenovirus-mediated gene transfer of GNMT or GFP was employed in mixed neuron-glial cultures and examined as to whether overexpression of GNMT was beneficial to neuronal cultures. Results showed that GNMT overexpression was neuroprotective, and was most likely mediated through non-neuronal cells.

Materials and methods

Materials

Culture media, fetal bovine serum (FBS), and horse serum were from Gibco (Carlsbad, CA). Culture flasks or multiwell plates were from Corning (New York, NY). Cell inserts (Millcell 1 μm PET) were from Millipore (Billerica, MA). A methylthiazol tetrazolium (MTT) kit was from Chemicon (Billerica, MA). Lipopolysaccharide (LPS; *E. coli* 0111:B4) was purchased from Sigma Aldrich Co. (St. Louis, MO). Unless stated otherwise, all other chemicals were purchased from Sigma-Aldrich Co. Antibodies used in this study are listed as follows: mouse or rabbit anti-GNMT (donated by Dr. Y.M.A. Chen); rabbit or mouse anti-myelin basic protein (MBP) and anti-GFP (Chemicon); rabbit or mouse anti-βIII tubulin (Covance, Princeton, NJ); mouse anti-MAP-2 (Upstate Biotechnology, Lake Placid, NY); mouse anti-ED1 (CD68) (Serotec, Poole, UK); biotinylated *Griffonia Simplicifolia* lectin 1 isolectin B4 (GSA-IB4; Vector Lab, Burlingame, CA); mouse anti-iNOS (BD Bioscience, San Diego, CA); mouse anti-SV2 (DSHB, Iowa City, IA); rabbit anti-phospho-protein kinase C (pan-) (phospho-PKC) (Cell Signalling, Danvers, MA); goat anti-actin (Santa Cruz Biotech, Santa Cruz, CA).

Preparation of recombinant adenoviruses

We used first generation E1-deleted adenoviral vector ($\sim 10^{10}$ plaque forming units (pfu)/ml) encoding GNMT under the control of a cytomegalovirus (CMV) promoter (Ad-GNMT). The adenovirus encoding green fluorescence protein (Ad-GFP) under the control of CMV was used as a mock control. Details for generation of Ad-GFP and Ad-GNMT were described previously.[2,14] Recombinant adenoviruses were purified to a high concentration using a two-step cesium chloride ultracentrifugation. The viral titers of the purified recombinant adenovirus were further determined by a plaque-forming assay.[8]

Mixed neuronal-glial culture

Mixed neuronal-glial cultures were prepared from the cerebrocortical regions of embryonic Sprague–Dawley (SD) rat fetuses at gestation 15–17 days, as described in Hung *et al.*[6] and Tsai *et al.*[17,18] Briefly, fetal cortexes were dissociated with mixtures of papain/protease/deoxyribonuclease I (0.1%: 0.1%: 0.03%) and plated onto poly-L-lysine coated multiwell plates at density $\sim 3 \times 10^5$ cells/cm^2. Cultures were maintained in Dulbecco's modified Eagle's medium (DMEM, Gibco) supplemented with N2 (Gibco, for serum-free condition) or with 10% fetal bovine serum (FBS, Gibco). The cells were incubated at 37°C in a water-saturated atmosphere of 5% CO2/95% air. Cultures were infected by Ad-GFP or Ad-GNMT on the second day after seeding. Mixed neuron-glial cultures were harvested 2–7 days after adenoviral infection.

Microglial cultures

Microglial cultures were purified from confluent mixed glial cultures. Mixed glial cultures were prepared from neonatal cortical regions of SD rats as described previously.[15,16] Briefly, triturated cortexes were passed through nylon meshes and maintained in DMEM supplemented with 10% FBS. The cells were incubated at 37°C in a water-saturated atmosphere of 5% CO_2/95% air. The medium was renewed every 2–3 days. Eight to ten days later, microglial cells were collected using the shake-off method,[11] and replated onto multiwell plates. More than 98% of the cells were microglia as identified by positive immunoreactivity for ED-1 (CD68) or *Griffonia Simplicifolia* lectin 1 isolectin B4 (GSA-IB4), microglial markers.

Transducing primary cultures with adenoviruses

About 5×10^4 pfu, each of Ad-GFP or Ad-GNMT, were added to mixed neuron-glial cultures or microglia in multiwell plates. Two to seven days after adenoviral transduction, cultured cells were either fixed by 4% paraformaldehyde for morphological examination or harvested for biochemical assays. To examine the functional expression of Ad-GNMT, cell lysates of Ad-GNMT-transduced cultures were further processed for RT-PCR and Western blot analysis.

Hydrogen peroxide or lipopolysaccharide exposure

Nontreated control, Ad-GFP- or Ad-GNMT-transduced cells were maintained in serum-free medium. Hydrogen peroxide (60 μmol/L) was then added to the culture medium for 24 h and the surviving cells were analyzed for the degree of MTT reduction,[1] while cultured media were collected for assay of lactate dehydrogenase (LDH). In the experiments of LPS exposure, nontreated, Ad-GFP- or Ad-GNMT-transduced cells were maintained in a serum-containing medium (DMEM + 10% FBS). During LPS treatment, the culture medium was switched to DMEM + 2% FBS + 2% horse serum. After 2 days, the medium was saved for nitrate/nitrite measures by Griess reagents, while cells were fixed for immunohistochemical staining.

Neuronal survival

Loss of cell viability after toxin treatment was determined by assaying (1) LDH release in medium; (2) the degree of MTT reduction. Assay of MTT reduction, which is reduced to a blue formazan product by viable cells, followed a method described in Tsai and Lee.[16] Neuronal survival was also evaluated by visual observation and counts of βIII tubulin (neuronal marker)-immunoreactive (IR) numbers using a Zeiss Axiovert fluorescent microscope.

Western blot analysis

The cultured medium was saved for biochemical assays. The cells were washed twice with phosphate-buffered saline (PBS) and solubilized in lysis buffer containing PBS, 1% NP-40, and a protease inhibitor kit (BM, Mannheim, Germany). Protein concentration of the resultant lysate was determined using the method of Bradford (Bio-Rad protein assay, Bio-Rad Laboratories Ltd., Montreal, Quebec). Equal amounts of proteins were loaded and separated using 8%–12% gels (SDS-PAGE) as previously described.[17]

Total RNA extraction and RT-PCR

Total RNAs from mixed neuron-glial cultures were prepared using a High Pure RNA isolation kit from Roche (Mannheim, Germany). Titan one tube RT-PCR kit (Roche) was further used for amplification. The concentration and purity of the RNA preparations were determined by measuring the absorbance at 260 and 280 nm using a spectrophotometer. The nucleotide sequences of the primers were based on published cDNA sequences of human GNMT (forward, 5′-GCAGCCTTCGGAGGTAAGTG-3′; reverse, 5′-CTAGCAGTGCCTGGGCAGAG-3′), having been provided and examined by Dr. Y.M.A. Chen and his co-workers.[7,19] After amplification, the products were separated on 1% agarose gels containing ethidium bromide. The bands (~157 base pair) were visualized under UV transillumination.

Biochemical assays

Activity of LDH in the medium was measured spectrophotometrically as the oxidation of NADH in the presence of pyruvate using a commercial kit from Sigma. The production of NO was assayed as the accumulation of nitrite in medium using colorimetric reaction with Griess reagents (1% sulfanilaminde /0.1% naphthyl ethylene diamine dihydrochloride/2% phosphoric acid) as described in Tsai et al.[17,18] Briefly, after 2 days of LPS (1μg/mL) treatment, the culture medium was collected. The cultured medium (150 μL) was mixed with 50 μL of Griess reagents and incubated at room temperature for 10 min. The absorbance of the resultant products was measured at 540 nm. Sodium nitrite ($NaNO_2$) was used as the standard to calculate nitrogen dioxide (NO_2^-) concentrations.

Immunohistochemical analysis

Primary cultures were plated on poly-L-lysine-coated plates and fixed in 4% paraformaldehyde solution for 20 min. Cells were then permeabilized with 0.2% Triton X-100. Cells were stained with primary antibodies and with the respective fluorescence-tagged secondary antibodies (Jackson ImmunoResearch Inc., West Grove, PA). Images of immunoreactive (IR) cultured cells were obtained with a fluorescent microscope equipped with fluorescence optics. Images of neurons or non-neuronal cells were taken with a charge coupled device camera. Neuronal numbers were quantified by blind counting of 10 adjacent microscopic fields at 100× magnification, in each of three wells per condition. Experiments were repeated 3–4 times.

Statistics

One-way ANOVA followed by Bonferroni *t*-test was used to determine statistical differences between treatments. A statistically significant difference was accepted at $P < 0.05$.

Results

Adenovirus prefers infection to non-neuronal cells

To optimize the infection condition and characterize the infection tropism of adenovirus, mixed neuron-glial cultures or glial cultures were infected by Ad-GFP (50 or 20 MOI, respectively). Two days after infection, cells were fixed and processed for immunohistochemistry. As shown in Figure 1A and B, Ad-GFP predominantly infected non-neuronal cells. Relatively rare (or almost none) MAP-2 immunreactive neurons were found to express GFP. By contrast, almost all cells expressed strong GFP-IR in mixed glial cultures infected by Ad-GFP (Fig. 1C).

Indentification of glycine *N*-methyltransferase in rat tissues and in adenoviral-GNMT-infected cultures

Adult rat tissues, including cortex, spinal cord, and livers were assayed for endogenous GNMT expression. Western blot analysis of these tissue homogenates showed that two CNS tissues (cortex and spinal cord) express minute (or undetectable) levels of GNMT. By contrast, rat livers expressed relatively high amounts of GNMT as shown in Figure 2A. Ad-GNMT encoding human GNMT was propagated in E1-inserted human embryonic kidney (HEK) 293 cells and was further purified by two-step cesium chloride ultracentrifugation. After the purified Ad-GNMT had been analyzed for correct GNMT insertion (data not shown), the protein/mRNA expression of GNMT was examined in ads-infected mixed neuron-glial cultures. As shown in Figure 2B, overexpression of GNMT protein (32 kDa) and human GNMT mRNA (~157 bp) was revealed in Ad-GNMT-infected mixed neuronal-glial cultures.

GNMT overexpression increased cell survival

The effect of overexpressing GNMT on cell survival was examined 5 days after Ad-GNMT infection to cultures. About 5×10^4 pfu, each of Ad-GFP (mock) or Ad-GNMT, were added to mixed neuron-glial cells in multiwell plates. Cultures were then processed for immunohistochemical staining for MAP-2 (neuronal marker), SV2 (synaptic marker) and MBP (oligodendroglial marker). As shown in Figure 3A–D, GNMT overexpression enhanced neuronal survival. More neurite connections of MAP-2-IR and SV-2-IR neurons in Ad-GNMT-infected cultures were found than in Ad GFP (mock) cultures. Concurrently, more mature MBP (+)-IR oligodendrocytes with longer processes were observed in Ad-GNMT-infected cultures. Cultures were also harvested at 22 h after Ad-GNMT or

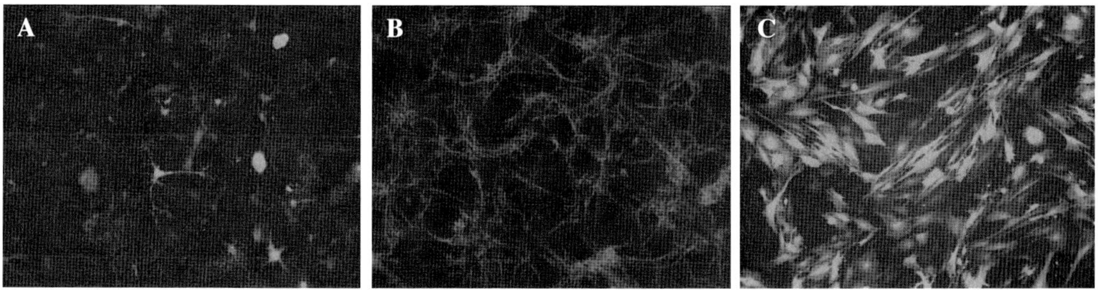

Figure 1. Infective tropism of recombinant adenovirus in mixed neuron-glial and glial cultures. Cells in (A) and (B) are Ad-GFP-infected mixed neuron-glial cultures, cells in (A) are stained for green fluorescence protein (GFP); cells in (B) are stained for MAP-2. (A) and (B) are double-labelled images. Cells in (C) are Ad-GFP-infected mixed glial cultures stained for GFP.

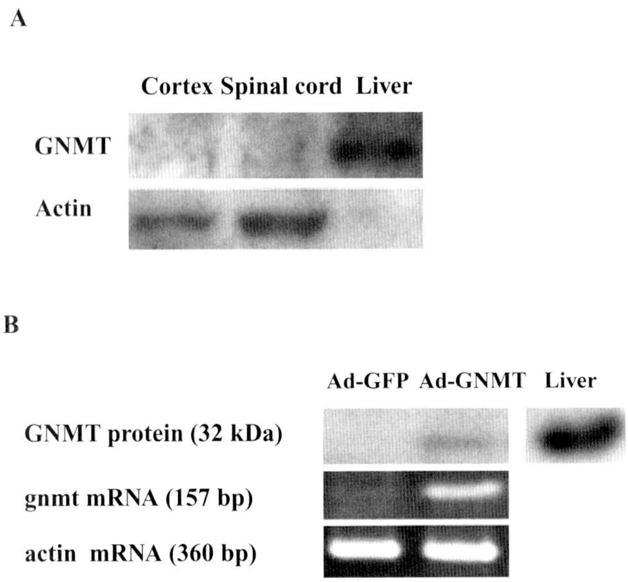

Figure 2. Identification of GNMT expression in rat tissues or in Ad-GNMT-infected mixed neuron-glial cultures. (A) Western blot analysis of endogenous expression of GNMT (~32 kDa) and actin (~42 kDa) in rat cerebral cortex, spinal cord, and liver. (B) Overexpression of GNMT protein and human gnmt mRNA (~157 bp) in Ad-GNMT-infected mixed neuronal-glial cultures. Note that because Ad-GNMT encodes human GNMT, human gnmt mRNA is not present in non-treated rat cultures.

Ad-GFP infection in order to probe the early cellular changes provoked by GNMT overexpression. As shown in Figure 4A, PKC phosphorylation was induced in Ad-GNMT-infected cells.

GNMT overexpression protected cells from H_2O_2 and LPS challenge

The neuroprotective effect of GNMT overexpression was examined by challenging cortical mixed neuron-glial cultures with H_2O_2. Treating cultures with H_2O_2 (60 μmol/L) for 24 h induced a decrease of MTT reduction and an increase of LDH release in all culture treatments (Figs. 4B and C). Ad-GNMT but not Ad-GFP infection significantly attenuated this H_2O_2 toxicity. The neuroprotective effect of GNMT overexpression was further examined by exposure of mixed neuron-glial cultures to an endotoxin, LPS, which is a cell wall component of gram-negative bacteria and is a powerful immune challenge. Treating mixed neuron-glial cultures with LPS (1 μg/mL; 2 days) significantly induced increases of both nitric oxide synthase (iNOS)-IR cells and NO (as nitrate/nitrite) release to medium (Figs. 5A and B). GNMT overexpression significantly inhibited LPS-induced increases of both nitrate/nitrite and iNOS (Figs. 5A and B).

Beneficial effects of GNMT overexpression in microglia

Microglial cultures were prepared and examined as to whether overexpressing GNMT in microglia was beneficial. Enriched microglia (>98% GSA-IB4-IR, Fig. 6A) was first seeded in a Millicell insert (1 μm PET; Millipore) and infected with Ad-GFP or Ad-GNMT (~10^4 pfu). These microglia-containing inserts were then transferred to a 24 well plate that had been seeded with cortical mixed neuron-glial cultures. The resultant co-cultures were maintained for 5 days. As shown in Figures 6B–D, Ad-GFP-infected microglia enhanced βIII tubulin(+) neuronal survival (6C compared to 6B) without direct cell–cell contact. Ad-GNMT-infected microglia further enhanced βIII tubulin(+) neuronal survival (6C compared to 6D). The Ad-GNMT-infected microglial cells alone were exposed to LPS (1 μg/ml) for 2 days. The resulting cultured media were collected and analyzed for nitrate/nitrite. Figure 6E shows that LPS strongly induced nitrate/nitrite release in microglial cultures. Ad-GNMT infection

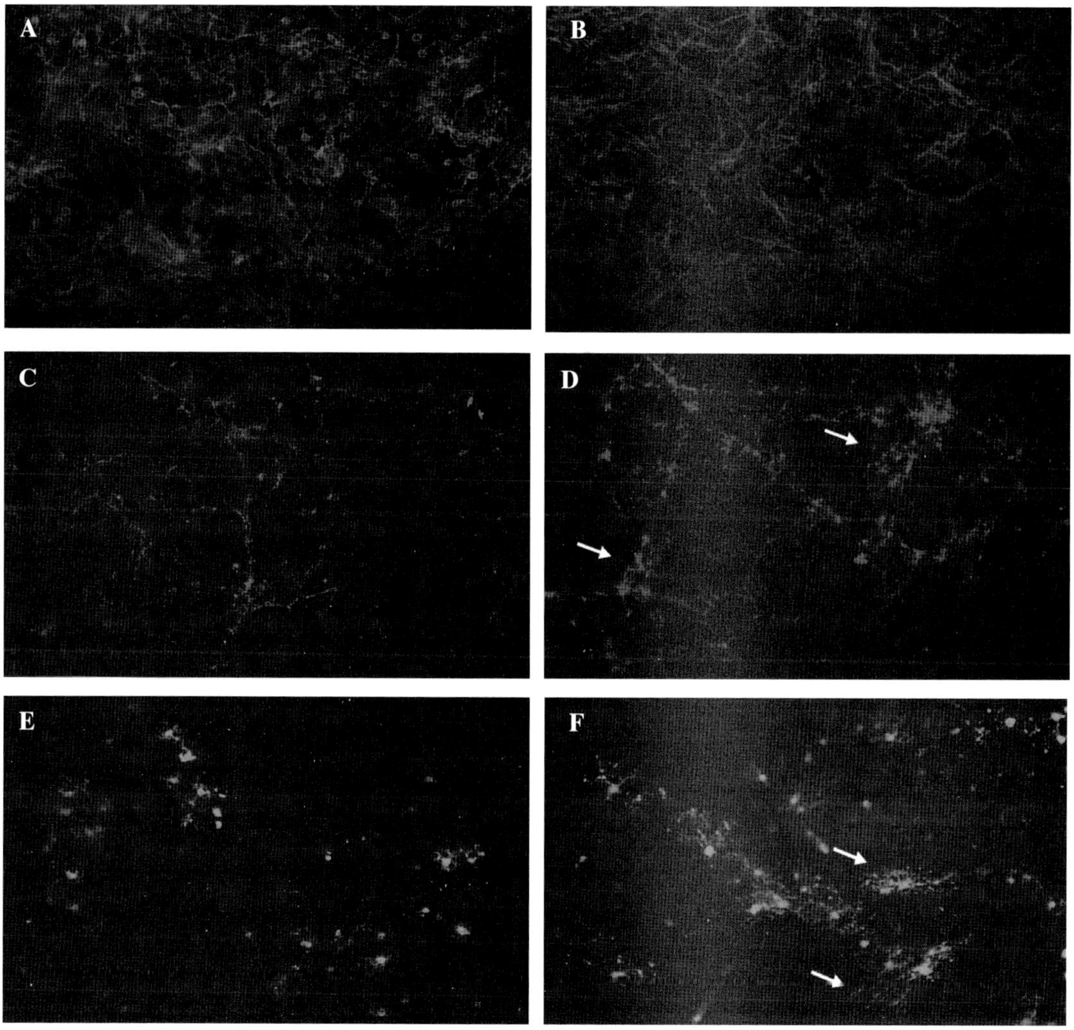

Figure 3. Ad-GNMT infection increases cell survival in cortical mixed neuron-glial cultures. Cells in the images have been treated as follows: (A), (C), and (E) are infected by Ad-GFP as a mock control, whereas (B), (D), and (F) are infected by Ad-GNMT. Cells in (A) and (B) are stained for MAP-2, a neuronal marker; cells in (C) and (D) are stained for SV2, a synaptic vesicle marker; cells in (E) and (F) are stained for myelin basic protein (MBP), an oligodendroglial marker. Arrows in (D) indicate more neurite connection; arrows in (F) indicate MBP (+) cells with longer processes.

significantly inhibited LPS-induced nitrate/nitrite release to the medium.

Discussion

GNMT is the most abundant hepatic methyltransferase and has been known to regulate the SAM:SAH ratio (i.e., methylation capacity). Because of the importance of GNMT in the liver and the small expression in the CNS, it is vital to understand its function in the CNS. We employed recombinant adenovirus encoding GNMT, allowing stable delivery of GNMT gene in primary CNS cultures. To our knowledge, this is the first time that GNMT has been shown to enhance neurite outgrowth in the CNS. Continuously enhanced GNMT expression not only increased neuronal survival but also protected cells from toxin challenge. This effect was, at least in part, mediated through PKC phosphorylation.

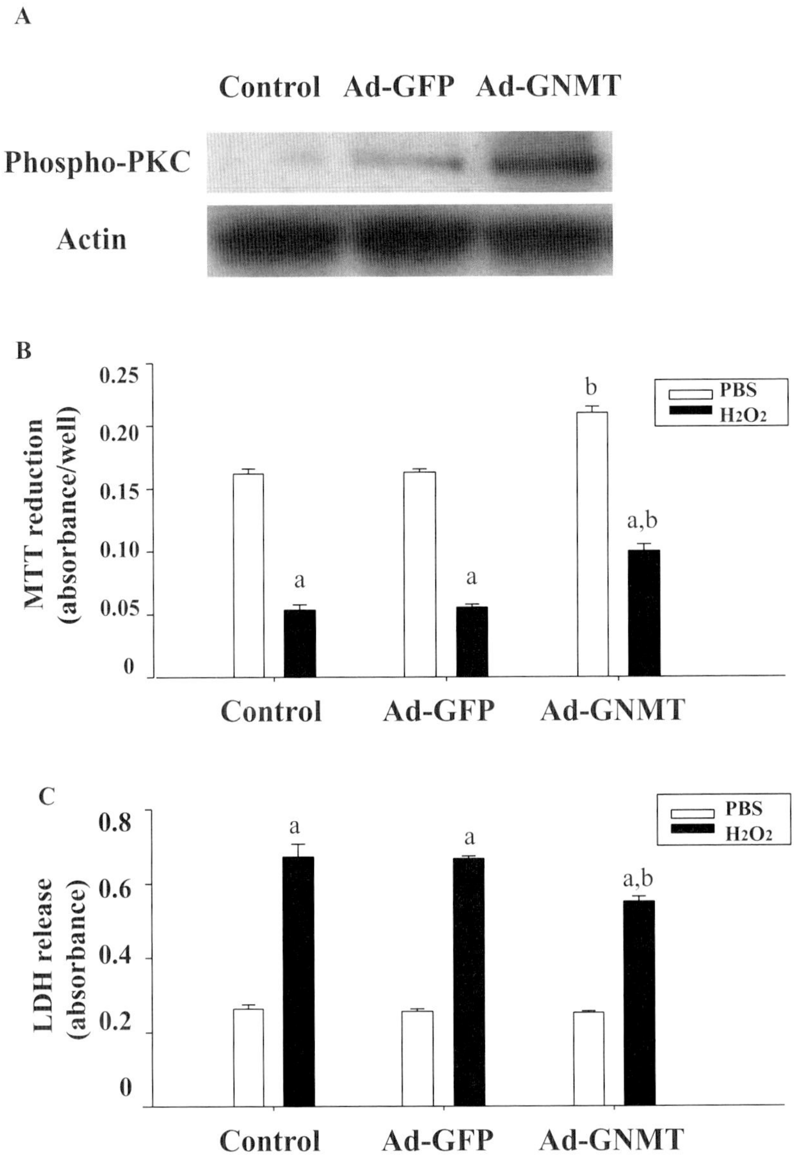

Figure 4. Ad-GNMT infection to mixed neuron-glial cultures increases the level of phosphorylated protein kinase C (pan phospho-PKC) and protects cells from H_2O_2-induced toxicity. (A) Western blot analysis phospho-PKC level in cultures 22 h after Ad-GFP or Ad-GNMT infection. (B) The degree of MTT reduction in cultures after exposing adenovirus-infected cells to H_2O_2 or vehicle. (C) Release of cytosolic lactate dehdyrogenase (LDH) in medium after treatment as in (B). [a]: $P < 0.05$ PBS versus H_2O_2-treated. [b]: $P < 0.05$ Ad-GNMT + H_2O_2 or Ad-GFP + H_2O_2 versus H_2O_2 only.

Expression of GFP or GNMT in Ads-infected cells is under the control of CMV promoter. About 18 h after recombinant adenoviral infection to cultured cells, the Ads-encoded proteins became detectable (our unpublished results). Consistent with this notion, phosphorylated PKC was selectively induced in Ad-GNMT-infected cells 22 h after adenoviral infection. This phosphorylated PKC was probed by antibodies against all pan-phosphorylated PKC. Because numerous isoforms

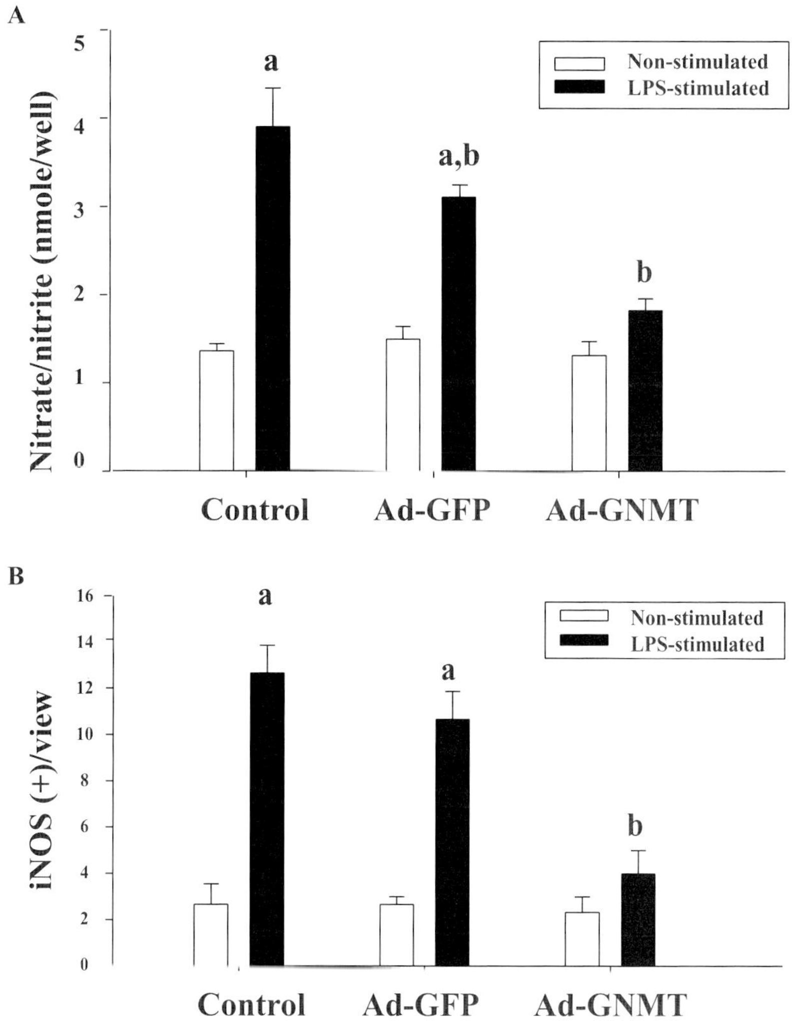

Figure 5. Ad-GNMT infection to mixed neuron-glial cultures reduces LPS stimulation. (A) Assay of nitrite/nitrate levels in cultured medium after exposing adenovirus-infected cells to LPS for 2 days. (B) Assay of nitric oxide synthase (iNOS) immunoreactive (IR) cells (per1.5 mm^2) in cultures after LPS stimulation. [a]: $P < 0.05$ non-stimulated versus LPs-stimulated. [b]: $P < 0.05$ Ad-GNMT/LPS or Ad-GFP/LPS versus LPS only.

of phosphorylated PKC have been reported, future work is required to identify the responsible PKC isoform.

Consistent with previous results,[17,18] in the present study recombinant adenovirus highly preferred infection to non-neuronal cells in mixed neuron-glial or glial cultures. The above-mentioned neuroprotective effect of Ad-GNMT infection was observed in a condition in which almost no neurons were infected in mixed neuron-glial cultures. In a transwell system that permits cell-contact-independent communication through diffusible soluble factors, Ad-GNMT-infected microglia promoted neuronal survival in co-cultures through diffusible soluble factors. Further, Ad-GNMT-infected microglia reduced LPS stimulation. This evidence suggests that GNMT overexpression might promote the release of neuroprotective agents from non-neuronal cells, thereby protecting neuronal cells. In order to obtain insights into the role of GNMT in neuroprotection and cerebral inflammation, further works will focus on proteomic analysis of diffusible soluble factors produced by Ad-GNMT-infected microglia.

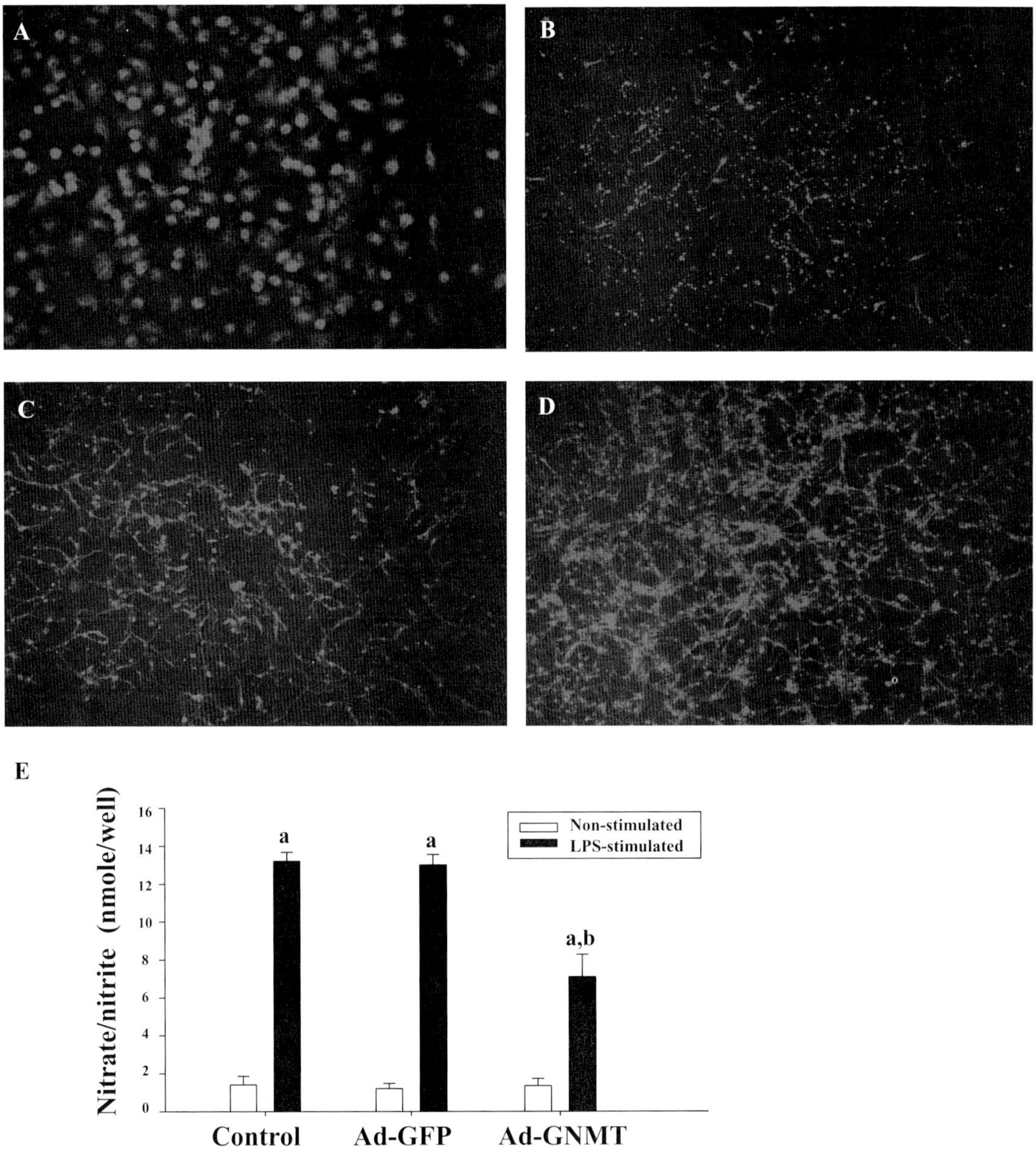

Figure 6. Beneficial effects of Ad-GNMT infection to microglial cells. Cells in the images have been treated as follows: (A) microglial cells only, stained for GSA-IB4; (B) mixed neuron-glial cultures after only 7 days *in vitro*; (C) mixed neuron-glial cultures co-cultured with microglial cells; and (D) mixed neuron-glial cultures co-cultured with Ad-GNMT-infected microglial cells. Cells in (B), (C), and (D) are stained for βIII tubulin, a neuronal marker. (E) Assay of nitrite/nitrate levels in cultured medium of Ads-infected microglia two days after exposure to LPS.[a]: $P < 0.05$ non-stimulated versus LPS-stimulated; [b]: $P < 0.05$ Ad-GNMT/LPS or Ad-GFP/LPS versus LPS.

Although the precise cellular targets for overexpressed GNMT remain to be determined, our data support an emerging new function of GNMT in the nervous system and will provide insight into the mechanisms of nerve regeneration. It would also bring us significantly closer to devising therapeutic approaches to encourage the growth of axons after, say, spinal cord injury.

Acknowledgments

This work was supported by grants from the Republic of China (ROC) National Science Council (NSC96-3112-B-010-018 & 97-3112-B-010-010), from Taipei Veterans General Hospital (V96S6-001 & V97S6-001) and a grant from the ROC Ministry of Education, Aim for the Top University Plan, Taiwan.

Conflicts of interest

The authors declare no conflicts of interest.

References

1. Berridge, M.V. & A.S. Tan. 1993. Characterization of the cellular reduction of 3-(4,5-dimethylthiazol-2-yl)-2,5-diphenyltetrazolium bromide (MTT): subcellular localization, substrate dependence, and involvement of mitochondrial electron transport in MTT reduction. *Arch. Biochem. Biophys.* **303:** 474–482.
2. Chen, S.Y. *et al.* 2004. Glycine N-methyltransferase tumor susceptibility gene in the benzo(a)pyrene-detoxification pathway. *Cancer Res.* **64:** 3617–3623.
3. Chen, Y.M. *et al.* 1998. Characterization of glycine-N-methyltransferase-gene expression in human hepatocellular carcinoma. *Int. J. Cancer* **75:** 787–793.
4. Fawcett, J.W. *et al.* 1992. Axonal growth on astrocytes is not inhibited by oligodendrocytes. *J. Cell Sci.* **103**(Pt 2): 571–579.
5. Goldberg, J.L. & B.A. Barres. 2000. The relationship between neuronal survival and regeneration. *Annu. Rev. Neurosci.* **23:** 579–612.
6. Hung, H. *et al.* 2000. Age-dependent increase in C7-1 gene expression in rat frontal cortex. *Brain Res. Mol. Brain Res.* **75:** 330–336.
7. Lee, C.M. *et al.* 2006. Benzo[a]pyrene and glycine N-methyltransferse interactions: gene expression profiles of the liver detoxification pathway. *Toxicol. Appl. Pharmacol.* **214:** 126–135.
8. Liou, J.Y. *et al.* 2000. Colocalization of prostacyclin synthase with prostaglandin H synthase-1 (PGHS-1) but not phorbol ester-induced PGHS-2 in cultured endothelial cells. *J. Biol. Chem.* **275:** 15314–15320.
9. Liu, H.H. *et al.* 2003. Characterization of reduced expression of glycine N-methyltransferase in cancerous hepatic tissues using two newly developed monoclonal antibodies. *J. Biomed. Sci.* **10:** 87–97.
10. Markus, A., T.D. Patel & W.D. Snider. 2002. Neurotrophic factors and axonal growth. *Curr. Opin. Neurobiol.* **12:** 523–531.
11. McCarthy, K.D. & J. de Vellis. 1980. Preparation of separate astroglial and oligodendroglial cell cultures from rat cerebral tissue. *J. Cell Biol.* **85:** 890–902.
12. McKerracher, L. & H. Higuchi. 2006. Targeting Rho to stimulate repair after spinal cord injury. *J. Neurotrauma.* **23:** 309–317.
13. Sandvig, A. *et al.* 2004. Myelin-, reactive glia-, and scar-derived CNS axon growth inhibitors: expression, receptor signaling, and correlation with axon regeneration. *Glia* **46:** 225–251.
14. Shyue, S.K. *et al.* 2001. Selective augmentation of prostacyclin production by combined prostacyclin synthase and cyclooxygenase-1 gene transfer. *Circulation* **103:** 2090–2095.
15. Tsai, M.J. & E.H. Lee. 1994. Differences in the disposition and toxicity of 1-methyl-4-phenylpyridinium in cultured rat and mouse astrocytes. *Glia* **12:** 329–335.
16. Tsai, M.J. & E.H. Lee. 1998. Nitric oxide donors protect cultured rat astrocytes from 1-methyl-4-phenylpyridinium-induced toxicity. *Free Radic. Biol. Med.* **24:** 705–713.
17. Tsai, M.J. *et al.* 2005. Effect of enhanced prostacyclin synthesis by adenovirus-mediated transfer on lipopolysaccharide stimulation in neuron-glia cultures. *Ann. N.Y. Acad. Sci.* **1042:** 338–348.
18. Tsai, M.J. *et al.* 2007. Dual effect of adenovirus-mediated transfer of BMP7 in mixed neuron-glial cultures: neuroprotection and cellular differentiation. *J. Neurosci. Res.* **85:** 2950–2959.
19. Tseng, T.L. *et al.* 2003. Genotypic and phenotypic characterization of a putative tumor susceptibility gene, GNMT, in liver cancer. *Cancer Res.* **63:** 647–654.
20. Wagner, K.A. *et al.* 1995. Effects of nonsteroidal antiinflammatory drugs on ulcerogenesis and gastric secretion in pylorus-ligated rat. *Dig. Dis. Sci.* **40:** 134–140.
21. Yeo, E.J. & C. Wagner. 1994. Tissue distribution of glycine N-methyltransferase, a major folate-binding protein of liver. *Proc. Natl. Acad. Sci. USA* **91:** 210–214.

Ann. N.Y. Acad. Sci. ISSN 0077-8923

ANNALS OF THE NEW YORK ACADEMY OF SCIENCES
Issue: *Neuroprotective Agents*

Neuromodulation

Advances in the next five years

Russell J. Andrews
NASA Ames Research Center (Smart Systems & Nanotechnology), Moffett Field, California
Address for correspondence: Russell J. Andrews, 50 East Hamilton Ave., Suite 120, Campbell, CA 95008.
rja@russelljandrews.org

Neuromodulation (deep brain stimulation; DBS) has become an established treatment for movement disorders (e.g., Parkinson's disease), and is in trials for refractory epilepsy, headache, and certain mood disorders. Two main themes will advance DBS significantly in the next five years: closed-loop DBS, that is, feedback from brain electrical activity to direct the stimulation; and computational analysis (CA)—electrophysiological modeling to enhance DBS. Closed-loop DBS is currently in clinical trials for refractory epilepsy. New imaging techniques offer preoperative modeling for DBS surgery, including nerve fiber tracts (diffusion tensor imaging), and imaging of volume of tissue activated by a specific electrode. CA techniques for DBS include mathematical models of the abnormally synchronized electrical activity which underlies epilepsy, movement disorders, and likely many mood disorders as well. By incorporating feedback loops and multiple recording and/or stimulating sites, the abnormally synchronized brain electrical activity can be desynchronized, then "unlearned" ("unkindling" in epilepsy). Characteristics of DBS utilizing CA include low frequency rather than high frequency stimulation; multiple stimulation and/or recording sites; likely 10-fold or more reduction in electrical current needs (much smaller "pulse generators"); more focused and less disruptive stimulation—fewer unwanted side effects; and potential to "cure" certain disorders by resetting abnormal firing patterns back to normal. These advantages of more sophisticated DBS techniques bring the following challenges, which may require a decade of research before reaching clinical practice because many brain disorders involve neurotransmitter abnormalities (e.g., dopamine in Parkinson's disease and certain mood disorders). Namely, how do we monitor and modulate neurotransmitters in addition to electrical activity? How do we get multiple microelectrodes into the brain in a minimally invasive manner? In the accompanying article, I address these two issues and offer some potential solutions.

Keywords: computational analysis; deep brain stimulation; depression; epilepsy; mood disorders; movement disorders; neuromodulation

Introduction

A major type of neuromodulation—deep brain stimulation (DBS)—has been reviewed (both historical development and current techniques) in previous *Annals* volumes and elsewhere.[1–3] To summarize: over the past 15 years DBS has become an established treatment for movement disorders (e.g., Parkinson's disease) refractory to medications alone. Clinical trials are ongoing with DBS in the treatment of refractory epilepsy, mood disorders (e.g., depression, obsessive-compulsive disorder), headache, and other nervous system disorders.

Current DBS techniques utilize an electrode 1.27 mm in diameter placed stereotactically into a specific nucleus or region of the brain, for example, in Parkinson's disease the subthalamic nucleus is the primary stimulation site (see Figs. 1A and 1B). The drawbacks of the current DBS technique have been discussed in a previous *Annals* volume.[3]

Two major advances in DBS technique over the next five years or so should markedly improve the effectiveness of neuromodulation for various nervous system disorders, well beyond the current indications of movement disorders, such as Parkinson's disease, essential tremor, and dystonia.

doi: 10.1111/j.1749-6632.2009.05379.x

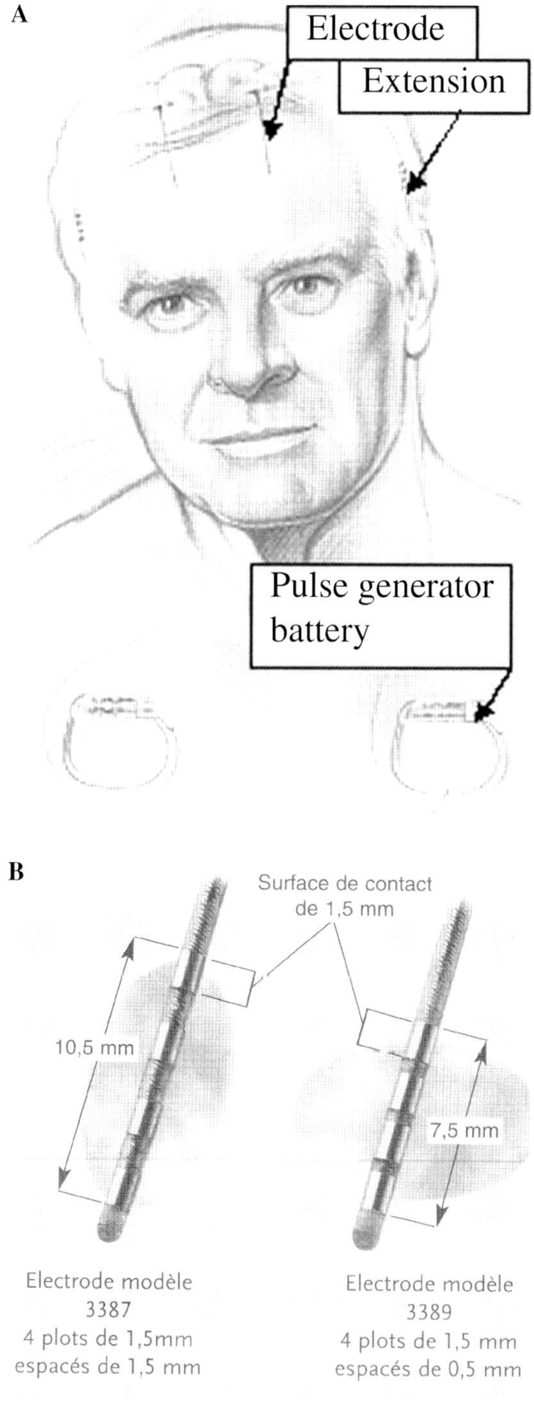

Figure 1. (A) Illustration of bilateral deep brain stimulator electrodes and pulse generators. (Courtesy of Medtronic Inc., Minneapolis, MN). (B) Close-up view of two deep brain stimulator electrode designs (1.27 mm diameter). (Courtesy of Medtronic Inc.).

Closed-loop deep brain stimulation

To date, DBS has employed constant stimulation to reversibly "jam" electrical activity in a volume of brain tissue defined by the electrode's location and the stimulation parameters, that is, which of the four electrodes are involved, type of stimulation (monopolar or bipolar), voltage, frequency (Hz), and pulse width (in ms). The stimulation is "dumb" in the sense that it is constant, and not guided by the changes in the brain's electrical activity relevant to the disorder being treated.

NeuroPace (Mountain View, CA) has developed a closed-loop DBS system for the treatment of refractory epilepsy (Figs. 2A–2C). Brain electrical activity is monitored by implanted electrodes (either cortical surface or depth electrodes) so that when an impending seizure is detected, a stimulating current can be given through an implanted electrode to abort the seizure. Although promising, closed-loop responsive neurostimulation for epilepsy has not yet identified the recording and stimulating sites that are effective in many patients with refractory epilepsy. However, the use of (abnormal) brain electrical activity to guide the stimulation is a clear advance over constant brain stimulation. Furthermore, implanting the "pulse generator" (battery and microprocessor) in the scalp/skull, rather than subcutaneously in the anterior chest wall, is also a significant advance in reducing a major source of complications, that is, infection and connector lead breakage.

Computational analysis and deep brain stimulation

Computational analysis (CA) in the form of computer modeling is already being used for planning optimal DBS electrode placement.[4–6] The marriage of (1) sophisticated imaging (MRI) with (2) data on electrical stimulation properties of brain tissue using standard DBS electrodes and parameters offers advantages in both planning electrode placement and in our understanding of DBS effects (e.g., on treating movement disorders) and unwanted side effects (Figs. 3A and 3B).

Much more significant for DBS in terms of efficacy in treating disorders of the nervous system is the incorporation of advanced stimulation techniques that are based on our present knowledge

A

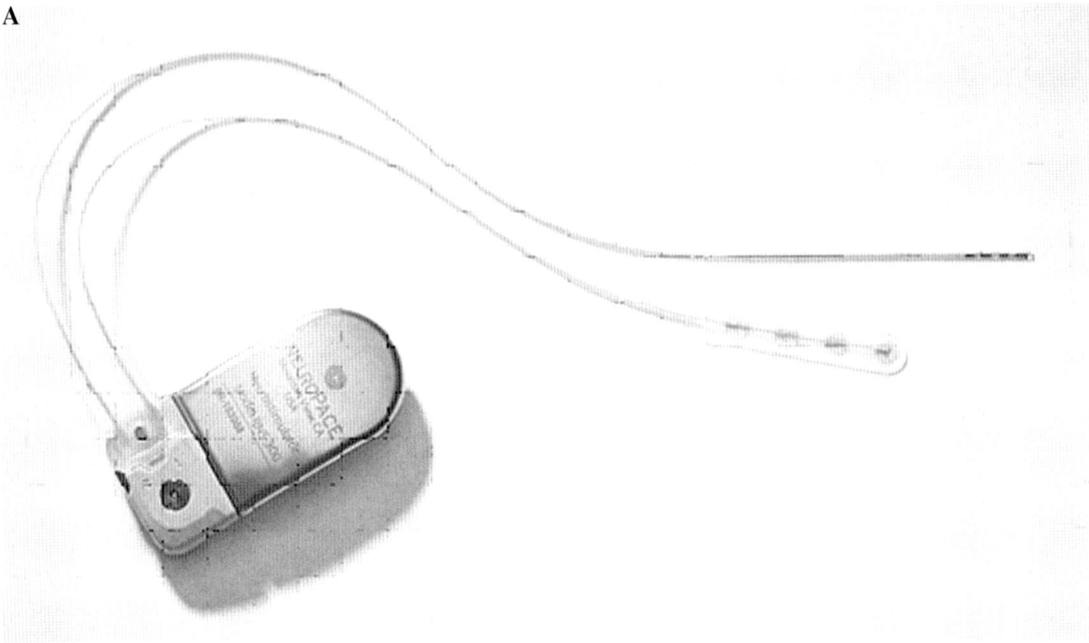

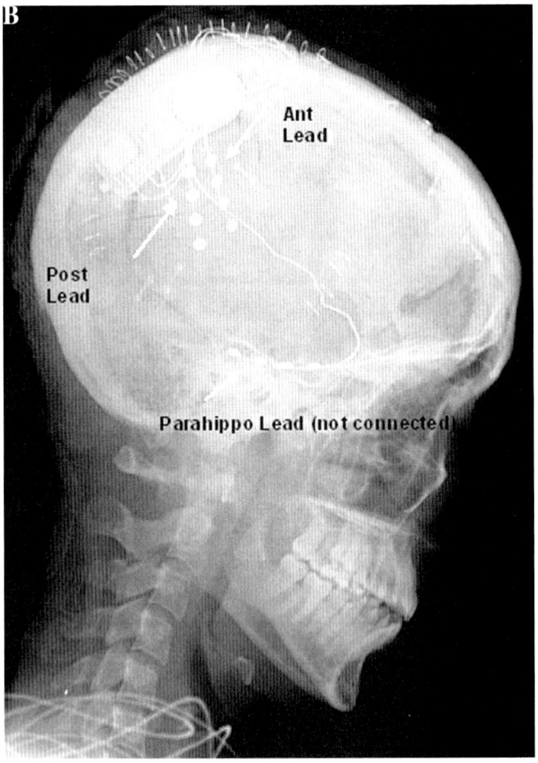

Figure 2. (A) NeuroPace responsive neurostimulation (RNS) device showing pulse generator plus recording and stimulating electrodes (Courtesy of NeuroPace Inc.). (B) Lateral skull radiograph showing NeuroPace RNS pulse generator implanted in the skull and electrodes (leads) (Courtesy of NeuroPace Inc.). (C) Electrocorticogram (ECoG) from implanted NeuroPace RNS system (Courtesy of NeuroPace Inc.).

C

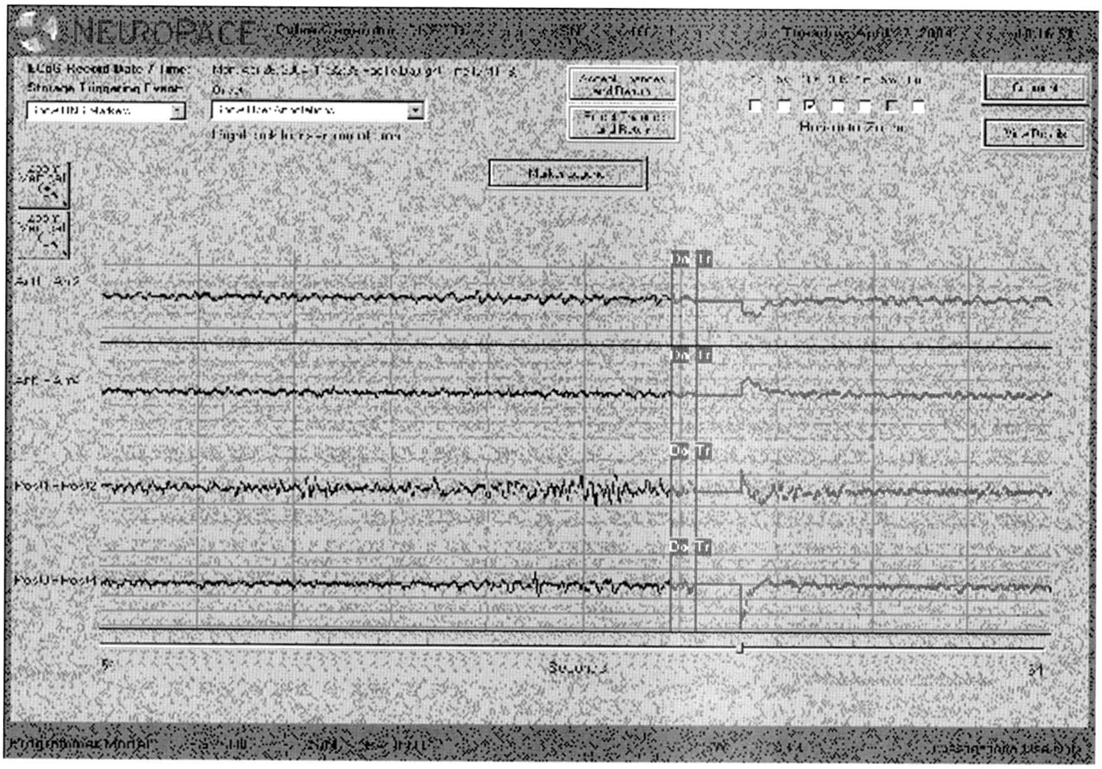

Figure 2. *Continued.*

regarding brain function in certain nervous system disorders. The use of (1) closed-loop feedback (as seen in the section above for epilepsy), (2) multiple stimulation electrodes, and (3) computational analysis techniques to maximize treatment efficacy while minimizing stimulation current requirements are all under investigation.[7–9]

Abnormal synchronization of brain electrical activity has been recognized in clinical syndromes, for example, epilepsy and movement disorders, for years. It has received more attention with the hypothesis that thalamocortical dysrhythmia (TCD)—an abnormal synchronization or coherence of brain electrical activity, particularly in the low-frequency (4 to 8 Hz) theta band—may underlie many nervous system disorders (Fig. 4).[10–12] Evidence from controls as well as patients with a variety of nervous system disorders—from epilepsy to Parkinson's disease to mood disorders to neurogenic pain—has shown that patients have an increase of coherence in the low-frequency range in particular, as shown on magnetoencephalography (MEG).[10] These findings, which are supported by EEG analysis in patients and intraoperative data from patients undergoing surgery for various disorders, offer a basis upon which to develop techniques of neuromodulation that might ameliorate the TCD.[13,14]

The present high-frequency DBS paradigm began two decades ago when Benabid in Grenoble found that a high-frequency (100 Hz or greater) current delivered through an electrode in the thalamus provided the same relief from tremor that an ablation in the same region provided.[15] Until the advent of computational modeling, little has changed regarding the electrode and the stimulation parameters. Several groups have recently shown that the use of (1) multiple stimulation electrodes, (2) closed-loop feedback, and/or (3) low-frequency stimulation may result in more effective and less costly (in terms of electrical energy consumed, yielding increased battery life) DBS.[7–9] Figure 5 shows the raster plot of the spike times for eight neurons in a model of the globus pallidus interna (GPi) in four conditions: normal, Parkinson's patient (untreated), Parkinson's patient (high-frequency DBS), and Parkinson's patient (low-frequency DBS determined by

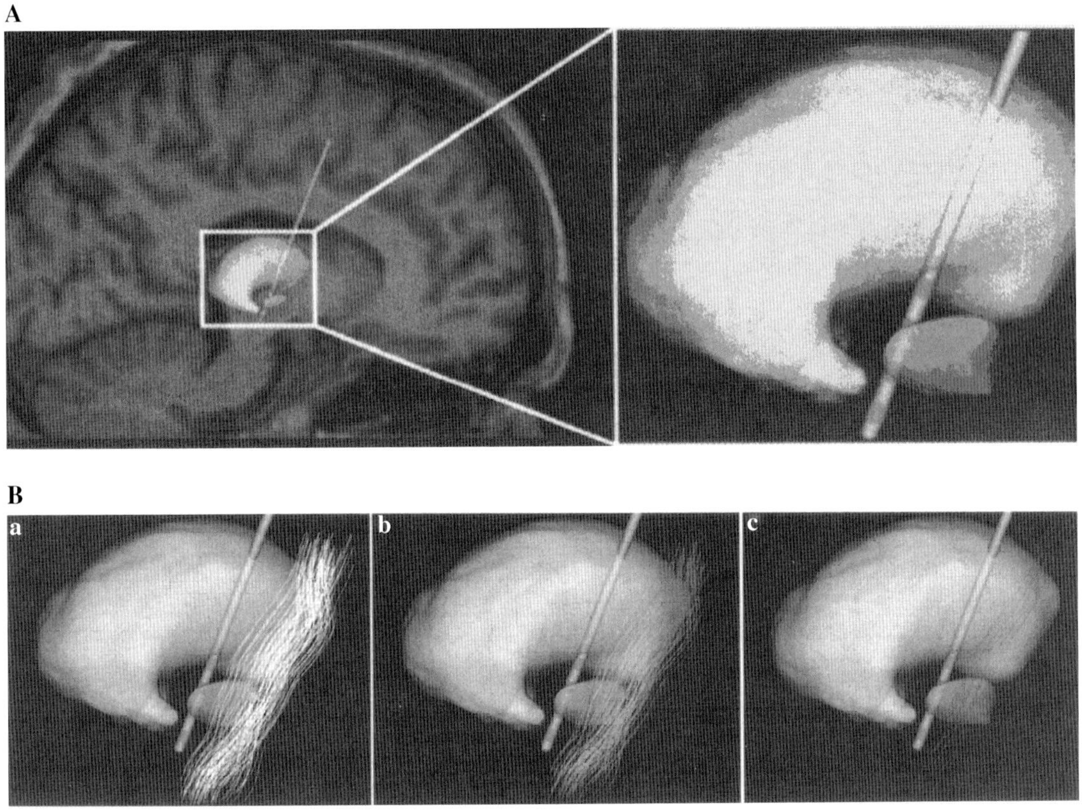

Figure 3. (A & B) A: MRI scan with 3D brain atlas thalamus (*yellow*), subthalamic nucleus (*green*), and DBS electrode superimposed. B: a – Thalamus, subthalamic nucleus, and DBS electrode with 100 corticospinal tract (CST) fibers (*white*). b – With the red contact (#2) active, the more highly stimulated CST fibers are in red, the less highly stimulated CST fibers are in blue. c – Only the more highly stimulated fibers are shown (9 of 100). (Reproduced from Ref. 5, with permission.)

a closed-loop feedback computational analysis algorithm). High-frequency DBS has a "jamming" function; low-frequency feedback DBS largely restores the spike pattern (compare with the normal spike pattern above) and requires considerably less current.

One group in particular has investigated modeling the brain for DBS using computational analysis techniques.[8,9] They have considered the effect of stimulation in regions where the neuronal output is inhibitory rather than excitatory, and have also developed models using either multiple stimulation electrodes (up to four) or closed-loop feedback to guide the stimulation (or both). The following quote summarizes the four basic techniques considered; Figure 6 illustrates the findings in the four techniques for DBS:

> . . .we considered four different stimulation techniques: the known standard high-frequency DBS (SDBS), the multisite coordinated reset stimulation (MCRS), the multisite coordinated delayed feedback stimulation (MDFS), and the nonlinear delayed feedback stimulation (NDFS). These techniques have in common the goal of reducing the synchronized activity of the target population either by re-establishing a normal physiological activity in a highly synchronized population of neurons (MCRS, MDFS, or NDFS) or by reversibly mimicking a tissue lesioning (SDBS). SDBS employs a high-frequency pulse train, continuously applied through one or more stimulation sites. MCRS uses short pulse trains to subsequently reset subpopulations of the neuronal network,

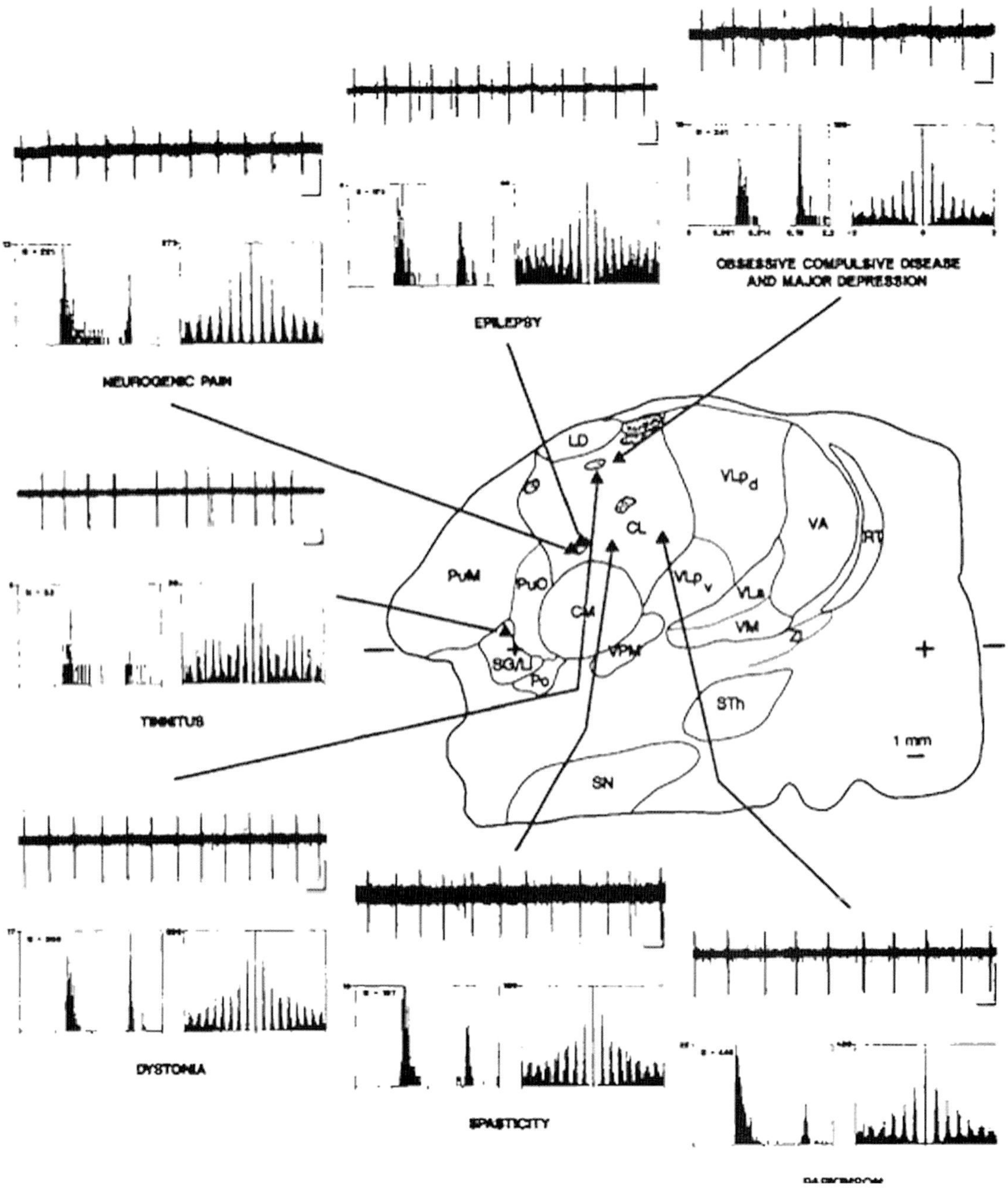

Figure 4. Examples of unit activities recorded in the medial thalamus (central lateral nucleus and suprageniculate-limitans complex) of 104 patients undergoing thalamotomy for one of the stated conditions (major depression and obsessive-compulsive disorder, epilepsy, neurogenic pain, tinnitus, dystonia, spasticity, and Parkinson's disease). The low-frequency (3 to 5 Hz) rhythmic bursting activity is analyzed by interspike interval (*left*) and autocorrelation histogram (*right*) in each disorder. Horizontal and vertical scale bars for unit activities are 200 ms and 100 mV, respectively. Further details are given in Ref. 12. (Reproduced from Ref. 12, with permission.)

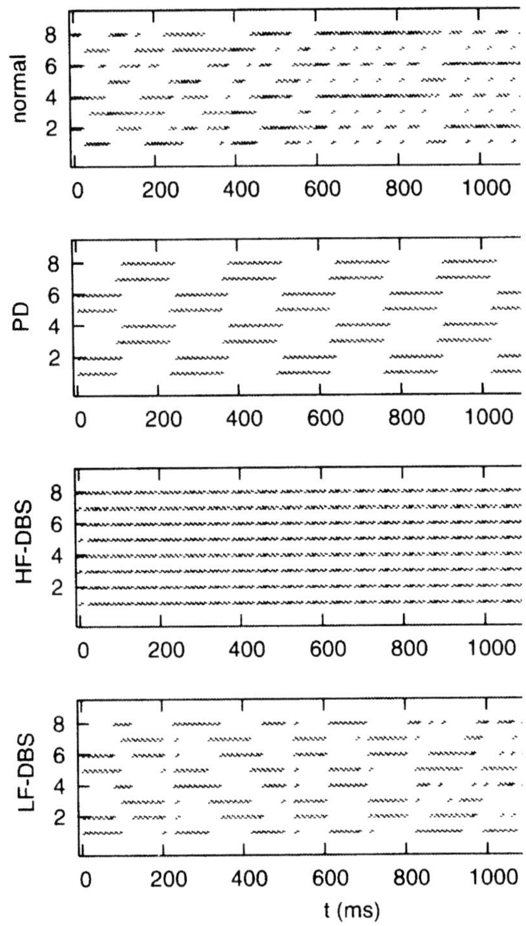

Figure 5. Raster plot of the spike times (firing patterns) in eight globus pallidus interna (GPi) neuronal cells under four different conditions: *Top* – normal; *Second* – Parkinson's disease; *Third* – Parkinson's disease with standard high-frequency DBS; *Bottom* – Parkinson's disease with low frequency closed-loop, computational analysis optimized DBS. (Reproduced from Ref. 7, with permission.)

> which induces a desynchronized state. Here, the stimulation was applied through a small number of stimulation sites that were equally spaced within the neuronal population. Desynchronization is achieved by MCRS by utilizing a self-organization principle, in particular, the slaving principle induced by the pathological neuronal interactions (i.e., interactions that have the potential to induce a pathological synchronization). The third and the fourth methods use delayed feedback for stabilizing a desynchronized state, which was intended to be as close to the physiological mode of action as possible. Here, the local field potential (LFP) of the target population was measured, amplified, delayed and fed back into the ensemble. (p. 634)[9]

Computational analysis is likely to provide significant advances in DBS efficacy because of the following:

- Low-frequency desynchronizing stimulation rather than high-frequency "jamming" stimulation increases efficacy and reduces electrical current requirements;
- Multiple electrodes for monitoring and/or recording facilitate resetting to normal neuronal firing patterns;
- Reduction in unwanted side effects due to more focused, precise stimulation techniques;
- Pulse generators located in the skull or scalp because electrical current requirements are reduced; and
- Potential "cure" for certain disorders by returning the abnormal neuronal firing patterns to normal.

Challenges for neuromodulation after the next five years

The advantages of closed-loop feedback and sophisticated computational analysis are quite straightforward in principal, although much laboratory and clinical research will be needed to realize their full potential. Additional challenges are apparent that will likely take longer to solve, but offer even more potential advantages for truly "curative" neuromodulation:

- Because the brain communicates both electrically and chemically (i.e., through neurotransmitters), the most effective treatments for disorders ranging from epilepsy to Parkinson's disease to mood disorders are likely to involve returning both neurotransmitters (concentration and distribution) and electrical firing patterns back to normal. Abnormalities in dopamine appear to underlie both Parkinson's disease and certain mood disorders.
- In order to precisely "retune" complex neuronal networks, large numbers of electrodes may be required. How will multiple electrodes be inserted into the brain in a

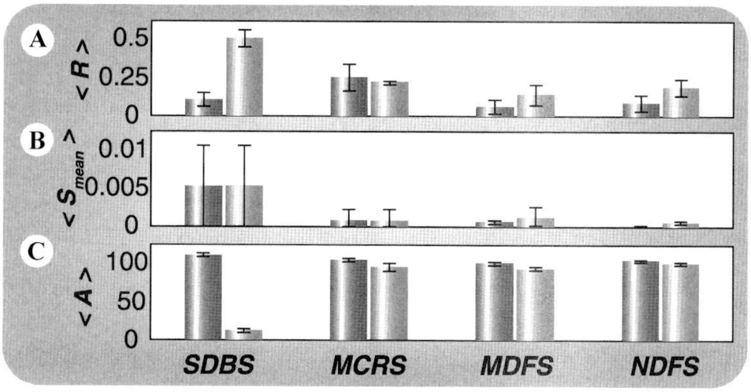

Figure 6. Comparison of four stimulation techniques. In each of the four, the left column is the result when the stimulation output or effect is excitatory and the right column the result when the stimulation output or effect is inhibitory. A: R = measure of synchronization. B: S = stimulation current required. C: A = measure of relative burst rate (percentage of bursting compared with unstimulated condition). SDBS: standard high-frequency DBS; MCRS: multisite coordinated reset stimulation; MDFS: multisite coordinated delayed feedback stimulation; NDFS: nonlinear delayed feedback stimulation. (Reproduced from Ref. 9, with permission.)

minimally invasive manner? In the accompanying article, we address these two issues and offer some potential solutions.

Conflicts of interest

The author declares no conflicts of interest.

References

1. Andrews, R.J. 2003. Neuroprotection trek—the next generation: neuromodulation I. Techniques—deep brain stimulation, vagus nerve stimulation, and transcranial magnetic stimulation. *Ann. N.Y. Acad. Sci.* **993:** 1–13.
2. Gildenberg, P.L. 2005. Evolution of neuromodulation. *Stereotact. Funct. Neurosurg.* **83:** 71–79.
3. Andrews, R.J. 2007. Neuroprotection at the nanolevel—Part II Nanodevices for neuromodulation—deep brain stimulation and spinal cord injury. *Ann. N.Y. Acad. Sci.* **1122:** 185–196.
4. McIntyre, C.C. *et al.* 2006. Optimizing deep brain stimulation parameter selection with detailed models of the electrode-tissue interface. In *Proc. 28th IEEE EMBS Conf.*: 893–895. IEEE. New York, NY.
5. Chaturvedi, A. *et al.* 2006. Subthalamic nucleus deep brain stimulation: accurate axonal threshold prediction with diffusion tensor based electric field models. In *Proc. 28th IEEE EMBS Conf.*: 1240–1243. IEEE. New York, NY.
6. McIntyre, C.C., S. Miocinovic & C.R. Butson. 2007. Computational analysis of deep brain stimulation. *Expert. Rev. Med. Devices* **4:** 615–622.
7. Feng, X.J. *et al.* 2007. Toward closed-loop optimization of deep brain stimulation for Parkinson's disease: concepts and lessons from a computational model. *J. Neural Eng.* **4:** L14–L21.
8. Hauptmann, C. & P.A. Tass. 2007. Therapeutic rewiring by means of desynchronizing brain stimulation. *Biosystems* **89:** 173–181.
9. Hauptmann, C., O. Popovych & P.A. Tass. 2007. Desynchronizing the abnormally synchronized neural activity in the subthalamic nucleus: a modeling study. *Expert Rev. Med. Devices* **4:** 633–650.
10. Llinas, R.R. *et al.* 1999. Thalamocortical dysrhythmia: a neurological and neuropsychiatric syndrome characterized by magnetoencephalography. *PNAS* **96:** 15222–15227.
11. Llinas, R.R. & M. Steriade. 2006. Bursting of thalamic neurons and vigilance. *J. Neurophysiol.* **95:** 3297–3308.
12. Jeanmonod, D., M. Magnin & A. Morel. 1996. Low-threshold calcium spike bursts in the human thalamus: common physiopathology for sensory, motor and limbic positive symptoms. *Brain* **119:** 363–375.
13. Sarnthein, J. *et al.* 2006. Increased EEG power and slowed dominant frequency in patients with neurogenic pain. *Brain* **129:** 55–64.
14. Sarnthein, J. & D. Jeanmonod. 2007. High thalamocortical theta coherence in patients with Parkinson's disease. *J. Neurosci.* **27:** 124–131.
15. Benabid, A.L. *et al.* 1987. Combined (thalamotomy and stimulation) stereotactic surgery of the VIM thalamic nucleus for bilateral Parkinson disease. *Appl. Neurophysiol.* **50:** 344–346.

Ann. N.Y. Acad. Sci. ISSN 0077-8923

ANNALS OF THE NEW YORK ACADEMY OF SCIENCES
Issue: *Neuroprotective Agents*

Neuromodulation

Advances in the next decade

Russell J. Andrews
NASA Ames Research Center (Smart Systems & Nanotechnology), Moffett Field, California
Address for correspondence: Russell J. Andrews, 50 East Hamilton Ave., Suite 120, Campbell, CA 95008.
rja@russelljandrews.org

Many nervous system disorders (e.g., Parkinson's disease, mood disorders) involve neurotransmitters as well as electrical activity. Pharmacologic treatment does not target the precise location(s) where neurotransmitter imbalances occur. Additionally, non-neuronal cells in the brain—notably astrocytes—influence neuronal activity through both electrical and neurochemical modulation of nearby neurons. Precise monitoring/recording and modulating/stimulating (both electrical and neurochemical) can optimize therapy in specific disorders and specific patients. Carbon-fiber microelectrodes (5 μm diameter) in freely moving rodents have shown that dopamine release is heterogeneous within various regions in the nucleus accumbens, a region involved in many mood disorders. Because neurons are only several microns in diameter (axons, dendrites, and synaptic clefts smaller still), ultramicroelectrodes will be essential to selectively monitor/modulate the cell body, the axon, or at the intracellular level. Nanoelectrode arrays can monitor both electrical activity and dopamine in real time with submicron resolution, and stimulate neurons with equal precision. Computational models indicate that precise monitoring/modulating (electrically and neurochemically) at the subnucleus or neuron level will be necessary to restore normal firing patterns and neurotransmitter levels in many brain disorders. Endovascular techniques can introduce ultramicroelectrodes (0.5 micron or smaller) into the brain via capillaries; such electrodes can stimulate/record neuronal tissue with a response virtually identical to extra-vascular microelectrodes. Within the next decade, hundreds if not thousands of submicron-sized monitoring/modulating electrodes can be placed wherever needed to restore brain function to normal. The term "neuromodulation" will likely replace deep brain stimulation (DBS) as both neurochemistry and electrical activity are included in the therapeutic modalities.

Keywords: carbon nanotubes; deep brain stimulation; dopamine; mood disorders; movement disorders; nanoelectrode arrays; neuromodulation; neurotransmitters

Introduction

A comprehensive explanation of many brain disorders, notably Parkinson's disease and severe depression, must consider the neurotransmitter abnormalities as well as the overly synchronized electrical activity described in the accompanying article. This has ramifications for treatment in that the current first-line interventions for Parkinson's disease and many mood disorders are medications taken orally that are intended to restore neurotransmitters in the brain, such as dopamine and serotonin, to more normal levels. Like the precision required for more accurate restoration of neuronal firing pattern abnormalities in brain disorders, more precise amelioration of neurotransmitter abnormalities will be necessary in the future.

Neuropharmacology as well as electrophysiology

Unfortunately, oral medications result in changes in neurotransmitters throughout the brain, whereas the abnormal concentrations are in discreet sites. This can produce unwanted side effects, much as slightly misplaced deep brain stimulation (DBS) electrodes can produce potentially serious side effects. The need for more targeted interventions

doi: 10.1111/j.1749-6632.2009.05380.x

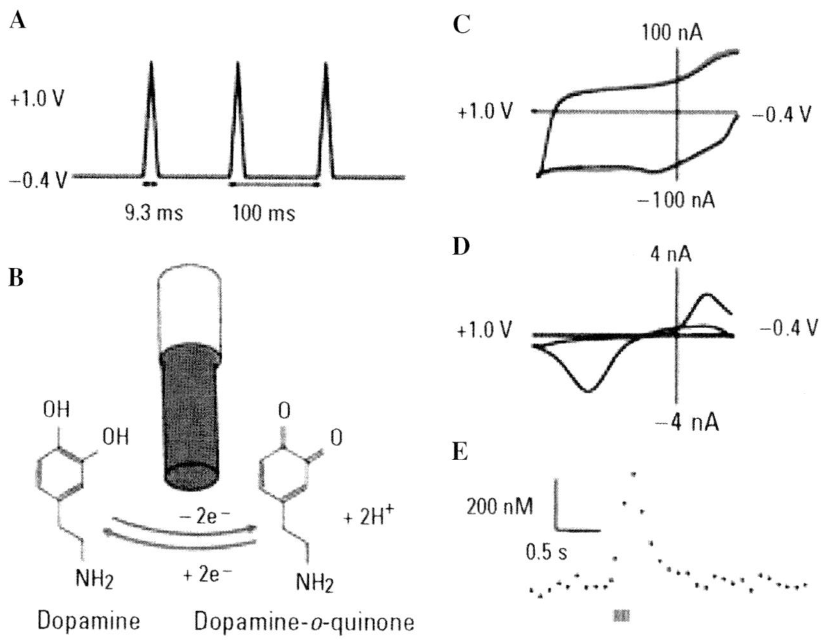

Figure 1. Fast-Scan Cyclic Voltammetry (FSCV). (A) Electrode potential is scanned from −1.4 to +1.0 V and back every 100 ms at 300 V/s. (B) Dopamine is oxidized to dopamine-o-quinone and then reduced back to dopamine. (C) *Black line:* large background charging current of the electrode. *Red line:* small changes in the presence of dopamine. (D) Subtracting the black line from the red line in (C) produces the cyclic voltammogram "fingerprint" for dopamine. (E) The current at the oxidation potential is converted to concentration (using an *in vitro* calibration value) which is plotted versus time to monitor dopamine concentration changes after brief electrical stimulation (4 pulses at 100 Hz, indicated by hash marks). (Reproduced from Ref. 3, with permission.)

affecting neurotransmitter abnormalities in Parkinson's disease and mood disorders has been addressed.[1] The need for models and computational analysis that takes into account pharmacological (including neurotransmitter) effects as well as electrophysiological effects has also been addressed.[2]

Continuous measurement of changes in neurotransmitter concentrations (notably dopamine, which is electrochemically active or oxidizable) *in vivo* has been made possible by fast-scan cyclic voltammetry (FSCV) using carbon-fiber microelectrodes as small as 5 μm diameter[3] (see Fig. 1). Severe depression is correlated with deficits in dopamine in the nucleus accumbens in the ventral striatum, a region which interacts with both the limbic and motor control systems.[1] It has recently been shown, using FSCV in awake and unrestrained rats, that within the nucleus accumbens there are variations in dopamine release depending upon location—such spatial and temporal heterogeneity being previously undocumented.[4] These findings argue that submillimeter precision may be necessary for optimal restoration of neurotramsmitter levels in mood disorders.

Glial cells as well as neurons

Neuromodulation techniques, such as DBS, have focused on brain electrical activity and neuronal firing patterns. However, a major portion of the brain is composed of glial cells, including astrocytes. A recent review documents the evidence that astrocytes may release neurotransmitters (notably glutamate) through a vesicular (non-synaptic) mechanism[5] (see Fig. 2). The importance of this finding is indicated by the electrical coupling of neurons (synchronization of firing patterns) in the region of these glutamate-releasing astrocytes. In several different experiments, blocking synaptic transmission with tetrodotoxin failed to abolish this synchronization.[5] This suggests that glial cells, notably astrocytes, are likely to play a very important role in the abnormal synchronization of neuronal

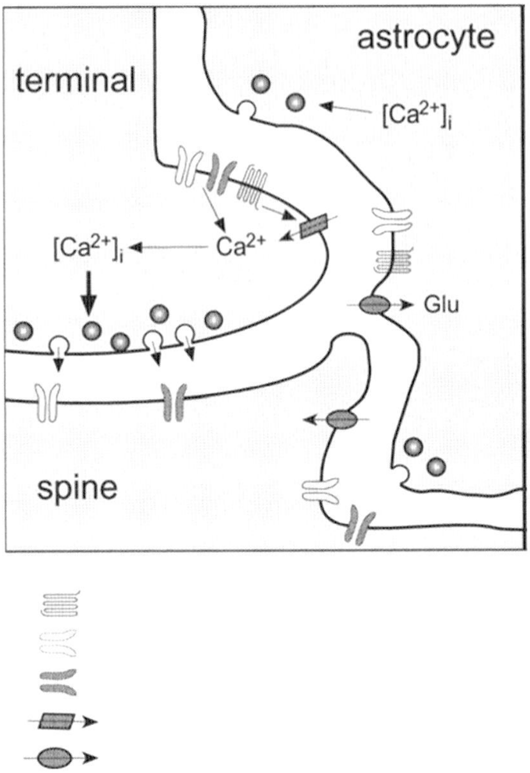

Figure 2. The tripartite synapse, bidirectional signaling between neurons and astrocytes. After Ca^{2+} entry into the presynaptic terminal, glutamate stored in vesicles is released and signals to the dendritic spine of a postsynaptic neuron. Glutamate can also reach astrocytic glutamate receptors leading to intracellular signaling, while a portion of this transmitter is taken up by surrounding astrocytes and stored, partially, in vesicular compartments. Vesicular glutamate is released by astrocytes upon an increase of $[Ca^{2+}]i$ via regulated exocytosis. The released glutamate can act on adjacent neurons through their pre- and postsynaptic glutamate receptors. Symbols: Top – Metabotropic glutamate receptors; 2nd – Non-*N*-methyl-D-aspartate (NMDA) receptors; 3rd – NMDA receptors; 4th – Voltage-gated Ca^{2+} channels; Bottom – Glutamate uptake. (Reproduced from Ref. 5, with permission.)

firing patterns that is a hallmark of many brain disorders (as described in the accompanying article).

The importance of astrocytes in neuronal firing patterns is already being considered in computational modeling. Data from experiments on the vesicular release of glutamate by astrocytes and its effect on paroxysmal depolarization shifts in surrounding neurons has been incorporated into a computational model.[6] Such complex models (more than a dozen parameters each for both the calcium oscillation and the vesicle cycles) represent a major advance in describing the complex interactions between glial cells and neurons. These interactions likely play a major role in the abnormal synchronization underlying many brain disorders.

Getting charged at the neuronal level

As described in the accompanying article, improved efficacy in neuromodulation (or DBS) will depend on multiple electrodes and more precise recording/stimulating electrodes. Several groups have recently reported dramatic improvements in both precision of stimulation (and recording) of neuronal activity using carbon nanotubes (CNTs).[7,8] This has included *in vitro* work with hippocampal neurons[7] and PC12 cells in neuronal networks.[8,9] Figure 3 is a scanning electron micrograph of the PC12 neural network on a bed of CNTs coated without (Fig. 3 *top*) or with (Fig. 3 *bottom*) a polypyrrole (Ppy) conductive polymer coating. The Ppy coating on the CNTs greatly reduces the $\sim$ 100 nm diameter fibrils that sprout from the PC12 cells, the fibrils being generally accepted as a response to local stress on the PC12 cell. As the close-up view (Fig. 4) shows, some CNTs actually penetrate the PC12 cell membrane which raises the possibility of intracellular recording.

The increase in precision that CNT arrays offer for neuromodulation will likely be overshadowed in importance by the increase in capacitance and decrease in impedance that Ppy-coated CNT arrays offer.[10–12] It was shown several years ago that CNT arrays coated with a conductive polymer, such as Ppy, could both (1) increase capacitance (or charge transfer, thus improving stimulation) on FSCV, and (2) decrease impedance (thus improving recording) by an order of magnitude or more in comparison with traditional metal microelectrodes.[9,10] This was taken a step further recently when standard microelectrodes were coated with CNTs (in turn coated with Ppy) and compared with uncoated microelectrodes both on impedance spectroscopy and FSCV as well as *in vivo*.[11,12] The CNT/Ppy coated electrodes showed a 23-fold decrease in impedance and a 45-fold increase in capacitance in comparison with gold microelectrodes (Fig. 5).

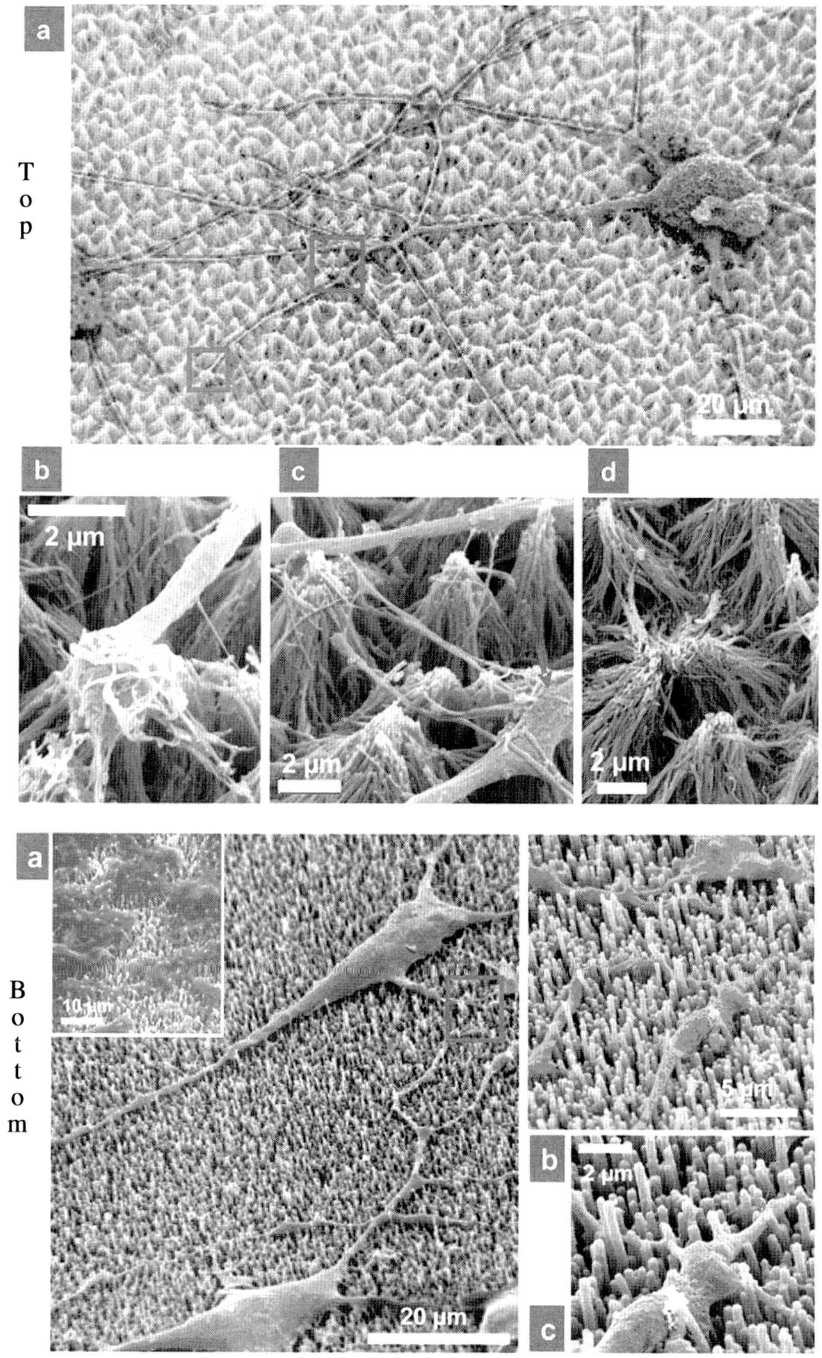

Figure 3. Scanning electron micrograph images of the PC12 neural network interpenetrating with free-standing carbon nanotubes (CNTs). *Top:* Collapsed microbundles of CNTs not coated with polypyrrole (Ppy). Note the abundance of ~100 nm diameter nanofibrils extending from the PC12 cell processes—a stress response. *Bottom:* A thin (~10 nm) coating of Ppy on the CNTs prevents their collapse into microbundles and also greatly reduces the nanofibrils seen in the top images. (Reproduced from Ref. 8, with permission.)

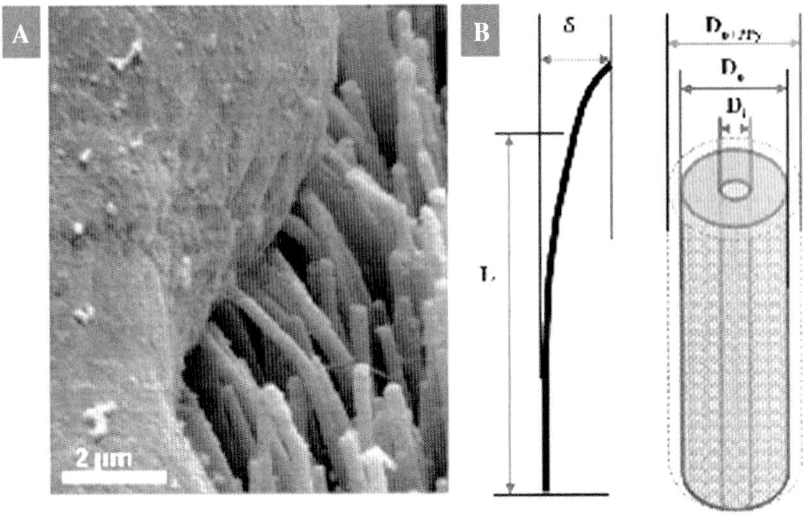

Figure 4. High-resolution scanning electron micrograph of interface between a PC12 cell and polypyrrole (Ppy)-coated carbon nanotubes (CNTs). (**A**) Ppy-coated CNTs maintain vertical alignment but are flexible enough to bend with the force of the cell body (and can penetrate the cell in some cases). (**B**) The parameters involved in the cell adhesion force derived from the bending of the CNTs. (Reproduced from Ref. 8, with permission.)

Measuring neurotransmitters as well as electrical activity

The importance of monitoring (and potentially modulating) neurotransmitter activity in the brain with anatomic precision has been noted above, for example, dopamine in Parkinson's disease and certain mood disorders. CNT arrays have been shown to be able to monitor dopamine levels with a detection level and response time far exceeding that of carbon-fiber microelectrodes.[9,12] Other electrochemically active or oxidizable neurotransmitters, such as serotonin, can be similarly monitored. The potential to monitor non-oxidizable neurotransmitters, such as glutamate—important in astrocyte-neuron interaction as noted above—is present with enzymatic functionalization of the CNT electrode.[12,13]

Addressing the brain precisely but minimally-invasively

A millenia ago—in the pre-wheel era especially—land travel for man was time-consuming, exhausting, and frequently dangerous. The waterways were utilized for efficient transport whenever possible. Similarly, trans-parenchymal "travel" in the brain for neuromodulation electrode placement is both inefficient and dangerous (risk of hemorrhage). The brain has "waterways" which reach every neuron and glial cell—the capillaries. As interventional neuroradiology becomes more sophisticated, utilizing the cerebral vasculature for minimally-invasive access to any region of the brain for electrode placement becomes more feasible. As described in the accompanying article, the future of neuromodulation likely depends on multiple—from dozens to hundreds or more—micron-sized electrodes placed with sub-nucleus, and possibly sub- or intracellular precision.

The use of capillaries for access to the nervous system for electrical recording and stimulating has been described.[14] Figure 6 illustrates the concept: sub-micron diameter catheter electrodes are placed in the regions of interest within the brain via the capillaries. Recording and stimulating from extracellular and intravascular electrodes yields remarkably similar results for both the peripheral nervous system (sciatic nerve) and the central nervous system (spinal cord) (Fig. 7).

Combining (1) the improvements in recording and stimulating obtained with conductive polymer (e.g., Ppy) coated CNT electrodes, with (2) minimally-invasive but precise access via the capillaries yields a major advance in neuromodulation.

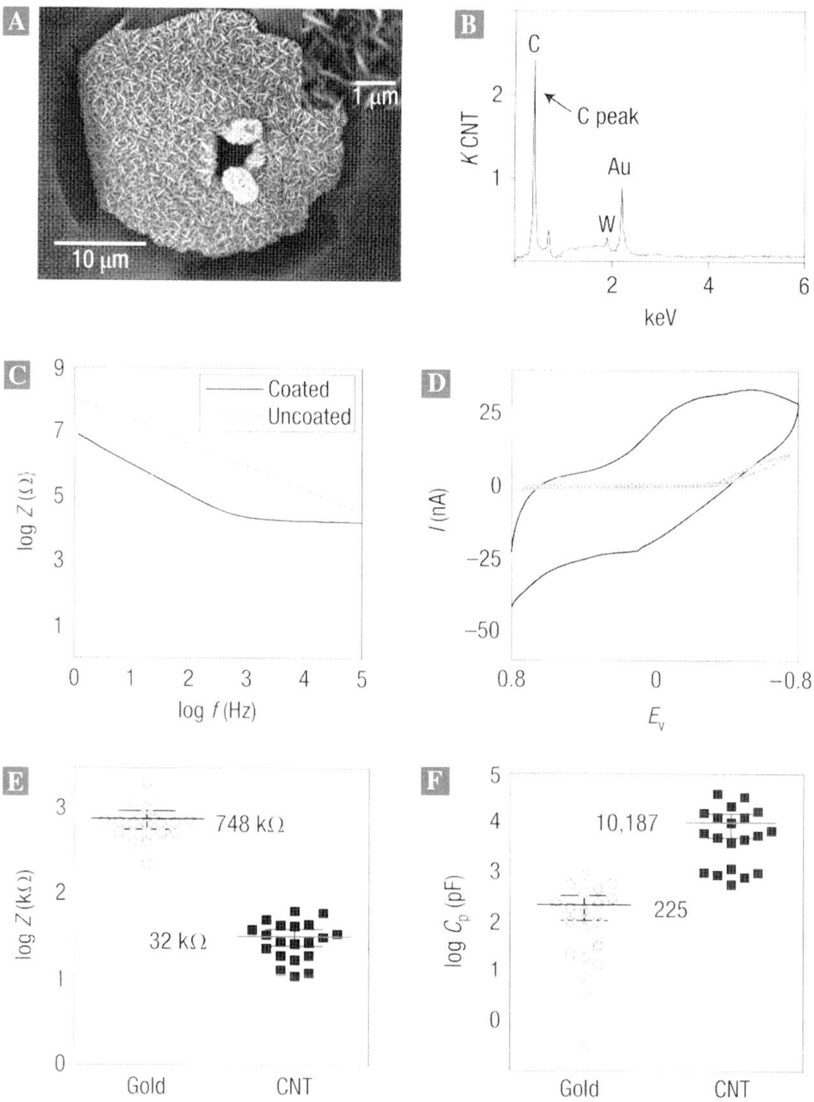

Figure 5. Impedance and charge-transfer characteristics of carbon nanotubes (CNT)-coated microelectrodes. (**A**) Scanning electron micrograph image of CNT-coated microelectrode. Crater formed by ablating the coating to access the iridium-tin oxide conductor. *Inset:* Porous character of the CNT coating. (**B**) Energy-dispersive x-ray analysis confirms carbon in the electrode coating. (**C**) Impedance spectroscopy scan shows decreased impedance at all frequencies (from 1×10^{-1} to 1×10^{5} Hz). (**D**) Fast-scan cyclic voltammetry (FSCV) shows a dramatic increase in charge transfer with CNT-coated microelectrodes. (**E**) 23-fold decrease in impedance with CNT-coated microelectrodes. (**F**) 45-fold increase in charge transfer with CNT-coated microelectrodes. (Reproduced from Ref. 11, with permission.)

It will allow a virtually limitless number of micron-sized electrodes to be placed with cellular-level precision wherever needed for neuromodulation. What remains is to integrate the computational analysis models of brain function (and dysfunction) with these novel electrodes.

Nonhierarchical neuromodulation

Another analogy may be helpful: the public dissemination of information by newspaper or television is both (1) hierarchical (there are only a handful of newspapers or TV channels) for

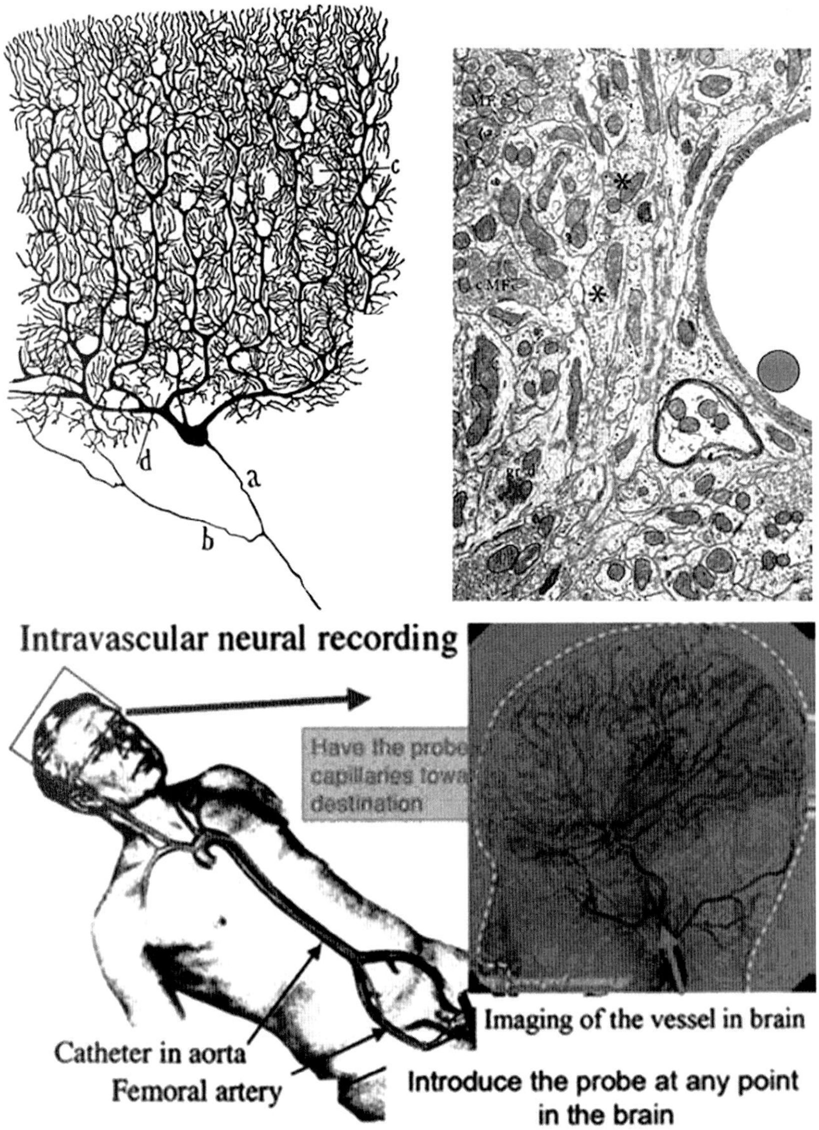

Figure 6. *Top: Left:* Purkinje cell showing spaces occupied by capillaries. *Right:* Electron micrograph through Purkinje cell dendrite including capillary (simulated electrode "dot" is 500 nm diameter). *Bottom*: Using endovascular neurointerventional techniques, nanoprobes may be delivered to capillaries anywhere in the brain. (Reproduced from Ref. 14, with permission.)

thousands to millions of individuals, and (2) unidirectional (apart from the "Letters to the Editor" or feedback polls, information flows from the editorial office to the populace—and not vice versa). This situation is similar to present-day single electrode, open-loop (no feedback) DBS. Computational analysis modeling indicates that next-generation neuromodulation will entail many electrodes guided by mutual feedback—there will be no single external pulse generator (battery and microprocessor), or in other words no "editor in chief." There will be constant fine-tuning among the many electrodes, each of which is constantly sampling and modifying at the cellular (neuronal and glial) level its

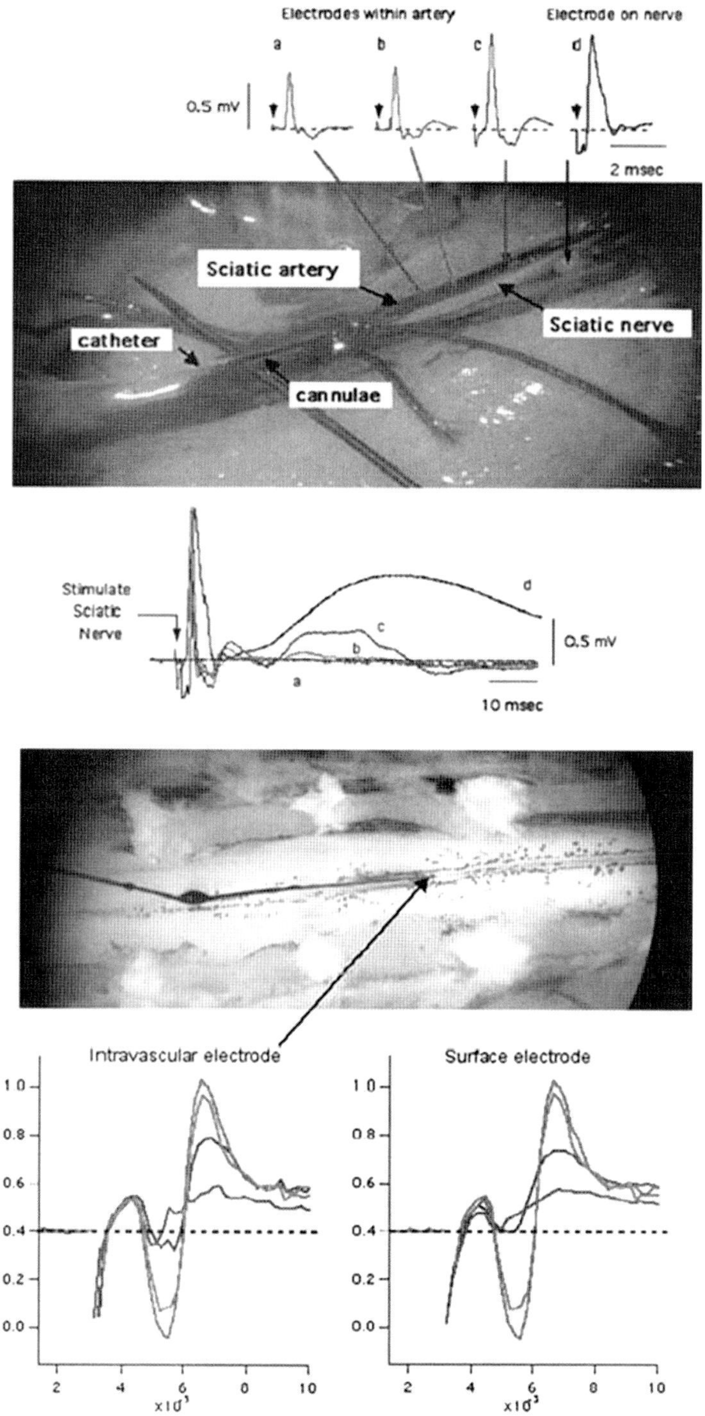

Figure 7. *Top:* Sciatic artery and nerve with intravascular (A,B,C) and surface extracellular (D) electrodes, with responses elicited by sciatic nerve stimulation. *Bottom:* Spinal cord with 1 μm intravascular electrode—comparing intravascular and extracellular recording as the stimulus amplitude is increased. Amplitude: mV, time: msec. (Reproduced from Ref. 14, with permission.)

particular electrical and chemical (neurotransmitter) environment.

To carry the analogy further, one may contrast centralized media (newspapers and TV) with the Internet (e.g., email, YouTube, MySpace, Twitter). In the latter, the communication is not via a central "clearinghouse" but rather individual to individual (or individual to group, or group to individual—in a feedback fashion). Nonhierarchical neuromodulation will use the "neural Internet" of computational analysis to provide constant information exchange between many (possibly thousands or millions) of electrodes which are monitoring local electrical and chemical activity at sites throughout the brain. The comparison has been made to the intelligence of "swarms" of robots, ants, bees, etc.[15,16]

By the end of the next decade we will likely relegate the stodgy "Encyclopedia Britannica" of brain atlases and fixed wiring diagrams dictating one-way neuromodulation to the Smithsonian Museum of Neuroscience. In its place will be a constantly interactive "Wikipedia" of electrical and chemical flux—a neuromodulatory "beehive" of activity guided by as yet undefined "swarm theories."

Conflicts of interest

The author declares no conflicts of interest.

References

1. Schlaepfer, T.E. 2008. Deep brain stimulation to reward circuitry alleviates anhedonia in refractory major depression. *Neuropsychopharmacology* **33:** 368–377.
2. Gillies A. & D. Willshaw. 2007. Neuroinformatics and modeling of the basal ganglia: bridging pharmacology and physiology. *Expert. Rev. Med. Devices* **4:** 663–672.
3. Venton, B.J. & R.M. Wightman. 2003. Psychoanalytical electrochemistry: dopamine and behavior. *Anal. Chem.* **75:** 414A–421A.
4. Wightman, R.M. *et al.* 2007. Dopamine release is heterogeneous within microenvironments of the rat nucleus accumbens. *Eur. J. Neurosci.* **26:** 2046–2054.
5. Ni, Y., E.B. Malarkey & V. Parpura. 2007. Vesicular release of glutamate mediates bidirectional signaling between astrocytes and neurons. *J. Neurochem.* **103:** 1273–1284.
6. Silchenko, A.N. & P.A. Tass. 2008. Computational modeling of paroxysmal depolarization shifts in neurons induce by glutamate release from astrocytes. *Biol. Cyber.* **98:** 61–74.
7. Wang, K. *et al.* 2006. Neural stimulation with a carbon nanotube microelectrode array. *Nano Lett.* **6:** 2043–2048.
8. Nguyen-Vu, T.D.B. *et al.* 2007. Vertically aligned carbon nanofiber architecture as a multifunctional 3-D neural electrical interface. *IEEE Trans. Biomed. Eng.* **54:** 1–8.
9. Andrews, R.J. 2007. Neuroprotection at the nanolevel—Part II Nanodevices for neuromodulation—deep brain stimulation and spinal cord injury. *Ann. N.Y. Acad. Sci.* **1122:** 185–196.
10. Nguyen-Vu, T.D.B. *et al.* 2006. Vertically aligned carbon nanofiber arrays: an advance toward electrical-neural interfaces. *Small* **2:** 89–94.
11. Keefer, E.W. *et al.* 2008. Carbon nanotube coating improves neuronal recordings. *Nat. Nanotech.* **3:** 434–439.
12. Parpura, V. 2008. Carbon nanotudes on the brain. *Nat. Nanotech.* **3:** 384–385.
13. Pantono, P. & W.G. Kuhr. 1993. Dehydrogenase-modified carbon-fiber microelectrodes for the measurement of neurotransmitter dynamics. 2. Covalent modification utilizing avidin-biotin technology. *Anal. Chem.* **65:** 623–630.
14. Llinas, R.R. *et al.* 2005. Neuro-vascular central nervous recording/stimulating system: using nanotechnology probes. *J. Nanopart. Res.* **7:** 111–127.
15. Beni, G. & J. Wang. 1989. Swarm intelligence in cellular robotic systems. *Proc. NATO Adv. Workshop Robots Biol. Sys.*
16. Miller, P. 2007. Swarm theory. *National Geographic* July 2007.

Ann. N.Y. Acad. Sci. ISSN 0077-8923

ANNALS OF THE NEW YORK ACADEMY OF SCIENCES
Issue: *Neuroprotective Agents*

Nanotechnology applications and approaches for neuroregeneration and drug delivery to the central nervous system

Gabriel A. Silva

Departments of Bioengineering, Ophthalmology and Neurosciences Program, University of California, San Diego, California

Address for correspondance: Dr. Gabriel A. Silva, MSc, PhD, UCSD Jacobs Retina Center, 9415 Campus Point Drive, La Jolla, CA 92037-0946. gsilva@ucsd.edu

Nanotechnology is the science and engineering concerned with the design, synthesis, and characterization of materials and devices that have a functional organization in at least one dimension on the nanometer (i.e., one billionth of a meter) scale. The potential impact of bottom up self-assembling nanotechnology, custom made molecules that self-assemble or self-organize into higher ordered structures in response to a defined chemical or physical cue, and top down lithographic type technologies where detail is engineered at smaller scales starting from bulk materials, stems from the fact that these nanoengineered materials and devices exhibit emergent mesocale and macroscale chemical and physical properties that are often different than their constituent nanoscale building block molecules or materials. As such, applications of nanotechnology to medicine and biology allow the interaction and integration of cells and tissues with nanoengineered substrates at a molecular (i.e., subcellular) level with a very high degree of functional specificity and control. This review considers applications of nanotechnology aimed at the neuroprotection and functional regeneration of the central nervous system (CNS) following traumatic or degenerative insults, and nanotechnology approaches for delivering drugs and other small molecules across the blood-brain barrier. It also discusses developing platform technologies that may prove to have broad applications to medicine and physiology, including some being developed for rescuing or replacing anatomical and/or functional CNS structures.

Keywords: nanotechnology; central nervous system; neuroregeneration; blood brain barrier

Introduction

Nanotechnology is in a broad sense the science and engineering concerned with the design, synthesis, characterization, and application of materials and devices that have a functional organization in at least one dimension on the nanometer (i.e., one billionth of a meter) scale, ranging from a few to about 100 nanometers. A nanometer is three orders of magnitude smaller then a micron, 10^{-9} versus 10^{-6}, respectively, and is roughly the size scale of molecules (e.g., a DNA molecule is about 2.5 nm long, while a sodium atom is about 0.2 nm). The potential impact of bottom up self-assembling nanotechnology, custom made molecules that self-assemble or self-organize into higher ordered structures in response to a defined chemical or physical cue, and top down lithographic type technologies where detail is engineered at smaller scales starting from bulk materials, stems from the fact that these nanoengineered materials and devices exhibit emergent mesocale and macroscale chemical and physical properties that are often different than their constituent nanoscale building block molecules or materials. As such, applications of nanotechnology to medicine and biology allow the interaction and integration of cells and tissues with nanoengineered substrates at a molecular (i.e., subcellular) level with a very high degree of functional specificity and control.

This article summarizes and is adapted from two previous reviews written by the author[1,2] and describes applications of nanotechnology aimed at the neuroprotection and functional regeneration of the central nervous system (CNS) following

doi: 10.1111/j.1749-6632.2009.05361.x

traumatic or degenerative insults, and nanotechnology approaches for delivering drugs and other small molecules across the blood-brain barrier (BBB). It also discusses developing platform technologies that may prove to have broad applications to medicine and physiology, including some being developed for rescuing or replacing anatomical and/or functional CNS structures. The interested reader is referred to other reviews and commentaries that discuss applications of nanotechnology to both basic and clinical neuroscience.[3–11]

Applications of nanotechnology to the CNS

Clinical nanotechnology applications to the CNS are further behind applications to other areas of medicine and biology, such as, for example, orthopedic applications, DNA/genomic sensors, and novel drug and gene delivery approaches (see for example Refs. 12–22). (The one exception to this are approaches for drug delivery across the blood-brain barrier,[23–26] which will be the subject of the next paper in this series.) This is in part due to some of the unique challenges imposed by the CNS, such as restricted and difficult anatomical access, an extremely heterogeneous cellular and molecular environment, and the complexities of the system's anatomical and functional "wiring" and associated information processing. Despite these challenges, the potential benefits of nanotechnologies for the treatment of both peripheral and CNS disorders are tremendous, and may eventually offer the patient and clinician novel therapeutic choices that simply do not exist today. True to the highly interdisciplinary nature of this area of research, it is important that technological advancements occur in conjunction with basic and clinical neuroscience advancements. Therefore, three things must occur in parallel for nanotechnology applications in neurology and neurosurgery to come to fruition: (1) advancements in chemistry and materials science that produce ever more sophisticated synthetic and characterization approaches; (2) advancements in the molecular biology, neurophysiology, and neuropathology of the nervous system; and (3) the design and integration of specific nanoengineered applications to the nervous system which take advantage of the first two points. As these areas develop in an integrated and parallel fashion, nanotechnology based applications for nervous system disorders should start to reach the clinic.

Neuroprotection

Free radical mediated injury is known to play a major role in the disease process of ischemic, traumatic, and degenerative disorders in the CNS.[27–35] Chemical species such as superoxide ($O_2^{-\bullet}$), hydroxyl ($^{\cdot}OH$), peroxynitrite ($ONOO^-$), and peroxide (H_2O_2) can produce a host of oxidative mediated deleterious changes in cells, including DNA fragmentation, peroxidation of cell membrane lipids, decreased mitochondrial energy production, and transporter protein inactivation.[29,33,35,36] One approach being developed to deal with this is the development of carbon-60 fullerene based neuroprotective compounds.[36–39] Fullerenes are molecules composed of large three dimensional arrays of evenly spaced carbon atoms, similar to the pattern produced by the rhombuses on a soccer ball. Fullerenols are hydroxyl (i.e., ^-OH) functionalized fullerene derivatives and have been shown to possess antioxidant and free radical scavenger properties that are able to reduce glutamate, *N*-methyl-D-aspartate (NMDA), α-amino-3-hydroxyl-5-methyl-4-isoxazole-propionate (AMPA), and kainite induced excitotoxic and apoptotic cell death.[36–39] The mechanism of fullerenol mediated neuroprotection is due at least in part to inhibition of glutamate channels, because neither GABA(A) or taurine receptors were affected. In addition, fullerenols appear to lower glutamate induced increases of intracellular calcium concentrations, a critical mechanism of excitotoxicity in neurons.[36–39]

Other approaches for neuroprotection, including pharmacological, gene therapy, and physiological, continue to be very active areas of research with significant clinical potential.[40–51] Fullerenols compliment these approaches by representing novel synthesis methods for the development of new neuroprotective compounds based on the controlled chemical manipulation and functionalization of these highly ordered synthetic structures. Given the proposed mechanism of fullerenol induced neuroprotection, it will be interesting to see what clinical applications develop for secondary injury following traumatic CNS disorders.

Neuroregeneration

The author's postdoctoral work in collaboration with colleagues focused on nanotechnology approaches for CNS regeneration following spinal cord injury and neural retinal degeneration.[52–55] Peptide amphiphile molecules, that is, peptide based molecules with a hydrophilic tail and hydrophobic head group, were designed to self-assemble into a network of nanofiber scaffolds only when present in physiological ionic conditions.[56–58] The surface of the nanofibers, made up of the hydrophilic head groups of aligned peptide amphiphile molecules, consisted of physiologically active peptide sequences designed to engage in cell signaling by acting as ligands for cell surface receptors. In our case the main peptide sequence we explored was the neuron specific extracellular matrix laminin-derived sequence isolucine-lysine-valine-alanine-valine (IKVAV),[53–55] which is known to promote the growth and development of neurites.[59–67] The peptide amphiphile molecules existed in a solution of water until they encountered physiological concentrations of cations, such as calcium, which triggered their self-assembly into nanofibers that "held" the water molecules in place, macroscopically forming a gel like substrate. Because of this unique property, we were able to encapsulate neural progenitor cells or neural retinal cells in these gels by mixing cell culture suspensions with peptide amphiphile solutions, trapping the cells in the interior of the gels. Because the functional peptide sequence formed the outer surface of the nanofibers, it allowed the functional signaling of encapsulated cells in three dimensions.

The results were quite dramatic, and in the case of encapsulated neural progenitor cells, included faster and more robust differentiation into mature neuronal phenotypes compared to controls. By 1 and 7 days *in vitro* 30% and 50%, respectively, of the neural progenitor cells expressed the mature neuron marker β-tubulin III.[53] We were also surprised to observe almost a complete exclusion of astrocyte development in these cultures (less than 1% and 5% at 1 and 7 days *in vitro*, respectively[53]), despite the multipotent nature of the progenitor cells. This suggests novel approaches for limiting the effects of reactive gliosis and glial scarring following traumatic or degenerative events by transplanting donor cells *in vivo* with the peptide ampiphile substrates. Similar results were observed with encapsulated retinal cells. The ultimate vision is for the peptide amphiphile solutions to be (minimally invasively) injected stereotaxically in combination with donor cells, have the nanofiber network form *in situ in vivo* and provide functional cellular signaling to both donor and host cells, while at the same time limiting the effects of reactive gliosis. This nanofiber system is currently being explored for spinal cord injury, stroke, and degenerative retinal disorders including age-related macular degeneration.

Platform technologies

In addition to nanotechnologies aimed specifically at replacing or rescuing CNS cells, which is still quite limited, a broader group of technologies being developed can be classified as platform technologies that have the potential for both basic neurobiology and clinical neurology/neurosurgery applications. One area that has received considerable attention is the growth and selected patterning of neural cell types on patterned surfaces. Still being explored on surfaces with microscale physical features or patterns of deposited macromolecules,[61,63,68,69] this approach has recently been extended to the nanoscale by photolithography etching on SiO_2 coated Si wafers characterized using atomic force and scanning electron microscopy[70] (see also Ref. 71). These authors determined that the ability of mixed primary cultures derived from the substantia nigra to grow and survive on surfaces with nanoscale features were closely linked to the physical dimensions of surface roughness, with optimal cell growth falling within a narrow window; features less then 10 nm or greater then 70 nm were associated with decreased cell adherence.

Other applications are taking advantage of some of the unique properties offered by carbon nanotubes to improve chronic CNS electrical stimulation. Clinically, functional electrical stimulation (FES) implants are being used more and more to treat intractable pain[72–76] and are also gaining momentum for the treatment of other disorders, such as urinary incontinence and Parkinsonian related disorders,[77–82] in most cases involving neurosurgical intervention. In addition, both stimulating and recording CNS electrodes are important neurophysiological and neuropathological experimental tools.[73,77,80,81,83–93] One of the most significant problems associated with the development of recording or stimulating chronic CNS electrodes is device failure associated with the fibrotic response mediated by glial and immune cells.[77,78,94–96] To address this, some groups are focusing on the development of novel carbon nanofiber based electrode arrays for CNS neuronal stimulation and recording.[8,11,97–104] In all cases the idea is to utilize the unique conductive electrical properties of carbon nanofibers for highly controlled focal stimulation.

Delivery of drugs and small molecules across the blood-brain barrier for CNS cancers

A significant amount of the work exploring nanotechnology approaches for crossing the BBB have focused on the delivery of antineoplastic drugs to CNS tumors. Primary CNS neoplasms are difficult to manage clinically and are associated with high rates of morbidity and mortality.[105–107] In one example of such work, radiolabeled polyethylene glycol (PEG) coated hexadecylcyanoarcylate nanospheres have been tested for their ability to target and accumulate in a rat model of gliosarcoma.[108] These authors observed a several fold increase in accumulation of nanospheres in the tumor relative to surrounding brain, although some accumulation in healthy tissue did occur. Another group has encapsulated the antineoplasitc drug paclitaxel in polylactic co-glycolic acid (PLGA) nanoparticles with impressive results. In *in vitro* experiments with 29 different cancer cell lines (including both neural and non-neural cell lines) they showed targeted cytotoxicity 13 times greater than with the drug alone.[109] Using a variety of physical and chemical characterization methods including different forms of spectroscopy and atomic force microscopy (AFM) they showed that the drug was taken up by the nanoparticles with very high encapsulation efficiencies and that the release kinetics could be carefully controlled. Research focusing on the delivery of many of the commonly used antineoplastic drugs is important because most of these drugs have poor solubility under physiological conditions and require less than optimal vehicles that can produce significant side effects. Paclitaxel, for example, must be administered as an adjuvant which can produce serious side effects including anaphylaxis, peripheral neuropathy, and hyperlipidemia.[110–112] In another example, various compounds including neuropeptides, such as enkephalins, the NMDA receptor antagonist MRZ 2/576, and the chemotherapeutic drug doxorubicin have been attached onto the surface of poly(butylcyanoacrylate) nanoparticles coated with polysorbate 80.[113–117] The polysorbate on the surface of the nanoparticles adsorb apolipoproteins B and E and are taken up by brain capillary endothelial cells via receptor-mediated endocytosis. Nanoparticle mediated delivery of doxorubicin is being explored in a rodent model of glioblastoma.[113,118] Importantly, recent work in a rat glioblastoma model has shown significant remission with minimal toxicity, setting the stage for potential clinical trials.[118]

Delivery of drugs and small molecules across the BBB for other CNS disorders and applications

In addition to antineoplastic drugs, the delivery of several other compounds are being explored using nanoparticle vehicles for a variety of CNS disorders and applications. Dalargin, a hexapeptide analog of leucine-enkephalin containing D-alanine that produces central analgesia when administered intracerebroventricularly, has no analgesic effects if administered systemically because it cannot cross the BBB.[12,119] [3H]-dalargin was conjugated to the same poly(butylcyanoacrylate) nanoparticles described above and injected systemically into mice and shown by radiolabeling to cross the BBB and accumulate in the brain.[12] Other similar studies have also shown the delivery of dalargin using polysorbate 80 coated nanoparticles.[120] Other polysorbate 80 nanoparticles have been chemically conjugated to the hydrophilic drug diminazenediaceturate (diminazene) and proposed as a novel treatment approach for second stage African trypanosomiasis (HAT).[121] In other work, PEG treated polyalkylcyanoacrylate nanoparticles were shown to cross the BBB and accumulate at high densities in the brain in experimental autoimmune encephalomyelitis (EAE),[122] a model for multiple sclerosis.[123,124] These authors have proposed this approach as a new delivery system for neuroinflammatory diseases.

In other applications, molecules other than drugs need to cross the BBB for therapeutic or diagnostic reasons, including oligonucleotides, genes, and contrast agents. Solid lipid nanoparticles consisting of microemulsions of solidified oil nanodroplets loaded with iron oxide injected systemically into rats have been shown to cross the BBB and accumulate in the brain with long lasting (i.e., slow clearance) properties.[125] Iron oxides are classic superparamagnetic MRI contrast agents which directly affect both T1 and T2 water molecule relaxation times, although they have a greater affect on the latter.[126,127] Because iron oxides are insoluble in water they must be delivered as modified colloides for clinical applications, usually achieved by coating them with hydrophilic molecules such as dextrans.[128] Therefore, the delivery vehicle used is critical in determining the functional properties of the contrast agent. By taking advantage of the ability of these solid lipid nanoparticles to cross the BBB, nanoparticles complexed with iron oxides may provide a novel approach to imaging the CNS by MRI. Other work has demonstrated proof of concept delivery of oligonucleotides across the BBB in an *in vivo* mouse model and an *in vitro* endothelial cell model aimed at developing novel treatments for neurodegenerative disorders.[129] These authors synthesized a nanogel consisting of cross-linked PEG and polyethylenimine that spontaneously encapsulated negatively charged oligonucleotides. They showed in their *in vivo* model that intravenous injections resulted in a 15-fold accumulation of oligonucleotides in the brain after one hour with a concurrent twofold decrease of accumulation in the liver and spleen when compared to freely administered oligonucleotides (i.e., not encapsulated in nanogel particles). A related area is the delivery of genes to the CNS for gene therapy. Tyrosine hydroxylase (TH) expression plasmid was delivered to the striatum of adult rats using PEG immunoliposome nanoparticles in order to normalize TH expression levels in the 6-hydroxydopamine rat model of Parkinson's disease.[130] Using specific antibodies to transferrin receptors conjugated to the nanoparticles, TH plasmids were shown to be expressed throughout the striatum.

Mechanisms of action and safety considerations for crossing the BBB

Although as summarized above there is a considerable and impressive amount of basic and preclinical work demonstrating the potential of nanoparticle approaches for the delivery of drugs and other molecules across the BBB following systemic administration, comparatively little is known about the molecular and cellular mechanisms by which nanoparticles cross the BBB or the safety considerations involved. To address this, other work is being carried out to understand these fundamental mechanisms. For example, poly(butylcyanoacrylate) nanoparticles coated with polysorbate 80 are thought to cross the BBB via plasma adsorption of apolipoproteins B and E resulting in receptor-mediated endocytosis by brain capillary endothelial cells, because these apolipoproteins naturally cross the BBB.[25,113–117,131] In some cases, *in vitro* models of the BBB have allowed investigating fundamental properties associated with nanoparticle translocation in a rigorously controlled experimental environment.[132,133] Using an *in vitro* model of the BBB consisting of brain derived endothelial cells and astrocyte co-cultures, the translocation of polyethylene glycol hexadecylcyanoacrylate derivitized nanoparticles by endocytosis was confirmed using confocal microscopy.[133] In some cases, translocation is achieved not by vesicular endocytosis but by facilitated transporter binding. By conjugating different ligands to nanoparticle carriers, different transporters could potentially be recruited to facilitate the translocation of specific molecules or compounds. For example, nanoparticles composed of polyoxyethylene 21 stearyl ether conjugated with thiamine on their surfaces have been shown to cross the BBB via specific interactions with thiamine transporters.[134]

Understanding and evaluating safety considerations associated with the use and application of these nanotechnologies is also a critical prerequisite to their clinical use. In general, preliminary work looking at nonspecific effects and toxicity of nanoparticle-drug systems designed to specifically target ligands or cells (e.g., tumor cells) of interest have demonstrated little adverse effects or toxicity in relevant animal models.[23,135] In addition to physiological safety considerations associated with the nanoparticles themselves, other practical safety issues will also have to be considered in order to properly protect both the patient and the health care professional. For example, detailed handling and administration protocols will have to be developed for the safe use of nanoparticles since there is growing evidence that inhaled particles can result in multiple negative effects, including nonspecific CNS effects, translocation from the lungs to the circulation, and both localized and systemic inflammatory responses.[136] By keeping safety considerations at the forefront, understanding the fundamental molecular and cellular mechanisms involved in nanoparticles crossing the BBB, and designing well controlled and appropriate preclinical and clinical translational studies, the use of nanotechnologies for safely, efficiently, and specifically delivering drugs and other molecules across the BBB may prove one of its highest impact contributions to clinical neuroscience.

Acknowledgments

This work was supported by funds from NIH grants NINDS NS054736.

Conflicts of interest

The author declares no conflicts of interest.

References

1. Silva, G.A. 2005. Nanotechnology approaches for the regeneration and neuroprotection of the central nervous system. *Surg. Neurol.* **63:** 301–306.
2. Silva, G.A. 2007. Nanotechnology approaches for drug and small molecule delivery across the blood brain barrier. *Surg. Neurol.* **67:** 113–116.
3. Blumling, J. & G.A. Silva. In press. Diagnostic and therapeutic nanotechnologies with applications to the retina and optic nerve. *J. Neuro. Ophthal.*
4. Jaiswal, J.K. *et al.* 2003. Long-term multiple color imaging of live cells using quantum dot bioconjugates. *Nat. Biotech.* **21:** 47–51.
5. Provenzale, J.M. & G.A. Silva. 2009. Uses of nanoparticles for central nervous system imaging and therapies. *Amer. J. Neuro. Radiol.* **30:** 1293-1301.
6. Silva, G.A. 2004. Introduction to nanotechnology and its applications to medicine. *Surg. Neurol.* **61:** 216–220.
7. Silva, G.A. 2006. Neuroscience nanotechnology: progress, opportunities and challenges. *Nat. Rev. Neurosci.* **7:** 65–74.
8. Pancrazio, J.J. 2008. Neural interfaces at the nanoscale. *Nanomed.* **3:** 823–830.
9. Suh, W.H. *et al.* 2009. Nanotechnology, nanotoxicology, and neuroscience. *Prog. Neurobiol.* **87:** 133–170.
10. Sharma, H.S. 2007. Nanoneuroscience: emerging concepts on nanoneurotoxicity and nanoneuroprotection. *Nanomed.* **2:** 753–758.
11. Malarkey, E.B. & V. Parpura. 2007. Applications of carbon nanotubes in neurobiology. *Neurodegener Dis.* **4:** 292–299.
12. Alyaudtin, R.N. *et al.* 2001. Interaction of poly(butylcyanoacrylate) nanoparticles with the blood-brain barrier *in vivo* and *in vitro*. *J. Drug Target.* **9:** 209–221.
13. Drummond, T.G., M.G. Hill & J.K. Barton. 2003. Electrochemical DNA sensors. *Nat. Biotechnol.* **21:** 1192–1199.
14. Hirosue, S. *et al.* 2001. Plasmid DNA encapsulation and release from solvent diffusion nanospheres. *J. Control Release* **70:** 231–242.
15. Hong, J.W. & S.R. Quake. 2003. Integrated nanoliter systems. *Nat. Biotechnol.* **21:** 1179–1183.
16. LaVan, D.A., T. McGuire & R. Langer. 2003. Small-scale systems for *in vivo* drug delivery. *Nat. Biotechnol.* **21:** 1184–1191.
17. Lee, K.B. *et al.* 2002. Protein nanoarrays generated by dip-pen nanolithography. *Science* **295:** 1702–1705.
18. Lyuksyutov, S.F. *et al.* 2003. Electrostatic nanolithography in polymers using atomic force microscopy. *Nat. Mater.*
19. Muller-Mai, C.M. *et al.* 1995. Nanoapatite and organoapatite implants in bone: histology and ultrastructure of the interface. *J. Biomed. Mater. Res.* **29:** 9–18.
20. Sham, J.O. *et al.* 2004. Formulation and characterization of spray-dried powders containing nanoparticles for aerosol delivery to the lung. *Int. J. Pharm.* **269:** 457–467.
21. Service, R.F. 2001. Self-assembling materials. Coated nanofibers copy what's bred in the bone. *Science* **294:** 1635–1637.
22. Zhang, S. 2003. Fabrication of novel biomaterials through molecular self-assembly. *Nat. Biotechnol.* **21:** 1171–1178.
23. Gelperina, S.E. *et al.* 2002. Toxicological studies of doxorubicin bound to polysorbate 80-coated poly(butyl cyanoacrylate) nanoparticles in healthy rats and rats with intracranial glioblastoma. *Toxicol. Lett.* **126:** 131–141.
24. Kreuter, J. 2001. Nanoparticulate systems for brain delivery of drugs. *Adv. Drug Deliv. Rev.* **47:** 65–81.
25. Kreuter, J. *et al.* 2002. Apolipoprotein-mediated transport of nanoparticle-bound drugs across the blood-brain barrier. *J. Drug Target.* **10:** 317–325.
26. Lockman, P.R. *et al.* 2002. Nanoparticle technology for drug delivery across the blood-brain barrier. *Drug Dev. Ind. Pharm.* **28:** 1–13.
27. Lo, E.H., T. Dalkara & M.A. Moskowitz. 2003. Mechanisms, challenges and opportunities in stroke. *Nat. Rev. Neurosci.* **4:** 399–415.

28. Blass, J.P. 2003. Cerebrometabolic abnormalities in Alzheimer's disease. *Neurol Res.* **25:** 556–566.
29. Wilson, J.X. & A.W. Gelb. 2002. Free radicals, antioxidants, and neurologic injury: possible relationship to cerebral protection by anesthetics. *J. Neurosurg. Anesthesiol.* **14:** 66–79.
30. Raghupathi, R., D.I. Graham & T.K. McIntosh. 2000. Apoptosis after traumatic brain injury. *J. Neurotrauma.* **17:** 927–938.
31. Verma, A. 2000. Opportunities for neuroprotection in traumatic brain injury. *J. Head Trauma Rehabil.* **15:** 1149–1161.
32. Gagliardi, R.J. 2000. Neuroprotection, excitotoxicity and NMDA antagonists. *Arq. Neuropsiquiatr.* **58:** 583–588.
33. Rosenberg, G.A. 1999. Ischemic brain edema. *Prog. Cardiovasc. Dis.* **42:** 209–216.
34. Mishra, O.P. & M. Delivoria-Papadopoulos. 1999. Cellular mechanisms of hypoxic injury in the developing brain. *Brain Res. Bull.* **48:** 233–238.
35. Mahadik, S.P. & S. Mukherjee. 1996. Free radical pathology and antioxidant defense in schizophrenia: a review. *Schizophr. Res.* **19:** 1–17.
36. Dugan, L.L. *et al.* 2001. Fullerene-based antioxidants and neurodegenerative disorders. **7:** 243–246.
37. Dugan, L.L. *et al.* 1996. Buckminsterfullerenol free radical scavengers reduce excitotoxic and apoptotic death of cultured cortical neurons. *Neurobiol. Dis.* **3:** 129–135.
38. Dugan, L.L. *et al.* 1997. Carboxyfullerenes as neuroprotective agents. *Proc. Natl. Acad. Sci. USA* **94:** 9434–9439.
39. Jin, H. *et al.* 2000. Polyhydroxylated C(60), fullerenols, as glutamate receptor antagonists and neuroprotective agents. *J. Neurosci. Res.* **62:** 600–607.
40. Kostrzewa, R.M. & J. Segura-Aguilar. 2003. Novel mechanisms and approaches in the study of neurodegeneration and neuroprotection. A review. *Neurotox Res.* **5:** 375–383.
41. Hendriks, W.T. *et al.* 2004. Viral vector-mediated gene transfer of neurotrophins to promote regeneration of the injured spinal cord. *Prog. Brain Res.* **146:** 451–476.
42. Petrova, P.S. *et al.* 2004. Discovering novel phenotype-selective neurotrophic factors to treat neurodegenerative diseases. *Prog. Brain Res.* **146:** 168–183.
43. Aruoma, O.I., T. Bahorun & L.S. Jen. 2003. Neuroprotection by bioactive components in medicinal and food plant extracts. *Mutat. Res.* **544:** 203–215.
44. Reyes, O., I. Sosa & D.P. Kuffler. 2003. Neuroprotection of spinal neurons against blunt trauma and ischemia. *P. R. Health Sci. J.* **22:** 277–286.
45. Neufeld, A.H. & B. Liu. 2003. Glaucomatous optic neuropathy: when glia misbehave. *Neuroscientist.* **9:** 485–495.
46. Klijn, C.J. & G.J. Hankey. 2003. Management of acute ischaemic stroke: new guidelines from the American Stroke Association and European Stroke Initiative. *Lancet Neurol.* **2:** 698–701.
47. Schapira, A.H. 2003. Neuroprotection in PD–a role for dopamine agonists? *Neurology* **61:** S34–42.
48. Muir, K.W. & K.R. Lees. 2003. Excitatory amino acid antagonists for acute stroke. Cochrane Database Syst RevCD001244.
49. Simpkins, N. & J. Jankovic. 2003. Neuroprotection in Parkinson disease. *Arch. Intern. Med.* **163:** 1650–1654.
50. Kaushik, S., S.S. Pandav & J. Ram. 2003. Neuroprotection in glaucoma. *J. Postgrad. Med.* **49:** 90–95.
51. Hinkle, J.L. & L. Bowman. 2003. Neuroprotection for ischemic stroke. *J. Neurosci. Nurs.* **35:** 114–118.
52. Service, R.F. 2003. American Chemical Society meeting. Molecular scaffolding helps raise a crop of neurons. *Science* **302:** 46–47.
53. Silva, G.A. *et al.* 2004. Selective differentiation of neural progenitor cells by high-epitope density nanofibers. *Science.* **303:** 1352–1355.
54. Silva, G.A. *et al.* 2002. Development of neural progenitor cells encapsulated in a peptide amphiphile substrate that is induced to self-assemble under physiological conditions. Soc. Neurosci. Abstracts.
55. Silva, G.A. *et al.* 2003. Nanoengineered peptide amphiphile network for photoreceptor replacement in degenerative retinal disorders. Ass. Res. Vis. Ophthal. (ARVO) Abstracts.
56. Hartgerink, J.D., E. Beniash & S.I. Stupp. 2001. Self-assembly and mineralization of peptide-amphiphile nanofibers. *Science* **294:** 1684–1688.
57. Hartgerink, J.D., E. Beniash & S.I. Stupp. 2002. Peptide-amphiphile nanofibers: a versatile scaffold for the preparation of self-assembling materials. *Proc. Natl. Acad. Sci. USA* **99:** 5133–5138.
58. Niece, K.L. *et al.* 2003. Self-assembly combining two bioactive peptide-amphiphile molecules into nanofibers by electrostatic attraction. *J. Am. Chem. Soc.* **125:** 7146–7147.
59. Yeung, C.K. *et al.* 2001. Modulation of the growth and guidance of rat brain stem neurons using patterned extracellular matrix proteins. *Neurosci. Lett.* **301:** 147–150.
60. Thiebaud, P. *et al.* 2002. PDMS device for patterned application of microfluids to neuronal cells arranged by microcontact printing. *Biosens. Bioelectron.* **17:** 87–93.

61. Wheeler, B.C. *et al.* 1999. Microcontact printing for precise control of nerve cell growth in culture. *J. Biomech. Eng.* **121:** 73–78.
62. Lauer, L. *et al.* 2002. Electrophysiological recordings of patterned rat brain stem slice neurons. *Biomaterials* **23:** 3123–3130.
63. Chang, J.C., G.J. Brewer & B.C. Wheeler. 2001. Modulation of neural network activity by patterning. *Biosens. Bioelectron.* **16:** 527–533.
64. Cornish, T. *et al.* 2002. Microcontact printing: a versatile technique for the study of synaptogenic molecules. *Mol. Cell Neurosci.* **20:** 140–153.
65. Kam, L. *et al.* 2001. Axonal outgrowth of hippocampal neurons on micro-scale networks of polylysine-conjugated laminin. *Biomaterials* **22:** 1049–1054.
66. Matsuzawa, M. *et al.* 1996. Directional neurite outgrowth and axonal differentiation of embryonic hippocampal neurons are promoted by a neurite outgrowth domain of the B2-chain of laminin. *Int. J. Dev. Neurosci.* **14:** 283–295.
67. Powell, S.K. *et al.* 2000. Neural cell response to multiple novel sites on laminin-1. *J. Neurosci. Res.* **61:** 302.
68. Chang, J.C., G.J. Brewer & B.C. Wheeler. 2003. A modified microstamping technique enhances polylysine transfer and neuronal cell patterning. *Biomaterials* **24:** 2863–2870.
69. Branch, D.W. *et al.* 2000. Long-term maintenance of patterns of hippocampal pyramidal cells on substrates of polyethylene glycol and microstamped polylysine. *IEEE Trans. Biomed. Eng.* **47:** 290–300.
70. Fan, Y.W. *et al.* 2002. Culture of neural cells on silicon wafers with nano-scale surface topograph. *J. Neurosci. Methods* **120:** 17–23.
71. Silva, G.A. 2004. Introduction to nanotechnology and its applications to medicine. *Surg. Neurol.* **61:** 216–220.
72. Richardson, D.E. 1995. Deep brain stimulation for the relief of chronic pain. *Neurosurg. Clin. N. Am.* **6:** 135–144.
73. Rushton, D.N. 2002. Electrical stimulation in the treatment of pain. *Disabil. Rehabil.* **24:** 407–415.
74. Sharan, A.D. *et al.* 2003. Precentral stimulation for chronic pain. *Neurosurg. Clin. N. Am.* **14:** 437–444.
75. Krames, E. 2002. Implantable devices for pain control: spinal cord stimulation and intrathecal therapies. *Best Pract. Res. Clin. Anaesthesiol.* **16:** 619–649.
76. Kumar, K., C. Toth & R.K. Nath. 1997. Deep brain stimulation for intractable pain: a 15-year experience. *Neurosurgery* **40:** 736–746; discussion 746–737.
77. Benabid, A.L. *et al.* 2000. Future prospects of brain stimulation. *Neurol. Res.* **22:** 237–246.
78. Barolat, G. & A.D. Sharan. 2000. Future trends in spinal cord stimulation. *Neurol. Res.* **22:** 279–284.
79. Pollak, P. *et al.* 2002. Intraoperative micro- and macrostimulation of the subthalamic nucleus in Parkinson's disease. *Mov. Disord.* **17**(Suppl 3): S155–161.
80. Benabid, A.L. *et al.* 2001. Deep brain stimulation of the corpus luysi (subthalamic nucleus) and other targets in Parkinson's disease. Extension to new indications such as dystonia and epilepsy. *J. Neurol.* **248**(Suppl 3): III37–III47.
81. Benabid, A.L. *et al.* 2000. Subthalamic stimulation for Parkinson's disease. *Arch. Med. Res.* **31:** 282–289.
82. Kupsch, A. & C. Earl. 1999. Neurosurgical interventions in the treatment of idiopathic Parkinson disease: neurostimulation and neural implantation. *J. Mol. Med.* **77:** 178–184.
83. Rousche, P.J. *et al.* 2003. Single electrode microstimulation of rat auditory cortex: an evaluation of behavioral performance. *Hear Res.* **179:** 62–71.
84. Rousche, P.J. *et al.* 1999. Examination of the spatial and temporal distribution of sensory cortical activity using a 100-electrode array. *J. Neurosci. Methods* **90:** 57–66.
85. Normann, R.A. *et al.* 1999. A neural interface for a cortical vision prosthesis. *Vision Res.* **39:** 2577–2587.
86. Rousche, P.J. & R.A. Normann. 1998. Chronic recording capability of the Utah Intracortical Electrode Array in cat sensory cortex. *J. Neurosci. Methods* **82:** 1–15.
87. Rousche, P.J. & R.A. Normann. 1999. Chronic intracortical microstimulation (ICMS) of cat sensory cortex using the Utah Intracortical Electrode Array. *IEEE Trans. Rehabil. Eng.* **7:** 56–68.
88. Starr, P.A. 2002. Placement of deep brain stimulators into the subthalamic nucleus or globus pallidus internus: technical approach. *Stereotact Funct. Neurosurg.* **79:** 118–145.
89. Hariz, M.I. 2002. Safety and risk of microelectrode recording in surgery for movement disorders. *Stereotact Funct. Neurosurg.* **78:** 146–157.
90. Deletis, V. & A. Bueno De Camargo. 2001. Interventional neurophysiological mapping during spinal cord procedures. *Stereotact Funct. Neurosurg.* **77:** 25–28.
91. Palmer, A.R. & A.Q. Summerfield. 2002. Microelectrode and neuroimaging studies of central auditory function. *Br. Med Bull.* **63:** 95–105.
92. Leopold, D.A. 2002. Visual neurophysiology: recordings from the human primate. *Curr. Biol.* **12:** R582–584.
93. Robinson, D.L. *et al.* 2003. Detecting subsecond dopamine release with fast-scan cyclic voltammetry *in vivo*. *Clin. Chem.* **49:** 1763–1773.

94. Mojarradi, M. *et al.* 2003. A miniaturized neuroprosthesis suitable for implantation into the brain. *IEEE Trans. Neural. Syst. Rehabil. Eng.* **11:** 38–42.
95. Kipke, D.R. *et al.* 2003. Silicon-substrate intracortical microelectrode arrays for long-term recording of neuronal spike activity in cerebral cortex. *IEEE Trans. Neural. Syst. Rehabil. Eng.* **11:** 151–155.
96. Beric, A. *et al.* 2001. Complications of deep brain stimulation surgery. *Stereotact. Funct. Neurosurg.* **77:** 73–78.
97. Kauffman, D.R. & A. Star. 2008. Electronically monitoring biological interactions with carbon nanotube field-effect transistors. *Chem. Soc. Rev.* **37:** 1197–1206.
98. Balasubramanian, K. & M. Burghard. 2006. Biosensors based on carbon nanotubes. *Anal. Bioanal. Chem.* **385:** 452–468.
99. Cellot, G. *et al.* 2009. Carbon nanotubes might improve neuronal performance by favouring electrical shortcuts. *Nat. Nanotechnol.* **4:** 126–133.
100. Mazzatenta, A. *et al.* 2007. Interfacing neurons with carbon nanotubes: electrical signal transfer and synaptic stimulation in cultured brain circuits. *J. Neurosci.* **27:** 6931–6936.
101. Lovat, V. *et al.* 2005. Carbon nanotube substrates boost neuronal electrical signaling. *Nano Lett.* **5:** 1107–1110.
102. Santos, R.M. *et al.* 2008. A comparative study of carbon fiber-based microelectrodes for the measurement of nitric oxide in brain tissue. *Biosens. Bioelectron.* **24:** 704–709.
103. Li, J. & R.J. Andrews. 2007. Trimodal nanoelectrode array for precise deep brain stimulation: prospects of a new technology based on carbon nanofiber arrays. *Acta Neurochir. Suppl.* **97:** 537–545.
104. Nguyen-Vu, T.D. *et al.* 2006. Vertically aligned carbon nanofiber arrays: an advance toward electrical-neural interfaces. *Small* **2:** 89–94.
105. DeAngelis, L.M. 2001. Brain tumors. *N. Engl. J. Med.* **344:** 114–123.
106. Nelson, D.F. *et al.* 1985. Survival and prognosis of patients with astrocytoma with atypical or anaplastic features. *J. Neurooncol.* **3:** 99–103.
107. Kornblith, P.L. & M. Walker. 1988. Chemotherapy for malignant gliomas. *J. Neurosurg.* **68:** 1–17.
108. Brigger, I. *et al.* 2002. Poly(ethylene glycol)-coated hexadecylcyanoacrylate nanospheres display a combined effect for brain tumor targeting. *J. Pharmacol. Exp. Ther.* **303:** 928–936.
109. Feng, S.S. *et al.* 2004. Nanoparticles of biodegradable polymers for clinical administration of paclitaxel. *Curr. Med. Chem.* **11:** 413–424.
110. Gelderblom, H. *et al.* 2001. Cremophor EL: the drawbacks and advantages of vehicle selection for drug formulation. *Eur. J. Cancer* **37:** 1590–1598.
111. Singla, A.K., A. Garg & D. Aggarwal. 2002. Paclitaxel and its formulations. *Int. J. Pharm.* **235:** 179–192.
112. Baker, M.T. & M. Naguib. 2005. Propofol: the challenges of formulation. *Anesthesiology* **103:** 860–876.
113. Gulyaev, A.E. *et al.* 1999. Significant transport of doxorubicin into the brain with polysorbate 80-coated nanoparticles. *Pharm Res.* **16:** 1564–1569.
114. Alyautdin, R.N. *et al.* 1997. Delivery of loperamide across the blood-brain barrier with polysorbate 80-coated polybutylcyanoacrylate nanoparticles. *Pharm Res.* **14:** 325–328.
115. Kreuter, J. *et al.* 1995. Passage of peptides through the blood-brain barrier with colloidal polymer particles (nanoparticles). *Brain Res.* **674:** 171–174.
116. Alyautdin, R.N. *et al.* 1998. Significant entry of tubocurarine into the brain of rats by adsorption to polysorbate 80-coated polybutylcyanoacrylate nanoparticles: an *in situ* brain perfusion study. *J. Microencapsul.* **15:** 67–74.
117. Friese, A. *et al.* 2000. Increase of the duration of the anticonvulsive activity of a novel NMDA receptor antagonist using poly(butylcyanoacrylate) nanoparticles as a parenteral controlled release system. *Eur. J. Pharm. Biopharm.* **49:** 103–109.
118. Steiniger, S.C. *et al.* 2004. Chemotherapy of glioblastoma in rats using doxorubicin-loaded nanoparticles. *Int. J. Cancer* **109:** 759–767.
119. Rousselle, C. *et al.* 2003. Improved brain uptake and pharmacological activity of dalargin using a peptide-vector-mediated strategy. *J. Pharmacol. Exp. Ther.* **306:** 371–376.
120. Schroeder, U. *et al.* 1998. Nanoparticle technology for delivery of drugs across the blood-brain barrier. *J. Pharm. Sci.* **87:** 1305–1307.
121. Olbrich, C. *et al.* 2002. Lipid-drug-conjugate (LDC) nanoparticles as novel carrier system for the hydrophilic antitrypanosomal drug diminazenediaceturate. *J. Drug Target* **10:** 387–396.
122. Calvo, P. *et al.* 2002. Quantification and localization of PEGylated polycyanoacrylate nanoparticles in brain and spinal cord during experimental allergic encephalomyelitis in the rat. *Eur. J. Neurosci.* **15:** 1317–1326.
123. Ercolini, A.M. & S.D. Miller. 2006. Mechanisms of immunopathology in murine models of central nervous system demyelinating disease. *J. Immunol.* **176:** 3293–3298.
124. Kanwar, J.R. 2005. Anti-inflammatory immunotherapy for multiple sclerosis/experimental autoimmune

encephalomyelitis (EAE) disease. *Curr. Med. Chem.* **12:** 2947–2962.

125. Peira, E. *et al.* 2003. *In vitro* and *in vivo* study of solid lipid nanoparticles loaded with superparamagnetic iron oxide. *J. Drug Target* **11:** 19–24.
126. Lovin, J.D. *et al.* 1985. Magnetic field dependence of spin-lattice relaxation enhancement using piperidinyl nitroxyl spin-labels. *Magn. Reson. Imaging* **3:** 73–81.
127. Wesbey, G.E. *et al.* 1985. Dilute oral iron solutions as gastrointestinal contrast agents for magnetic resonance imaging; initial clinical experience. *Magn. Reson. Imaging* **3:** 57–64.
128. Dupas, B. *et al.* 1999. Electron microscopy study of intrahepatic ultrasmall superparamagnetic iron oxide kinetics in the rat. Relation with magnetic resonance imaging. *Biol. Cell.* **91:** 195–208.
129. Vinogradov, S.V., E.V. Batrakova & A.V. Kabanov. 2004. Nanogels for oligonucleotide delivery to the brain. *Bioconjug Chem.* **15:** 50–60.
130. Zhang, Y. *et al.* 2003. Intravenous nonviral gene therapy causes normalization of striatal tyrosine hydroxylase and reversal of motor impairment in experimental parkinsonism. *Hum. Gene Ther.* **14:** 1–12.
131. Goppert, T.M. & R.H. Muller. 2003. Plasma protein adsorption of Tween 80- and poloxamer 188-stabilized solid lipid nanoparticles. *J. Drug Target* **11:** 225–231.
132. Ma, S.H. *et al.* 2005. An endothelial and astrocyte co-culture model of the blood-brain barrier utilizing an ultra-thin, nanofabricated silicon nitride membrane. *Lab. Chip.* **5:** 74–85.
133. Garcia-Garcia, E. *et al.* 2005. A relevant *in vitro* rat model for the evaluation of blood-brain barrier translocation of nanoparticles. *Cell Mol. Life Sci.* **62:** 1400–1408.
134. Lockman, P.R. *et al.* 2003. Brain uptake of thiamine-coated nanoparticles. *J. Control Release* **93:** 271–282.
135. Kreuter, J. *et al.* 2003. Direct evidence that polysorbate-80-coated poly(butylcyanoacrylate) nanoparticles deliver drugs to the CNS via specific mechanisms requiring prior binding of drug to the nanoparticles. *Pharm. Res.* **20:** 409–416.
136. Borm, P.J. & W. Kreyling. 2004. Toxicological hazards of inhaled nanoparticles—potential implications for drug delivery. *J. Nanosci. Nanotechnol.* **4:** 521–531.